DANA THORNOCK'S

LEAN&FREE
2000 PLUS™

ULTIMATE WELLNESS / WEIGHT CONTROL LIFESTYLE

"I highly recommend this program because it is based on sound principles of good health and nutrition. As an obstetrician, I have many women desperate to lose those extra pounds gained during pregnancy. Thank goodness there is finally a program that deals not only with the physical but also the psychological aspects of weight control."
—*Mark R. Bitner, M.D., FACOG*

"This program is not a fad diet, or a diet of extremes but a nutritionally balanced eating plan. Take charge of your life today and capture the same excitement, enthusiasm, and success that Dana feels."
—*Mary K. Beard, M.D., FACOG*

"I have been concerned with the current surgical approaches and numerous popular approaches to fat loss for many years. I have studied the LEAN & FREE program and have recommended it to many of my patients. It is not a quick-fix approach, and I am convinced that it is the safest and most effective program available for the achievement and maintenance of ideal body composition, appearance, and health."
—*Dr. James L. Hopkins, M.D., General Surgeon*

I always wondered if there were two sets of rules—one set for people who are naturally lean and another set for people with excess body fat. But after reading Dana's book, I'm convinced there are not two sets of rules—just one healthy way to live.

I recommend this program to my patients with diabetes, hypoglycemia, high cholesterol, high blood pressure, eating disorders, chronic fatigue, depression, and people who want to lose body fat.
—*Sheryl Swain–Aguilar, Registered Dietitian*

"From age fourteen on, I tried everything—starvation diets, diet pills, diet shots. Nothing worked. Finally, out of desperation, I had my stomach stapled but only lost forty pounds." *So Janelle stopped dieting at a size 50 and 325 pounds and began eating over 2,000 calories a day.* "After just eighteen months on the program I weigh 165 pounds; I have gone from a size 50 to a size 10. My cholesterol dropped from 301 to 170. It is really wonderful to eat like a normal person. For the first time, I really like myself." *Janelle has lost 160 pounds and has no visible excess skin!*
—*Janelle, age 40*

Anorexia and bulimia no longer plague Lisa's life. She used to fluctuate between a size 0 and size 14. Now she has been stable for six years at a size 5, eating over 2,000 calories a day. Before beginning this program, after many medical tests, Lisa was told she could never bear children. Now she has born two beautiful children and is pregnant with her third.

"I cannot describe well enough the incredible changes that have occurred in my life because of Dana's program. I often look back and wonder if that sickly, ninety-pound fanatic was really me. My life is so full and meaningful. Very rarely do I spend time thinking about food, weight, calories, or size."
—*Lisa, age 26*

Charlene has lost 126 pounds, seen a reduction in size from a size 50 to a size 8 and is down to 14 percent body fat. She no longer has any problems with bulimia. She has been lean for four years now. Charlene just had her ninth child. She has beautiful skin.

When I was dieting, I felt Crabby and awful. After a while, I could't even lose weight on an 800-calorie diet. I've dropped from 266 pounds to 140. I love to eat. I've learned to nurture and love my body. I've **dropped 105 points on my cholesterol** (in addition to losing 126 pounds)."

—Charlene, age 37

"The LEAN & FREE 2000 program has changed my life. All symptoms of diabetes have disappeared totally. "Additionally, I've lost 25 pounds and reduced my pant size from 24 to 18. I know I'm just going to keep losing on this wonderful program."

—Clarise, age 36

Julia lost ninety-two pounds and reduced from a size 28 to a size 10. She has been weight stable for three and a half years.

"I'm **saving** a ton of **money**. Diets don't teach you to eat, they just want you to buy their high-priced foods. I eat real food now. I no longer feel panic stricken or obsessed with food because I know I can have all I want."

—Julia, age 36

*Gib's **blood pressure** has decreased from 160 over 105 to 128 over 84. His waist has dropped from 48 to 40 inches along with forty pounds in weight.*

"I'm retired and it's just wonderful to feel so good."

—Gib, age 60

Carol Ann reduced from a size 24 to a size 10 and lost eighty-eight pounds.

"Once I discovered Dana's program, I started eating good food and quit beating myself up emotionally when I wanted to eat goodies. I not only have freedom from excess body fat, I feel free to eat the foods I love to eat."

Carol Ann has maintained a size 10 for over four years.

—Carol Ann, age 46

- *For more inspiring success stories, turn to page 176.*
- *For answers to the most frequently asked health and weight-control questions, turn to page 157.*
- *To find out how easy this program is to live, turn to pages 207 and 241.*

ACKNOWLEDGMENTS

*T*his book was generated from my own experiences and studies, and it has received its inspiration from the work of many teachers and researchers and the thousands of students in my own nutrition and aerobics classes. I am especially appreciative to my first husband, Nyle, now deceased, and my current husband, Marty.

For their contributions to the success of this program, I would also like to express my gratitude to:

- ❑ each of our children, who inspired me to adapt this program to personal tastes and to the demanding, busy schedules of modern life.
- ❑ my devoted sisters, who helped with housekeeping, meals, chauffeuring, and editing.
- ❑ my parents and grandparents, whose lives serve as examples of true service and love.
- ❑ Dr. Mary Beard for her wisdom, counsel, and excellent medical editing.
- ❑ Thail and Dave Steffen and Gary Scothern for their countless hours at the computer.
- ❑ Evelyn Scothern, whose secretarial skills are matched only by her cheerfulness.
- ❑ Judith Nielsen Crocker, Jack Lyon, and Stew Nohrnberg for their exceptional editing.
- ❑ Publishers Press for their professionalism, promptness, and devotion to quality.
- ❑ Cheryl Young and Lisa Jones for their many hours with menus and recipes.
- ❑ Michael Lewis for his professional food photography and Lisa Jones for her art direction and food styling.
- ❑ Marie Barber, Ruth Ann Evans, LeAnn Gerber, Lisa Meiling, Win Peterson, Karla Porter, and Denise Simon for their dedicated teaching and willingness to test recipes.
- ❑ My LEAN & FREE students for their love, enthusiasm, and all that they teach me about happiness and life.
- ❑ Richard Bird for his masterful design work and years of dedicated service to this project; and Beth Bird for her tremendous help, patience, and support.

THIS BOOK IS AFFECTIONATELY DEDICATED TO

all those who have lived through many of the same diet nightmares I have, including:

- [ ] **waking up each morning with one question in mind: "What will I or won't I eat today?"**
- [ ] **looking withered and starved skinny from the waist up and fluffy from the waist down after dieting.**
- [ ] **stuffing themselves with two batches of chocolate-chip cookie dough after starving for days and then wishing to or succeeding in throwing it all up.**
- [ ] **remembering the cruel childhood nicknames and peer rejection.**
- [ ] **suffering from chronic fatigue, depression, light headedness, and extreme weakness.**
- [ ] **keeping twenty to sixty pounds after each pregnancy.**
- [ ] **putting all the lost weight back on plus more after every diet.**
- [ ] **letting the bathroom scales rule their lives.**
- [ ] **virtually living on antibiotics for constant illnesses.**

Here's to health and hearty appetites! Here's to the *freedom* to be the size that's ideal for you, eating all you want to eat (including goodies) and never worrying about your weight again. And here's to a life filled with *energy* and lived in service and joy!

Here's to the
EDUCATED CHOICE OF ABUNDANCE
and normal food.

Copyright © 1994
Danmar Health Corporation
All rights reserved

Published by
Danmar Health Corporation
P.O. Box 2000
Kaysville, Utah, 84037
1-801-546-3262

Library of Congress Cataloging-In-Publication Data
Thornock, Dana, 1958—
    Lean & Free 2000 Plus:
    Ultimate Wellness/Weight Control Lifestyle.
    Revised Edition
    Includes bibliographical references.
    1. Weight Control.   2. Nutrition.   3. Health.
    4. Diet.   I. Title.

ISBN 1-56684-034-1
613.25 1992,
Printed in the United States of America

10 9 8 7 6 5 4

NOTICE: The information in this book is true and complete to the best of our knowledge. This book is intended only as an informative guide for those wishing to know more about nutrition, fitness, emotional and physical health, and excess body fat loss. Although the advice given is similar to that recommended by many knowledgeable health professionals, the information is meant to complement the advice of your physician, not to replace, countermand, or conflict with it. We strongly recommend that you follow your doctor's advice in dealing with all health issues and problems. Diet, exercise, mental health, and medication decisions should be made between you and your doctor. Accordingly, either you or the professional treating you must take full responsibility for any use made of the information in this book. Information in this book is general and is made with no guarantees by the author or publisher. The author and publisher disclaim all liability in connection with the use of this book.

DANA THORNOCK'S

LEAN&FREE 2000 PLUS™

ULTIMATE WELLNESS / WEIGHT CONTROL LIFESTYLE

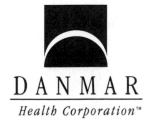

DANMAR
Health Corporation™

By Dana Thornock
Published by Danmar Health Corporation

LEAN&FREE 2000 PLUS™

THE ULTIMATE WELLNESS/WEIGHT CONTROL LIFESTYLE

LEAN&FREE 2000 PLUS™

THE 14 DAY COOKBOOK SAMPLER

LEAN & FREE 2000 PLUS Product order information, extra Right & Left-Brain Success Planner Sheets, Menu Planner Sheets, and Personal Progress Mail-in Forms are found in the back of this book.

FOREWORD

*I*n the past five decades, the industrialized nations of the world have seen spectacular changes in disease statistics. Before the discovery of antibiotics and the development of vaccines, thousands of people died each year from infectious diseases such as whooping cough, cholera, scarlet fever, smallpox, and influenza. As a result, the life expectancy was only in the mid-forties.

Today, because of advances in health care, the life expectancy for men and women is well into the seventies and rising. The leading causes of death are no longer viral (except for the current rise in the death rate by AIDS) or bacterial infections but heart disease, cancer, stroke, chronic obstructive lung disease, diabetes, cirrhosis of the liver, atherosclerosis (hardening of the arteries), and kidney disease. Nutritional and lifestyle factors contribute to the development of these diseases. Each one of us needs to take a look at our behavior patterns to see how we eat and drink and, whether we smoke, as well as how we live, work, and spend our leisure time.

To be healthy with lots of energy is everyone's desire. To achieve that goal requires us to take charge of our lives.

There are certain factors over which we have no control—such as our age, sex, family history, ethnic background, environment, and the quality of available health care. However, we do have choices as to our lifestyle and nutrition. We can prevent obesity and decrease the risk of developing high blood pressure, high cholesterol, adult onset diabetes, and degenerative arthritis of the weight-bearing joints. Proper nutrition, including increasing fiber, reducing fat, and exercising, as well as eliminating tobacco, caffeine, and alcohol, will reduce the risk for developing many of the diseases that today are the leading causes of death in the American population.

Dana has set forth in this text guidelines for healthy eating, exercising, and her formula for positive thinking. This program is not a fad diet, or a diet of extremes, but a nutritionally balanced eating plan, high in complex carbohydrates and moderate, but not excessively low in fat and protein. The principles set forth in this program can be followed by everyone regardless of age. Dana's counsel to eat a nutritionally balanced diet with optimal calories and exercise in moderation in order for the body to perform at its best is sound advice.

By following Dana's instructions, taking charge of your life, and making a commitment to becoming a healthy, "lean," positive-thinking person, you should experience the excitement of a new you. Before beginning any new eating and exercise program, be sure to discuss it with your doctor. Do not stop or change the medications prescribed by your doctor without consulting him or her first. Take charge of your life today and capture the same excitement, enthusiasm, and success that Dana feels. Good luck!

Mary K. Beard, M.D., FACOG
Private practice in obstetrics, gynecology, and infertility: associate clinical professor, University of Utah, Salt Lake City

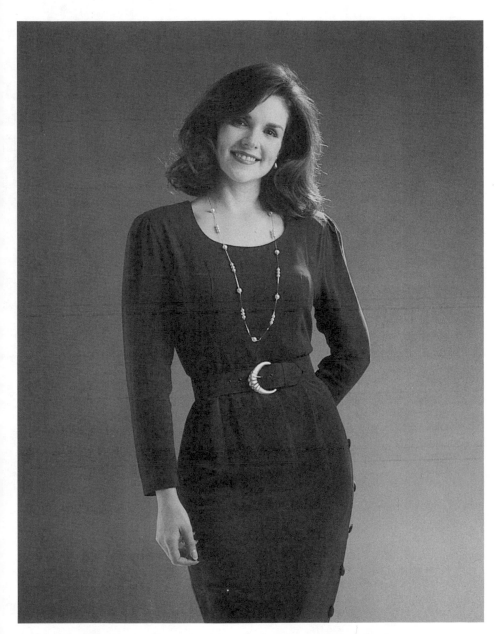

As I decreased from a size 18 to a size 4, I gradually increased my calories from less than 1,000 a day to more than 2,000 a day and learned to eat balanced meals comprised of normal, healthy, real-world food. And I implemented all of the principles of the LEAN & FREE LIFESTYLE.

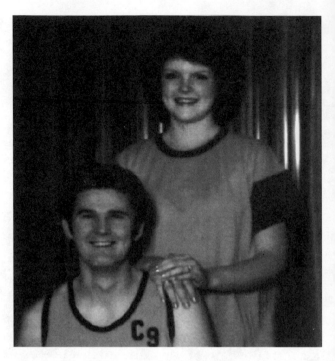

At a size 18 and 204 pounds, I had tremendous lower-back and stomach trouble, along with fatigue and depression. And I was starving!

Introduction

As a teenage girl I was fat, unhealthy, and frustrated. I had one dream, a very simple dream. I dreamed of being naturally lean and healthy, able to eat all the food I wanted, free from the horrible bondage of dieting.

At the time, it seemed an impossible dream. Now I know differently. I know, because I've made my dream come true. For the past eleven years I have been the lean and healthy person I dreamed of. I look better than I ever have, and I feel better, full of vitality and confidence. I have achieved all this, not by dieting but by eating.

Every day I eat about 2,000 to 3,500 calories of delicious and varied foods. Every day I follow the principles of health and eating that I uncovered after years of research, experimentation, and learning. These are the principles of the LEAN & FREE 2000 PLUS ULTIMATE WELLNESS/WEIGHT CONTROL LIFESTYLE, principles that not only restructured my body but, more importantly, restructured my inner self. Now, instead of focusing on my self and my own anxieties, I have found a way to channel my new energy toward being the loving, caring person I always hoped to be. Doing this has made my life so much more rich and expansive that I now have a new dream: to share my discovery with others who suffer the same guilt and frustrations that I did.

I'm well acquainted with this guilt and frustration, with the physical and emotional torture of obesity and failed diets. There was a time when I weighed 204 pounds, when I was barely able to squeeze into a size 14 dress or size 18 pants, when each thigh measured greater than my waist. The only diminutive thing about me was my self-esteem. I struggled with extreme depression and self-consciousness. I tried diet after diet and, as each one failed, I blamed myself. The only thing I seemed to lose on these diets was my health. I suffered overwhelming fatigue, constant illness and infections, and nearly intolerable back pain brought on by a desperate program of high-impact exercise.

In those days I was obsessed by thoughts about weight and food. My only purpose in life was to become thin, and that purpose consumed every ounce of my energy. At the same time, I resented the tyranny of those thoughts. So I began to hate my body and lose more and more confidence in myself. It seemed a hopeless situation, but it was not hopeless. There was a solution, a solution based on knowledge, and when I found it my entire life changed.

This knowledge can empower you, as it did me, to become the lean, healthy person you've always wanted to be, without ever having to diet or go hungry again. What you'll learn in the LEAN & FREE LIFESTYLE is based on scientific research and fact, and on thousands of personal experiences. This program isn't based on miracles or fables; it offers no gimmicks or quick fixes. It offers only truths — truths that work.

The "2000 PLUS" in the program name refers to the common sense of the past combined with the advanced technology of the present and future. It also stands for 2,000 plus calories. The majority of people who have become LEAN & FREE eat about 2,000 to 4,000 calories each day. However, some eat less and some more. This program is not about calorie numbers. It's about listening to your body and completely satisfying your body's hunger and energy needs.

If you diet or skip meals, you can trigger your body's starvation response, encouraging it to store fat. By eating an abundant amount of delicious, nourishing foods each day, you relieve your body of the starvation threat, making it possible to burn what you eat for energy rather than storing it as fat.

You can easily understand the principles in this program if you consider your favorite houseplant. To keep that plant vital and lush, you give it water and food and sunlight. Deprive it of these, and it withers and dies. Your body works the same way. That's why even people who have dieted "successfully" look gray, wrinkled, drawn, and tired.

In this program you will reverse everything you've been told about losing weight. You won't diet your way to an unhealthy, starved body. You will eat your way to health. You won't look wrinkled and drawn; you'll have much more energy and be less susceptible to illness. You'll actually reduce your risk of heart disease, stroke, cancer, diabetes, and many other diseases that plague people with high percentages of body fat and those who have starved themselves. You'll look great, you'll feel great, and you'll have the abundant vigor that frees you to be of service to all around you.

If you've dieted in the past, you probably think becoming lean by eating to full satisfaction on delicious, nourishing food is an outlandish idea. You've been conditioned to believe that the only way you'll ever lose weight is by eating small portions of bland, monotonous food. Yet you may also know that every time you finish a diet like this, you end up weighing more than you did before! So you become even more desperate, and when the next miracle diet comes along, you try again. It's a pattern I know very well. I rode the diet roller coaster for eight years, in spite of the fact that I never really believed in diets.

Even as a child I doubted the "logic" behind the theory that being overweight was simply the result of overeating. I saw too many thin people who ate far more food than I ever did and never gained an ounce. "They have naturally high metabolisms," I was told. But I sensed there was more, that there were uncovered secrets to being lean that I had yet to discover. Still, without the proper knowledge, I too fell into the diet trap. And it wasn't until I fully understood how and why my body stored and burned fat that I was able to say good-bye to diets forever and hello to a lean, healthy life.

During the past eleven years I have proven to myself and to thousands of others that eating, not starving, is the secret to successful weight management and optimal health. Now I eat what I want and as much as I want when I want. And I stay lean, but not because I'm one of those lucky people who was born with a high metabolism that burns off fat. I stay lean and healthy because I discovered the secrets of body-fat and health management you'll learn in this book.

The LEAN & FREE 2000 PLUS ULTIMATE WELLNESS/WEIGHT CONTROL LIFESTYLE is a direct result of my personal experience with body-fat problems, of my desperate desire to be lean, my repeated, discouraging experiments with diets, and finally my own determination to find out the truth about my body and how it works. It's the result of a personal odyssey that began when I was only a child.

As a little girl I was what my grandmother called "pleasantly plump." She was only half right. I was plump, but it was far from pleasant. Because of my extra weight, it took me three years to learn to ride a bicycle. Because of my weight and my lack of coordination, I was usually the last one picked for any team sport in school, so I became insecure and shy. I was also called nicknames, like "chubby," names that got worse during the junior-high-school years. In those years, when young people are so quick to target a weakness in others, I was often ridiculed because of my shyness and awkwardness.

My weight even interfered with my academic goals. Every term I would receive straight A's except for one devastating C in gym, even though I was making an all-out effort to succeed in my PE classes. But I was unhealthy and unfit. I would run hard in class, then have spells of nausea or dizziness. Sit-ups left me with purple bruises up and down my spine. I would often walk back to my locker room with a piercing side ache. My knees would buckle under me from extreme shakiness and weakness.

Still, I pushed on, until in eighth grade I received B's in PE and in the ninth grade I finally got A's. There was a new reason for this sudden capability. I had grown four inches between the eighth and ninth grade, and my body had stretched out to be slimmer and more graceful. When I returned to school after summer break I was 5'8 1/2" and weighed only 119 pounds. I was hardly recognizable. Friends asked me if I had been on a diet, but at that time I barely knew what a diet was. I was soon to find out. It was exhilarating to be slim and graceful, to be able to achieve my goals, and to receive the admiration of others. But it was not to last. My weight problems were just beginning.

By my sophomore year I had gained ten pounds. By my junior year I had gained ten more. In my senior year I gained ten pounds in just the first half of the year. The new slim me had disappeared nearly as quickly as it had come. Now I was a tight-fitting size 13-14. And I was concerned.

That's when I made the big mistake—I began to diet. Up until then I had been neither a fussy nor an obsessive eater. I had loved everything from broccoli to hot fudge cake. I had never experienced strange associations with food or uncontrollable cravings. When I began to diet, that all changed. I became preoccupied with foods, particularly those that were "taboo," like fats and sweets.

Far more agonizing than my desire for food were the disappointing results of my diets. After every low-calorie diet I gained more weight. I started dieting at 148 pounds and dropped to 140. Then I gained to 150 and dropped to 141. Finally, I gained to 152 and then dropped to a miserable 145. Desperate, I was soon eating only 600 calories per day. And still the weight stayed. Frantic, I began to deprive myself of even more calories. I became an habitual meal skipper and an intensive, exhausted exerciser.

The terrible cycle of eating, guilt, and punishment took over. One day I would eat 295 calories; the next I would binge to well above 4,000. I might binge on one and a half cups of chocolate-chip cookie dough for lunch or a half gallon of ice cream with chocolate syrup for dinner. Afterward, I felt stuffed but certainly not happy or satisfied. After such binges, I felt out of control and consumed with self-hate.

I was in the middle of my weight crisis when I entered college, where I majored in child and family studies with an emphasis on nutrition and communication. That choice was an attempt to master what I felt were my two greatest weaknesses: uncontrolled eating and extreme self-consciousness and shyness.

I was married at the beginning of my junior year in college, and the following spring my husband, Nyle, and I found we were expecting a baby. It was the first of four pregnancies, and each one would further affect my weight, my nutrition habits, and my self-image.

As with many new mothers, I felt my first baby seemed to bring life to an abrupt and screeching halt. Suddenly I was confined to home, surrounded by four walls, the cries of an infant, and 180 pounds of myself. I felt overwhelmed and I felt unattractive. This was not the fault of my husband, who was sweet and understanding and never criticized me. Still, I couldn't help but imagine how much delight he might take in a wife who was a size 9, as I had been in ninth grade.

Depressed by the pounds pregnancy had added to my already overweight body, I launched another diet while still nursing my baby, even though I'd had nothing but negative experiences with diets. As a result of that diet, little Aaron suffered from extreme constipation and is my only child with a tendency toward chubbiness.

A year after Aaron's birth, through calorie cutting and meal skipping, I had reduced to 136 pounds. Then I discovered I was pregnant again. During this pregnancy it seemed I only had to breathe to gain weight. Even though I was averaging no more than 1,200 calories per day, I gained about eight pounds between each visit to the doctor.

After I had Tyson, my second son, I weighed more than 200 pounds for six months. I tried everything to lose weight: six tiny meals per day; 800 calories per day; then 500 calories; then 300; even skipping meals altogether. I was also struggling with what I know now are the side effects of dieting: extreme depression, fatigue, strep throat, mononucleosis, ear infections, and intolerable back pain brought on by high-impact exercises and low blood sugar (hypoglycemia).

Frustrated and discouraged, I finally sought help. I contacted a college professor who performed a treadmill test on me, which revealed a resting pulse rate of 110, a severe electrolyte imbalance, and an erratic heartbeat. He then told me something that seemed incredible, impossible. It was something that would start me on the search that would eventually lead to the permanent solution to my weight and health problems. What he told me was this: *Recent scientific research indicates the body can't tell the difference between starving and dieting, so the answer to a lean, healthy body may be eating more, not less.*

I already knew that every time I dieted, I only seemed to get fatter. I knew that traditional diets and weight-loss methods were ineffective, even counterproductive. So his theory intrigued me, and it seemed worth investigating. I began a phase of intensive research and learning. I read all the literature I could find from all the experts: the World Health Organization, the National Institutes of Health, the American Cancer Society, the American Diabetic Association, and the American Heart Association. I studied the Pritikin weight-loss system and read many other reputable books. I kept thinking that one of these sources would have all the answers. Yet while they all made contributions to my understanding of good health and body-fat management, each fell far short of the complete solution. There was only one choice: I must develop something that worked for me or remain fat and unhealthy.

I began by incorporating into my lifestyle the two or three scientifically valid principles from each source that seemed to make the most sense for me. And, because I strongly believe in the importance of sharing and teaching new, invaluable discoveries, I began teaching these principles several times each week, and have since taught thousands of nonprofit nutrition and aerobics classes.

After a year, I felt that the principles of my new program had been fully integrated into my own life. I was eating between 2,000 and 3,500 calories per day, a dramatic increase over my previous habits. I was exercising moderately, my body fat was down, and I looked and felt great. Still I wasn't confident I had the complete answer.

I was still having occasional binges, then compensating with an extra hour or two of exercise. However, even though some of the pieces to the puzzle were missing, I was still aware of some amazing benefits. My former health problems had virtually disappeared. My resting pulse rate had dropped to fifty-five. I was excited about life. I still lacked complete faith in my "eat more and lose weight" philosophy, but the evidence was mounting. Every time I doubted and cut my calorie intake to less than comfortable satisfaction, I maintained or gained body fat.

Further proof came during my last two pregnancies. With my third son, Riley, I adhered strictly to my eating and exercise plan and gained only twenty-eight pounds, pounds that I lost quickly after he was born. Then I betrayed my own learning in my fourth pregnancy with son Chase. I felt if I had done so well with Riley, I might do even better this time by eating less. But instead I gained thirty-five pounds, and after his birth I didn't lose a single pound for four months.

These results left me confused, and I stayed confused until I heard about a fat-loss program run by a very reputable organization that promoted eating all you want. I was elated. I was sure this must be the final piece to my weight-management puzzle. My picture of easy, lifetime leanness and good health would at last be complete.

As it turned out, I had been set up for yet another disappointment in my ongoing battle with weight solutions and diets. Although this program did refer to abundant eating, in reality the program was based on another restricted diet of approximately 1,000 to 1,200 calories. For me this theory of weight loss had already been proven false and antiquated. I felt as if it were the year 1491 and I was sitting in a geography class being told the earth was flat. And I felt pain and empathy for the others in the class who probably weren't aware of the truths I had been lucky enough to discover.

I went home that night, took the food-recording sheet from class, and restructured it completely. I added categories for water, vegetables, grain, protein, and fruit. I replaced the column reading "why you are eating" with "snacks." I continued to attend class, but now I was following my own program. At the end of the nine-week course, I had dropped nineteen pounds and reduced from a size 10 to a size 4, the biggest improvement in the class. And, I was eating around 4,000 calories a day and still nursing a baby. Other students were eating about one-fourth what I was without any results, and many of them were nursing mothers too. They continually asked me how I was doing so well.

On the last night of class, the director of this organization, who was struggling with post-pregnancy fat-loss resistance, asked me if I would like to teach my program to the follow-up classes of students. She said my philosophy of balanced eating and abundant calories was exactly what their organization was trying to implement, but it had no one trained to teach such principles. With her full support, I rewrote most of the handouts and began teaching the class.

Teaching this course proved to be the validation of all the research and study I had completed and the system I had created. It proved to me conclusively that not only had my new lifestyle made me lean, healthy, and attractive but also that it would help do the same for everyone.

My first rule was that no class members were to weigh themselves, because success on this program is not measured by pounds lost. The woman that lost the most body fat during my ten-week course lost only one pound of weight. Yet she reduced forty inches and three dress sizes. And she did so while eating more than 2,000 calories a day. Most telling, she had just come off a medically supervised 800-calories-a-day diet in which she had gained eight pounds!

She is only one example of the millions of Americans who struggle with the frustration and disappointment of traditional diet plans. After the success of these classes, I had many people ask me to start my own classes, so I did. I expected only 30 people at my first class. There were more than 150. Since then I've had thousands of students of all types and sizes from all walks of life, and even the most conservative doctors have praised my program. But the bottom line for me is how I look and, even more important, how I feel. The program has given me strength, freedom, and the confidence that I can triumph over any obstacle or challenge, qualities that were put severely to the test when I lost my husband, Nyle, in a traffic accident.

In March of 1989, Nyle, our four boys, and I traveled to California for a vacation. I remember thinking on that trip, as I had many times before, how lucky I was to have a husband who was so supportive, so fun, and so attractive. That world of contentment and security was soon to be shattered.

While we were driving home at night across the desert, a large elk suddenly appeared on the road before us. The car hit the side of the animal, then left the road. When I steered it back onto the pavement, the damaged bumper caught the shoulder of the road, and we flipped end-over-end four times.

We had always been seat-belt fanatics, but that night the kids had been forced to sit up for hours. They were tired and unhappy. We had bedded them all down in the station wagon except the youngest, who was buckled into his car seat. Nyle had just unclasped his seat belt to reach back and give the baby his bottle.

Unrestrained, Nyle was thrown from the car. He hit the pavement and suffered fatal head injuries. Riley was lying next to Nyle on the road and was not expected to live through the night. Aaron had a crushed leg, with thirty breaks from the hip down to the knee, and a broken arm. Tyson had a crushed foot and ankle. Chase, my youngest, was unhurt. My head had slammed into the side window, and I was unconscious. I suffered a concussion and an injured neck.

Miraculously, after body casts and numerous surgeries, every one of the boys fully recovered. My own emotional recovery was slow but steady, and I believe it was achieved only because of the emotional and physical strength I had developed by following the principles of this program.

At first I began living my life one hour at a time. I couldn't imagine being happy for a week, so I tried to be happy for an hour. I read inspiring literature, listened to motivational tapes, and continued to follow the principles I had learned, which are the basis of Lean & Free 2000 Plus. For the first time in my life, I ate not because I was hungry but because I knew I must. I felt no hunger, just complete, consuming emptiness. I exercised because it gave me a welcome respite from grief. I didn't watch television or videos because they inevitably depressed me. Even a light-hearted story like *The Music Man* filled me with self-pity. Marian the Librarian's life was just beginning, and mine was over.

There is only one way to break the shackles of grief. It is by shifting your focus to others. I channeled my energy toward my children and my church, into community service, and into the service of teaching others about the principles of my program. Finally, with the loving support of family and friends, my boys and I recovered fully. I began to be happy for more than an hour at a time, for a week, for a month, then for several months.

I have no doubts that I would have struggled much harder and longer with my grief had this program not prepared me with physical and emotional health. It is a benefit of the Lean & Free Lifestyle.

Lean & Free is not really about food or body fat or exercise. It is about happiness—the happiness that comes from being strong, capable, and free to love and give. It is about breaking the ties that hold us down and prevent us from being all we can be, whether those ties are food obsessions, self-doubt, or grief. It's about making your life something more than just day-to-day survival. Ultimately, it's about love and our highest, greatest purpose.

Today I am happily remarried with eight children in my home, my four and the four children of my new husband, who lost his first wife to cancer about five weeks after the accident that took Nyle. I feel capable of handling life's biggest challenges, and the Lean & Free Lifestyle is largely responsible for that feeling.

In the past few years, the success of the program seems to have exploded. Its success is growing rapidly, chiefly through word-of-mouth. People tell their friends about an incredible system that lets you lose excess body fat through eating rather than dieting. The dramatic difference in how these people look and feel speaks for itself. In my community alone, fifty thousand people have benefited from this program. And now word of its success is spreading throughout the country.

The LEAN & FREE LIFESTYLE has worked for me and tens of thousands of other people—people just like you who had tried traditional, ineffective diets and who had nearly given up on themselves.

In this book you'll learn about some of these people and how the revolutionary principles in this program have finally released them from the miserable cycle of dieting, guilt, and self-hate. Now they are free, free to live and enjoy life at their highest level of potential.

You'll also learn the principles that freed these people, principles based on my many years of personal experience and researching the latest studies on health, nutrition, and weight management. This experience and study has led to the development of what I call the Eight Step LEAN & FREE 2000 PLUS ULTIMATE WELLNESS/WEIGHT CONTROL LIFESTYLE. Each of the eight steps is detailed in the following chapters.

Step 1: Knowledge

The key to having power over your own body lies in knowledge, the knowledge of how your body functions—specifically, how it stores and burns fat. To obtain that knowledge, I studied the latest scientific research available on the topic, becoming informed on nutrition, fitness, and fat loss. Once I understood how my body worked, I knew what needed to be done to create a fat-burning, energetic, attractive body. In chapter 1, I'll share this knowledge with you so you too can optimize your health and leanness.

You'll learn there are three types of bodies: (1) fat storing; (2) neutral; and (3) fat burning. Most important, you'll learn about your body's survival system and how you can work with it, not against it, to transform your body into a lean, fat-burning machine, one that is approximately 15 to 25 percent fat for a woman and 10 to 20 percent fat for a man.

This survival system operates very simply: If your body perceives a threat to its survival, it sets up defense mechanisms. And the biggest threat your body knows is the threat of starvation. As soon as you begin to deprive your body of plentiful food and nutrients, as happens when you diet or eat poorly balanced meals, those defense mechanisms may kick in. Your body may slow its metabolism and store fat in an aggressive attempt to protect itself from starvation. Excess fat storage is simply a symptom of a body under stress. Therefore, controlling stress becomes the first step in creating a healthy, high-energy, fat-burning body.

To do that, you must first stop dieting. Dieting may be the number-one cause of fat storage. There are other causes, too. I've isolated the twelve leading fat-storing stressors and will describe each one in this chapter, then provide you with methods for controlling them.

With this knowledge you will have the key to personal transformation. Perhaps for the first time in your life, you'll be able to understand how your body works and why it's in the shape it's in. This understanding will help give you control and trigger deep within you a sense of hope and belief. As you begin to understand many of the reasons for your excess body fat and poor health, you'll develop the power to change your life!

Step 2: Commitment

After step 1, you will have broken through the barrier. You'll finally have understanding, and with understanding comes the possibility for change. In chapter 2 you'll learn how to channel that hope into commitment, and commitment is essential if you are to succeed.

Unlike traditional diets, with their false promises of quick, easy results, the LEAN & FREE ULTIMATE WELLNESS LIFESTYLE requires time. It requires time simply because it takes time for your body to change from a fat-storing chemistry to a fat-burning chemistry. It cannot and will not happen magically overnight. Since this transformation will be gradual, you'll need to learn patience and perseverance. You will discover how to expand short-term goals into long-term goals. In this chapter you'll learn the key to keeping motivated while you gradually unveil the new you. You will already have achieved part of what's necessary to do that. After chapter 1, you'll have a belief in the possibility of change, a belief based on your new knowledge and understanding of your own body. Next, I will help you create a vision of your future as a lean, healthy, and happy person, a vision that is believable, attainable, and powerful. You'll know how you'll look, how you'll feel, and how your life will change. From this vision, you'll draw the emotional strength you need to successfully see yourself through the process of change.

To further inspire you, I'll offer stories, true stories, about people just like you who have transformed their bodies through the principles in this program. Their stories will motivate you even further, reinforcing your hope, belief, and commitment.

Your own transformation may happen more quickly or more slowly than theirs; every person is different. But after completing this chapter, you'll know unequivocally that you too can become lean, and stay lean, without ever having to diet or go hungry again.

Step 3: Nurturing

In the struggle against fat, we are often our own worst enemies, but not for the reasons we think. We think it is our own weakness, our lack of willpower, that causes us to remain fat. Ironically, it may not be our lack of willpower but our guilt and self-blame that is one of the major reasons for fat storage.

Fat-storing people are often filled with self-hate or a great dislike for the way their bodies look. They may end up despising their bodies and themselves, creating a virtual war in which their body is the enemy. This self-dislike creates a feeling of desperation that may encourage extreme dieting behavior and, in some cases, total starvation. As a result the body slows its metabolism during starvation or diet periods and greatly increases fat and sugar cravings. Then, when these foods are eaten, the body stores all it can in the fat cells because it is starved for nourishing calories and nutrients. Therefore, the more you hate your body, the more despair you'll feel. The more despair you feel, the more likely you are to go to extreme measures to change your body, setting up a vicious, compounding cycle of self-hate, desperate behavior, and excessive fat storage.

In chapter 3, you'll learn how to break this destructive cycle, first through knowledge and then through control. You'll learn how to become friends with your body, how to release it from blame, and how to forgive it. Until now, your body has only been a victim, a passive victim of your own lack of knowledge. You can now take active control of your life. You can sign a peace treaty with your body and begin to work with it, not against it. You'll learn how to nourish and nurture it, how to praise it, so that the major stress of self-hatred is eliminated. The relationship you'll have with your body will be one of teamwork, you and your body working in unison toward the common goal of health and fitness.

Step 4: Nourishment

By now it should come as no surprise to you that a basic principle in the LEAN & FREE LIFESTYLE is this: *eat.* Once you begin to feed and nourish your starving body, it will gradually drop its defense mechanisms against starvation. Unthreatened, it can cease to store fat in the stubborn way it did when you dieted.

Just as in chapter 3 you will learn to see your body as a friend and not an enemy, in chapter 4 you'll learn to see food in the same way. The right foods contain all the vitamins, minerals, complex carbohydrates, proteins, and essential fats your body requires to feel fully nourished and guaranteed of survival. In response to these foods, your body will trigger the fat-burning mechanisms that will reshape you and fill you with energy and vitality. On this program you will be feeding your body more good food than you've probably ever eaten in your life, for many people at least 2,000 calories of it a day. But you increase these calories *gradually.*

In chapter 4, you'll be introduced to the delicious, easy-to-prepare foods that can help transform your body from a fat-storing warehouse to a fat-burning machine.

Step 5: Movement

Our bodies have a built-in survival system that also served our ancestors. Before the Industrial Age, our ancestors were often under threat of famine, starvation, and death. Ironically, many of us today no longer worry about starving. Our major concern is dieting. Times have changed, but our bodies have not. So to fully understand how our bodies function, we must first understand the origin of those functions.

Before the Industrial Age, our ancestors, from whom we inherited our survival system, depended on hard physical labor to stay alive. Depending on their environment, their activities included hunting, fishing, gathering foods, tilling soil, harvesting crops, scrubbing clothing and floors by hand, building shelters, walking, running, and horseback riding, and the list goes on and on. The point is, they had to physically toil to maintain their very survival.

Although people still perform many of these same labors today, most of us do not engage in extensive amounts of vigorous physical activity. We're often emotionally and physically exhausted by our hectic schedules. So, we don't enjoy the relief from stress often provided by vigorous physical activity. Our ancestors had to move a lot to survive. Most of us do not.

Our ancestors' bodies stored fat when food was scarce as a way to protect against famine. Their metabolism slowed, so they burned fewer calories while at work and at rest.[11-15] However, when food was plentiful, their metabolisms quickened, and they burned many more calories throughout the day. Their energy increased as their fat stores decreased. They had more desire to move and were able to hunt, fish, plant, harvest, gather, and walk with more zest, further encouraging their bodies to burn fat. This fat loss increased their ability to obtain food. This further aided their survival.

In chapter 5 you'll learn seven simple movements that duplicate those of our ancestors and that help trigger your body's fat-burning systems. These movements are low in impact, based on efficiency, not intensity. When included in an easy-to-follow exercise routine, they will help you stay lean and tone your body to give it a supple, healthy look. These movements will also help create lean body tissue and produce fat-burning enzymes. And, as an extra bonus, you'll discover that these movements will help produce "feel-good" hormones, hormones that actually help crystallize your thinking, provide a buffer against emotional stress, and put you in a positive state of mind. No matter what your level of fitness, you'll

14

learn how to adapt these movements to the level of intensity and duration that is right for you.

Step 6: Service

In chapter 6, we'll explore the greater implications of being lean and free, its link with your life purpose.

The ultimate purpose of food is to translate fuel into active energy. For the early ancestors we've talked about, that purpose was mainly survival, survival of self and family. Their energy was focused almost exclusively on staying alive. Today we live in a different environment, but, as you've learned, the body's mechanisms remain the same.

To provide you with energy, your body needs to have a purpose for that energy. Since we no longer gather and hunt for food, since we no longer fight for our daily survival and strive constantly to ward off starvation, we must find purpose in something else.

It is the theory of the LEAN & FREE LIFESTYLE that the human purpose, free of the fight for survival, has been elevated to new, more universal realms. As the final step in this program, you'll learn how to redirect new-found energy from survival to a higher purpose.

The only purpose that remains to us is that of service, loving and selfless service to others. This purpose manifests itself differently for everyone. It can be expressed within a family or a community, or on a national or global scale. The ultimate goal of the LEAN & FREE LIFESTYLE is to free each of us to be healthy and energetic enough to focus not on our own worries and fears but on ways to be of greater service to others. That purpose will signal our bodies to generate energy and to remain healthy, lean, and strong. Without it, there is simply no reason to survive. With it, we do more than survive. We flourish.

Step 7: Planning

In chapter 7, I'll give you a system that integrates all you've learned in the previous chapters into a complete fat-reduction program. Included is a simple, daily planning sheet that will show you exactly what to do each day. There are also success sheets that employ all the principles of the program and enable you to grade your own progress. You won't need all A's to succeed! Even an average in the low B's will bring some results. You'll be free to eat pizza without failing. You'll be free to indulge in cookies without loathing yourself for hours afterward. You'll be free to eat, to enjoy life, and to take pride in your own ability to reshape your body and your life. You'll be given my easy-to-follow individually adustable meal plans, a "menu of plenty" that provides you with many delicious meals (breakfasts, lunches, dinners, and snacks). This menu plan is almost exactly the plan my family and I follow daily and most of the meals take five or ten minutes to prepare. They also work well with very tight budgets.

Step 8: Action

By chapter 7, you will be fully prepared to embark on your new program of health and fitness. You'll be ready for action! With a plan for that action now charted, I'll show you how to start the program and how to keep it going until these principles are a permanent part of your life.

First, I'll show you how to measure your progress, measurement that will no longer depend on that dreary and disheartening scale. Instead I'll identify ten signs of success that will help you know your body is making the appropriate changes, changes that will inspire you and fuel your commitment even further.

QUESTION: *Dana, these eight steps sound great, but I want to get started right now. What should I do today?*

ANSWER: *Simply start with the eating. Read pages 239 through 244 very thoroughly so that you understand exactly how to personalize the simple and delicious LEAN & FREE menus to your individual time schedule, calorie needs, and lifestyle. Then, follow the sample menus beginning on page 245. It's that simple. If you own a can opener, you can do this program!*

Gradually add in the other elements of your new LEAN & FREE LIFESTYLE over the next few weeks and months at a pace that is comfortable for you. But start with the eating!

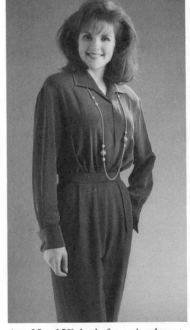

Age 35 – 15% body fat – size 4 pant

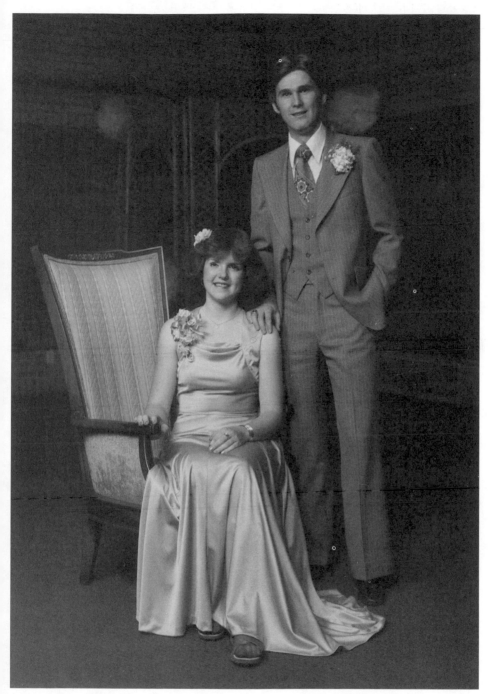

At age 19 I wore a tight size 14 pant and was about 34 percent body fat. I weighed 150 pounds. Today at a size 4 and 15 percent body fat, I weigh 150 pounds— amazing!

1. KNOWLEDGE

UNDERSTANDING YOUR BODY'S SURVIVAL SYSTEM

*I*n the introduction, I told you how I gained control of my body and my life, not by dieting but by gradually increasing my calories. I eat an average of more than 2,000 calories of delicious food every day.

Then I introduced you to the LEAN & FREE LIFESTYLE and its unique eight-step, fat-reduction system that teaches you to feed yourself lean and healthy rather than starve yourself thin.

While many people use the terms *lean* and *thin* interchangeably, there is a critical difference between them. People who are thin because they have lost significant amounts of weight through calorie deprivation (or starvation) programs also look unhealthy. They can appear gaunt, drawn, and wrinkled. They often experience lethargy and low energy.

Through dieting or starving, they have lost bone strength, muscle, and body water, three essentials of good health. But lean people are the opposite. They have smooth skin, well-defined muscles, and strong bones. They look healthy, vital, and vibrant. They radiate vibrancy and energy.

The LEAN & FREE LIFESTYLE can help you become naturally lean and let you feel and reflect all the benefits of a healthy and happy life. This program combines my eleven years of study and personal experience with the experiences of others who have successfully followed these principles and have attained leanness, inner well-being, and permanent freedom from dieting.

Now it's time for you too to take the first step, to begin accumulating the knowledge you need to transform your body. It is the lack of knowledge, not willpower, that has kept you from succeeding. Knowledge is the first critical step because it empowers and motivates you to take action. Once you know how your body works and what you need to do to change it from a fat-storing warehouse to a fat-burning machine, you will be able to accept the responsibility for changing your life. You will have the confidence that comes with knowing you are doing exactly what is needed to meet your goals. Later in the program, after you've attained this knowledge, I'll provide you with a specific plan of action. And that action will be based on the truths you've learned in this chapter.

Until now, you have been making decisions and taking actions based on information that was false, including the misconception that the less you eat, the leaner you'll be. You have been a victim. You have been a victim of popular trends, misleading advertising, ill-devised products and programs, and inadequate research about the human body.

Because you were guided in your actions by false information, those actions were ineffectual and futile. When success eluded you, you became disappointed and frustrated, and you blamed yourself. This self-hatred only increased your body's resistance to burning fat, so your goal became even more elusive.

There is only one way to break this vicious cycle of ignorance, failure, and despair. It is to replace ignorance with knowledge.

With information that is accurate, you can take actions that are appropriate and effective. You can cease to be a victim and can become instead the manager of your own body. When your actions are based on knowledge, on accurate information, you will get results. Those results, in turn, will increase your confidence and sense of empowerment. Your positive sense of self will then work in harmony with your body's survival system to increase your health and energy and decrease your stress level and excess body fat.

And, these results will become more and more noticeable, and your sense of control will strengthen even further.

The positive results and the confidence they inspire all spiral upward from that solid foundation of knowledge. It is knowledge alone that can free you from the desperate role of the victim and provide you with the power to design your own destiny.

To begin building your knowledge base, I'd first like to explain the term *metabolism,* because it's a term that plays an important role in any program designed to restructure the human body. You've probably heard people talk about metabolism all your life, but you may not be fully aware of what it really means. First of all, in spite of myths to the contrary, metabolism is not something lean people have that fat people don't. Everyone has a metabolism. Metabolism is simply the process your body goes through to transform the food you eat into energy. Its only purpose is to create energy to sustain life. This energy is used to maintain vital body functions, to perpetuate the species through reproduction, and to gather food for continued survival. People with lean, healthy bodies have fat-burning metabolisms. Their bodies burn more of what they eat for energy. And this energy is active and is used in purposeful ways. People who have excess body fat generally have fat-storing metabolisms. Their bodies store more of the food they eat as fat or stored energy. This stored energy is dormant, not active.

Right now your body is in either a fat-burning state, a neutral state, or a fat-storing state.

If it's in a fat-burning state, your body can convert virtually everything you eat into energy. If it's in a neutral state, your body is weight stable. That is, you can eat large amounts of food without gaining significant amounts of weight. You may gain ten pounds in a year but certainly not in a weekend. If you're in a fat-storing state, your body is under stress; for one reason or another there is a threat to your body's health and survival system.

In response to this stress, your body may be defending itself by storing a high percentage of what you eat as fat. As a result, you have little energy and crave quick-energy foods such as sweets and fats—foods that can encourage even more fat storage.

Having the ability to store fat is not a curse; it's a blessing. In fact, it is the key to the survival of our species. This survival system holds the important secret to how and why your body stores and burns fat. It is critical that you understand the system.

All the principles in this program are based on the functions of your body's survival system and its effect on your health. The survival system is not technical or complex. You need to understand only a few basic facts about it, and you will have the knowledge you need to develop habits that will promote fat loss and physical and emotional well-being.

❑ You must know first that this survival system works the same for us as it did for our great-grandparents. In spite of dramatic changes in the external world, our basic physiological processes remain unchanged. This system protected our great-grandparents from starvation the same way it protects us against low-calorie diets.

❑ Your survival system is organized around one dominant goal: to protect your body against starvation. This is because starvation was the most common cause of death throughout history and continues to be so even today, especially in third-world countries. So, historically, starvation is the biggest threat to our survival. And you have inherited that legacy; your body is intently focused on protecting you from starvation and cannot always recognize what you can, which is that starvation is no longer a threat to a large segment of the more affluent societies.

❑ Your body has three primary ways to protect you from starvation. It can store fat. It can reduce your ability to expend energy, so that fat can be saved. And it can increase your craving for quick-energy foods, such as sweets and fatty foods.

❑ There are different signals that your body may receive as threats of famine, drought, or starvation. When it receives these signals it may begin triggering its protective mechanisms of storing fat and reducing energy.

❑ Of these signals, a decrease in food or caloric intake is the strongest signal to store fat. That is why diets actually promote fat gain. But there are other signals too, some of which may surprise you, some of which have psychological or emotional causes.

Your Survival System:

1. functions the same as it did for our ancestors.
2. has one dominant goal—to protect your body against starvation.
3. regulates your (1) fat-storage, (2) energy level, (3) fat and sweet cravings.
4. may encourage your body to store fat and reduce your energy level if your health is threatened by famine or drought.
5. interprets dieting and meal skipping as a threat of famine and as the strongest signal to store fat.

Many people, particularly those who live in northern climates where the daily hours of sunlight are reduced in winter, experience a form of depression. Their survival system signals them to become lethargic; there is a dramatic decline in their energy; and they experience an increase in their cravings for sugar and fat as the availability of direct sunlight diminishes. This condition, in its most severe form, is called Seasonal Affective Disorder (SAD). SAD is caused when the body's survival system interprets the decreasing availability of light as a sign that food will soon be scarce, and that it must store fat to assure its survival. Many SAD victims gain considerable amounts of weight in the winter.

This weight gain is not their fault. Their bodies are simply responding to a threat to life. Any time your survival system is signaled by such a threat, it may begin increasing your fat stores to protect you. And such threats can take many forms, a shortage of food being the most powerful one.

If you have excess fat, it is probably because your body has been put under stress, stress that can signal your survival system that your health is being threatened. The stresses we are going to talk about in this chapter are all health threatening. As your body becomes less healthy, your survival system may reduce your energy level, slow your metabolism, and store more of the food you eat as fat because it is not being burned for energy.

Through my years of study and counseling, I have identified twelve key fat-storing stressors that can trigger your body's survival system to store excess fat. These key stressors may keep your body locked in a fat-storing zone for an extended length of time. Yet each of these stressors is avoidable—they should be eliminated, or at least moderated, for you to become optimally healthy and lean.

The Twelve Avoidable Fat-Storing Stressors

1. Dieting

The first and by far the most significant avoidable fat-storing stressor is dieting, or limiting your intake of food and skipping meals. Why? Because your body cannot tell the difference between starvation and a limited intake of food. All your body knows is that the ideal amount of food is not available and that it must switch into its life-saving mode by conserving energy and producing an insatiable appetite for sweets and fats. Any program that restricts your caloric intake to anything less than full satisfaction for you is a *diet*, no matter what it is called. And your body interprets calorie deprivation as starvation and reacts accordingly:

❑ You lose energy. You feel tired and lethargic.

❑ You crave fat and sugar-laden, quick-energy foods.

❑ Your body gradually converts lean muscle tissue to glucose to be used as energy. In other words, a highly muscled person would probably die much more quickly during total starvation than a high-fat person. So the body adapts to prevent death by starvation. Your body clings to fat stores by reducing the number of calories you burn at rest and during daily activity.[1-6*]

❑ Your body increases its number of fat-storing enzymes that act like little magnets to catch and store fat.[7-9]

❑ Without adequate complex carbohydrates in the diet, your body loses excessive amounts of water—resulting in gray, wrinkled, and dehydrated skin. Vitamin and mineral intake is restricted, resulting in a devitalizing of skin, hair, and nails and a loss of brightness in the eyes.

❑ You become depressed, a natural side effect of chemical changes taking place within your brain. This occurs when your body sets up its defenses against what it perceives as starvation and a threat to its health and well-being.
References begin on page 221.

22

Diets also have a long-term effect on weight gain. With each diet, your body may store more fat than before in an effort to protect you from future diets. So at first, you may lose weight on 1,500 calories per day. But then your body will begin to gradually slow your metabolism and reduce your energy level until you find you are only maintaining your new weight level at 1,500 calories.

At that point you may decrease to 1,200 calories per day. Again you will lose weight, but only until your body adjusts. Then you may maintain the weight and eventually even gain weight. In response, you may decrease your intake yet again, to 900 calories. The same pattern repeats itself: you lose, then maintain, then gain. Finally, you may get as efficient as one woman I know who gained thirteen pounds during two weeks of a 300-calorie-a-day diet. Your body has a tremendous capacity to adjust and store fat when caloric amounts are too low to guarantee its safety!

The inevitable conclusion that people who diet are fatter than those who don't is confirmed by many studies. Recently, the *American Journal of Clinical Nutrition* observed forty women who consumed approximately 1,500 calories per day (these women were labeled as "small eaters"). They also observed another forty who were considered "large eaters"; they consumed 2,400 calories per day. (Both the small and large eaters were nonexercisers.)

Since the "small eaters" averaged 33 percent body fat, we might assume that the "large eaters" would top the 40-percent mark. But we'd be wrong. The so-called "large eaters" averaged just 22 percent body fat![10] Why? Because they were eating enough food to satisfy the body's survival system, and it therefore felt no need to trigger fat-storing processes.

Another study of dieters and non-dieters showed that even though dieters ate 410 fewer calories per day than non-dieters, they were significantly fatter. The same study showed that dieters burned 620 fewer calories per day while involved in similar activities as the non-dieters.[6] This means that when a dieter moves, he or she may burn fewer calories than a non-dieter who is doing exactly the same activity at the same pace and duration. Remember, diets reduce your ability to turn the food you eat into energy by triggering your body's defense against starvation.

These are some of the many reasons that diets simply do not work. And there are many studies to prove it. In one study published by the National Institutes of Health, it was reported that of every two thousand people who diet, only ten lose all the weight they desire, and only one of that ten keeps the weight off for any appreciable length of time!

Those who do "succeed" pay a high price. You can easily identify such dieters in any crowd. They're the gaunt, skinny ones with dull, hollow eyes; graying complexions; dry, thinning hair; and flabby-skinned necks. The other "lucky 999" put all their weight back on plus approximately 8 to 20 percent more. As an example, if a dieter initially loses fifty pounds, chances are excellent that he or she will gain back anywhere from fifty-four to sixty pounds. When you multiply that by a lifetime of diets, it's easy to understand how some people attain weights of 400 pounds and even more.

These studies show why dieting is the number-one fat-storing stressor and why, by itself, it may even be more powerful than the other eleven stressors combined. By signaling your body that a famine is imminent, dieting triggers your body's survival system, causing it to store a high percentage of what you eat as fat, to reduce your energy level, and to crave quick-energy foods high in fat and sugar.

To reverse this fat-storing trend, you must quit starving yourself. And to do that, it is essential that you *gradually* increase your calories if you've been a dieter or a meal skipper. In chapter 4, I'll tell you about the delicious, normal foods you get to eat—foods you may have thought were absolute no-no's. I'll also teach you how to listen to your body's hunger signals. Remember, dieting to cure obesity and poor health is as counterproductive as drinking alcohol (a depressant) to cure depression.

2. Dehydration

The second avoidable fat-storing stressor is dehydration, because it can also seriously threaten your survival. When your body is low in water, your survival system may detect a drought/famine situation. Water cleanses your body. Without adequate amounts of it, your body cannot effectively rid itself of wastes and toxins.[12] The membranes surrounding your body's cells (the process of metabolism takes place within the cells of your body) become impaired and interfere with metabolic processes such as your muscles' ability to burn fat. For optimum health, your body should consist of approximately two-thirds water at all times.

3. Excess or Insufficient Fat Intake

The third avoidable fat-storing stressor is created by an imbalance in fat consumption.[13-18] In such cases, you may eat either too much fat or too little. If you eat too much fat, your body can store this excess in your fat cells, much more easily than it can store carbohydrates in the form of glycogen.[19,20] If you eat too little fat, your body may feel that it is in a starvation circumstance, because fat is an essential nutrient. And insufficient fat intake can weaken your immune system and negatively affect the growth and repair of muscles and all organs of the body. In both cases, the body feels threatened, is under stress, and activates its powerful survival system.

Fats are essential for health and provide your body with many benefits. They supply a highly concentrated source of energy, enhance the flavor and aroma of foods, cushion vital body organs, protect against temperature extremes, are broken down into fatty acids for prostaglandin and cell membrane formation, carry fat-soluble vitamins A, D, E, and K, and help you feel fuller longer after a meal.

However, excess dietary fat is easily deposited in your body's fat cells, leading to obesity. It has been tied to the increased risk of degenerative diseases such as heart disease, diabetes, high blood pressure, and cancer,[13-15,18,21-24] and certain fats may even encourage people to bleed excessively. Eskimos, known for their large intake of whale fat, have difficulty stopping even nosebleeds.

Insufficient fat intake can also create problems. Diets that are less than 10 percent fat may result in the weakening of cell walls and reduced resistance to infection and disease as well as a host of other maladies, including weakness and fatigue (also a symptom of *too much* dietary fat).

In order to de-stress your body and signal your survival system to increase your body's fat-burning capacity, it is essential to follow an eating program in which your fat intake, along with other nutrients, is completely balanced. I will fully describe a balanced eating plan later in this book. For now, know that the principles you'll learn in this program can accelerate your permanent reduction of excess body fat.

4. Excess Refined Carbohydrates and Insufficient Complex Carbohydrates

A diet too high in concentrated sugar and white-flour–based foods[28-34] (refined carbohydrates) combined with a low consumption of vegetables, grains, legumes, and fruits[35-46] (complex carbohydrates) is the fourth avoidable fat-storing stressor.

Sugar, honey, and other forms of refined carbohydrates require little time to digest and are quickly absorbed into the bloodstream, supplying quick, short-term energy that dissipates in a hurry. Your survival system may therefore increase your cravings for such refined carbohydrates when you eat too few nutritional calories to defend you against starvation. The consumption of large amounts of refined carbohydrates (especially on an empty stomach) may result in a marked rise in insulin, which can drive the glucose in your bloodstream into your fat cells. If high insulin levels persist, hypoglycemia may result.

Complex carbohydrates (vegetables, whole grains, legumes, and fruits) take a longer time to digest and provide energy at a slower, steadier, and more even rate. When supplied with plenty of complex carbohydrates, your survival system is assured of ample food. It can then relax and release excess stored fat. The vitamins and minerals from these foods are also necessary for efficient metabolism. When they are available, complex carbohydrates are more readily converted to energy rather than being stored as fat.

The LEAN & FREE LIFESTYLE will show you how to create a perfectly and easily balanced diet to eliminate this stressor. The elimination of this fourth stressor doesn't mean that you have to give up sweets. Quite the contrary. It means instead that you must learn when to eat them. This is wonderful news!

5. Excess Protein or Insufficient Protein

The fifth avoidable fat-storing stressor is excess protein or insufficient protein intake.[47-62] Protein is necessary for the growth and repair of muscle tissue and all organ systems. Since muscle provides the furnace where fat is burned, many people have the mistaken notion that the more protein they eat, the more fat they'll burn. However, your body can use only 10 to 15 percent protein in a complete eating program for muscle building. Whenever your menus include more than that from animal protein, combined with overall calorie restriction, your liver converts those proteins to glucose to be used for energy.

This process is very stressful to your body and may trigger the loss of significant amounts of water and muscle tissue. This explains why a high-protein, low-carbohydrate diet can produce immediate, dramatic weight loss. Your body is receiving insufficient amounts of carbohydrates needed for energy. So your liver must convert the protein you've eaten to glucose to be used for energy instead of allowing it to be used for growth and repair of muscle tissue. Therefore, you are destroying your fat-burning machinery—your muscle tissue—instead of burning fat. The scales go down while you dehydrate and lose muscle. And all of this signals your body's survival system to store even more fat.

The LEAN & FREE LIFESTYLE will easily provide the protein balance that eliminates the threat of either excessive or inadequate protein intake.

6. Excess Salt

The sixth avoidable fat-storing stressor is heavy salt consumption, which may result in an electrolyte imbalance and fluid retention.[63] If you occasionally consume excessive amounts of salt, increase your water intake to restore a fluid balance to your cells and help flush excess salt from your body. Heavy salt consumption signals your body that you are attempting to store water, and therefore a drought or famine is indicated. Too much salt also weakens cell membranes and impairs your cells' ability to carry nutrients in and waste products out of the cell.

Too little salt intake can also stress the body, leading to muscle cramps and mental apathy. However, salt deficiency is extremely rare.

7. Artificial Sweeteners and Unnecessary Drugs

The seventh fat-storing stressor is the use of any of the following: artificial sweeteners, caffeine, alcohol, tobacco, or illegal drugs. All of these alter your body's normal functioning and serve to threaten your health and survival system. This puts your body under stress, triggering its survival system to store excess fat.

Artificial sweeteners. According to many current studies, people who use artificial sweeteners gain more weight than those who do not. This is because the highly sweet taste of sweeteners fools your body into thinking you are storing energy for an impending famine.

If you drink diet soda, your favorite foods are probably cookies, ice cream, cake, donuts, pastries, and candy. Research shows that 150 million Americans use artificial sweeteners, such as those in diet sodas, to replace sugar. Yet at the same time, sugar consumption is up from 118 pounds per person per year to 127 pounds per year. That is because such sweeteners probably increase our cravings for sugar. NutraSweet (Aspartame), the most common artificial sweetener, seems to do just the opposite of what it promises (to control weight). Some studies suggest that it may promote weight gain even more than regular sugar.

❑ Studies suggest that artificial sweeteners: [64-76]
Are addictive: they produce a tremendous increase in cravings for
❑ both sugar and artificial sweeteners.
Promote depression: can severely alter the natural chemicals in the
❑ brain; can encourage extreme irritability, insomnia, and phobias.
Promote eye problems: May lead to flashes, pain, dryness, decrease
❑ in vision, and, in severe cases, blindness.
Promote hearing problems: ringing, buzzing, hearing loss, and noise
❑ intolerance.
Promote head and brain problems: headaches, dizziness, confusion, convulsions, severe drowsiness, slurred speech, hyperactivity, numbness,
❑ and facial pain.
Promote chest problems: rapid heartbeat, shortness of breath, and
❑ high blood pressure.
Promote gastrointestinal problems: nausea, diarrhea, and swal-
❑ lowing pain.
Promote skin and allergy problems, hair loss, and severe menstrual
❑ changes.
❑ Can promote hypoglycemia and diabetes.

In a recent issue of *Flying Safety*,[76] pilots were warned "Research shows us that artificial sweeteners (Nutrasweet) could cause problems in the form of flicker vertigo, sudden memory loss, dizziness during instrument flight and gradual loss of vision. We must be alert for [these] potential in-flight problems."

Some of the most dramatic health improvements I have seen while working with people have occurred within a very short time after they have discontinued their habit of drinking three or four 32-ounce diet colas per day.

Alcohol. Alcohol is a glamorously advertised drug, not a food. It may load the liver with fat, reduce the oxygen and blood supply to the heart and brain, and actually destroy brain cells. In excess, it may depress the immune system, worsen arthritic pain, and irritate the urinary tract and prostate.[77-83] If you choose to drink, be extremely moderate in your consumption. The best solution is to eliminate alcohol all together.

Caffeine. Caffeine is found not only in coffee but also in some teas and soft drinks. The use of caffeine may increase your risk of heart disease up to nine times. Caffeine may also promote changes in the normal heartbeat, leading to acute heart problems and elevated blood cholesterol.[84-93] Decaffeinated coffee is not necessarily the solution either. One study of 13,000 patients showed that heart disease risks were the same for regular coffee drinkers as for caffeine-free coffee drinkers because of harsh acids in both types of coffee that are so stressful to the body.

But it is cola caffeine, not coffee, that is the number-one addiction in many people's lives. I've seen people lose two inches around their waistlines in one week when they've eliminated colas from their lives.

If you are addicted to caffeine, you will probably suffer from withdrawal when you discontinue its use. You may experience headaches, irritability, fatigue, shaking, depression, or nausea. But after only three to ten days of abstinence, you'll be completely free. And you'll feel wonderful! You'll have eliminated another source of stress that can activate your body's fat-storing survival system and prematurely age your body.

Tobacco. This substance is well known for its association with heart disease and cancer.[94,94.5] Although it is not always linked to weight gain, it can certainly be associated with a loss of muscle tissue. Premature aging and poor skin tone may also be associated with this highly shackling drug.

Illegal drugs. These can create serious physical and emotional stress, thus activating your body's survival system to store excess fat. Your body must turn its attention to eliminating these poisons from your system rather than to burning fat, much as it does when you are battling an illness. The constant use of drugs can seriously threaten your physical and emotional health and well-being.

8. Sedentary Lifestyle

The eighth avoidable fat-storing stressor is a sedentary life-style.[95,95.5,96] Your body was designed to move. Even though our ancestors developed the ability to store fat, there was little obesity because they led an active life-style. They couldn't get their food at the corner store; they had to hunt for it or plant it and harvest it. To do so, they pushed, pulled, ran, sprinted, stretched, reached, and bent over. And when they traveled, they walked. They used their entire bodies every day to stay alive.

Your heritage is to be active. If you don't move, you lose lean muscle tissue, which burns fat and requires lots of calories. You'll learn to incorporate the most effective fat-burning movements possible into your life-style. These movements are directly patterned after the physically laboring movements of great-grandparents. They are non-strenuous and will gently encourage your survival system to release its excess stores of fat. These movements will also promote the release of endorphins by the brain, which are natural chemicals that can markedly reduce negative stress and depression, clarify your thinking, and elevate your mood. And, you'll be developing lean muscle, which serves as a furnace where your body can naturally burn fat. And remember, lean muscle has a high metabolic rate of its own.

These special patterns of movement not only improve your mental health and self-esteem, but they also help diminish your cravings for sweets, strengthen your bones, increase your energy level, improve your sleep, and reduce your risk of heart disease, cancer, stroke, and diabetes. Low-impact, sustained, nonstrenuous exercise is an essential part of your LEAN & FREE LIFESTYLE. In fact, this is the only type of exercise that effectively burns fat! Strenuous exercise of the "no-pain, no gain" variety mainly burns sugar, encourages injury, and causes fatigue.

9. Excess or Insufficient Sleep

Too little or too much sleep is the ninth avoidable fat-storing stressor.[97,98] Without proper amounts of sleep, your body cannot sufficiently recover from the stresses built up during the day. Much of the growth and repair of your lean muscle tissue, as well as emotional rejuvenation, occur while you sleep. If your body remains unrested and stressed, it may continue to store fat because your muscles may not build and repair enough to become effective at burning fat. Also, your body is unable to adequately rid itself of wastes and toxins. This may result in a decreased metabolic rate.

Each night, your body goes through two types of sleep. First, there are two to three hours of heavy sleep that rejuvenate your body. Then you need five to six hours more of light sleep to rest and refresh your mind. Without adequate amounts of both types of sleep, your body remains fatigued mentally and physically. This weakens your muscles and triggers your survival system to store excess fat by slowing you down both physically and emotionally. Weakened muscles and subsequent lethargy both contribute to fat storage. Lack of sleep may also trigger cravings for sweets and fats as your body searches for a quick energy boost to overcome fatigue.

I've known several people who reached a point on this program where they seemed to be floundering, although they were following the basic principles of nutrition and movement. When I went through their daily activities with them, I found they were not getting enough sleep. But once they began to sleep seven to eight hours per night, all the other elements of the program began to work. Muscular and emotional rejuvenation began to occur, and their bodies' ability to burn fat dramatically increased.

Too much sleep, regularly more than ten hours per night, may also signal your body to store fat because your metabolism may slow down and you may move less and lose muscle tissue—the same result as with too little sleep. Moderation is a great concept.

10. Self-Hate

The tenth avoidable fat-storing stressor is self-hate. Self-hate takes many forms. For a lot of people, it is the anxiety brought on by the scales, the mirror, and possibly by comments made about them by others. If you are overly fat and cannot bear to look at your body, this is a form of self-hate. And until you can resolve these feelings, your ability to reduce body fat will be minimized, even stifled. When you hate your body, you may feel desperate or angry about the way you look, which could result in your starving yourself and then craving and eating large quantities of fats and sweets.

When you hate your body, you set up psychological and physiological barriers against becoming lean and healthy, severely limiting or completely eliminating your progress, even if you are following the other principles of LEAN & FREE. You and your body have to work together. You must realize that being overly fat is not your fault. You simply haven't had the knowledge or the tools to solve your fat problem, and dieting, although based on good intentions, has made the problem much worse. Once you fully integrate what you're learning in this program, you'll begin to transform your body into the shape it was intended to be. You'll become more active, healthy, and loved by both yourself and others. And you'll realize that what you weigh has little to do with how fat or lean you are.

In chapter 3, I'll show you how to end the war with your body, how to nurture it, and how to begin to love yourself and your body for life.

11. Anger or Unresolved Disputes

Anger or unresolved disputes between you and members of your family, close friends, or associates is the eleventh avoidable fat-storing stressor. Until these difficulties are resolved, you will experience continued anxiety. This negative stress may signal your survival system to store excess body fat because the tension you feel may cause you to move less, skip meals, and perhaps even forget to eat. This may signal your survival system to increase your fat and sugar cravings and slow your metabolism.

I know a young woman who weighed more than 280 pounds. She followed correct fat-loss principles and reduced to around 200 pounds, but no matter how hard she tried, she couldn't lose more. Then she married and moved away from home. Within a few months, remarkably, she dropped to an ideal percent of body fat. I found out later that she had been under constant stress from her relationships with her mother and sister. This stress may have slowed her metabolism and decreased her energy level significantly. Once this conflict was removed, her metabolism and energy level greatly increased, and she dropped her excess body fat.

In chapter 3, I'll discuss several essential ways to resolve personal conflicts that might be affecting your efforts to be lean and free.

12. Lack of Life's Purpose

The twelfth and final avoidable fat-storing stressor is a lack of purpose in life. Lean, high-energy people are motivated by a reason to live. They have interests that go far beyond their own personal needs and that require active involvement in life. And the more active they are, the more energy they need. This needed energy is produced generously and freely by a body that is well fed, emotionally balanced, and free of avoidable fat-storing stress.

In contrast, those without a life's purpose, without a compelling reason to live, have nowhere to direct their energy other than to fulfill survival needs. Their energy becomes passive and stored. Their body resists movement. And, because they don't move, their survival system perceives that it is in a fat-conserving mode (inactivity doesn't burn fat) and responds by storing fat, reducing energy, and developing cravings for sweet and fatty foods.

Your body has an amazing ability to determine whether you need energy and how much you need. It responds to the signal that you need energy by burning fat and granting you your wish. Those who take pleasure in life, those who are driven by purpose, require the most energy of all. For the lean, high-energy person, that pleasure is derived most strongly through service to others. I'll talk more about this in chapter 6.

Now let's review some key points we've learned in this chapter.

Your body has a built-in survival system. Its role is to optimize your health and defend against starvation by regulating energy level and fat stores.

You inherited the invaluable ability to store fat from your ancestors. Fat helps your body defend itself against the number-one killer of mankind: starvation. Dieting, skipping meals, and lack of nutritional balance can all signal your survival system to respond as if a caloric or nutritional famine is present. Excess fat storage may then occur. Energy is reduced. And fat and sugar cravings can develop.

There are twelve avoidable fat-storing-stressors that signal the body's survival system to store excess fat. They are:

Dieting and Meal Skipping. Dieting and meal skipping is by far the most potent fat-storing stressor to which you can subject your body. Studies show that low-calorie diets work to create a high-fat, low-energy body. The first and most significant change you can make in your life is to stop dieting and skipping meals today!

Dehydration. Water is needed for efficient metabolism, muscle increase, and fat loss. Dehydration affects the efficiency of fat burning and may cause toxins to be stored in the body, further stressing the survival system.

Excess or Insufficient Fat Intake. An eating program heavy in dietary fat or too low in fat may encourage your body to store excess fat. Excess fat is easily stored in your fat cells, and too little fat may encourage destruction of muscle tissue and weaken the immune system.

Excess Refined Carbohydrates and Insufficient Complex Carbohydrates. Excessive sugar and white-flour-based foods (quick-energy foods) trigger your body's survival system to defend against starvation by storing excess fat. A meal plan featuring vegetables, grains, legumes, and fruits with moderate amounts of low-fat dairy products and lean meats signals your body that there is a ready abundance of calories and nutrients. These foods also provide the vitamins and minerals necessary to create a fat-burning metabolism, bounteous energy, and optimum health.

Excess or Insufficient Protein. A diet too high or too low in animal protein may encourage both muscle and water loss. Muscle is your body's fat-burning machinery. The LEAN & FREE LIFESTYLE will help you design an eating plan of moderate, not excessive or deficient, protein.

Excess Salt. Eating high concentrations of salt may signal your body that it needs to store water and that therefore a drought or famine is imminent. Excess salt may also weaken cell membranes and impair your cells' ability to convert food into energy.

Artificial Sweeteners and Unnecessary Drugs. Artificial sweeteners are highly concentrated sweets that may heighten your desire for sweet foods.

Artificial sweetener consumption may be more stressful to your body than regular sugar consumption, thus encouraging more excess fat storage than regular sugar.

Drugs such as caffeine and alcohol threaten your body's good health and may create nutritional deprivation.

A Sedentary Lifestyle. Your body was designed to move. A sedentary lifestyle may encourage excess fat storage by decreasing your muscle tissue, slowing your metabolism, and increasing your fat and sweet cravings. When you diet and exercise you are not giving your body the building blocks (calories and nutrients) it needs for growth and repair of fat-burning muscle tissue. This may signal your survival system to hang onto excess fat. When you fully nourish your body and follow specifically designed movements that are fun and gentle, you can de-stress your body and promote a fat-burning metabolism. Exercise markedly improves your body shape and your state of mind. You look and feel tremendously better when you exercise.

Insufficient or Excess Sleep. Too little or too much sleep can create stress that signals your body to store fat by decreasing muscle mass, activity level, and metabolism. Most people need seven to eight hours each night.

Self-Hate. Self-hate can keep you from becoming lean and healthy. Until you learn to love your body and not to blame it for excess body fat, you set up physiological and psychological barriers that can keep your body from changing from a fat-storing warehouse to a fat-burning machine.

Anger or Unresolved Disputes. Anger or unresolved conflicts with significant people in your life may need to be resolved before you can become lean and healthy. If these conflicts are upsetting you, they are probably perceived by your body as a threat to survival, causing it to store fat. They can provide the same kinds of psychological and physiological barriers as self-hate.

Lack of Purpose in Life. Food provides energy to sustain life and direct meaningful activity. Lean, healthy people have a life's purpose to which they direct the energy derived from food. Food becomes a source of energy to fuel their ambitions, hopes, and dreams, and the activities necessary to make them a reality. People without a life's purpose do not have a focal point at which to direct their energy. Their energy is passive and may be stored in their bodies as excess fat. The lack of purpose or a reason to live results in a dull and sedentary lifestyle that can trigger your body's survival system, signaling it to store fat, to reduce energy, and to create a desire for foods high in sugar and fat. Lean and healthy people are driven by a sense of purpose and a zest for life that ideally translate into service to others.

Now you have completed the first important step of the LEAN & FREE LIFESTYLE, the step of knowledge. You have become familiar with your body's remarkable and efficient survival system, a system designed to protect you from critical threats and particularly the threat of starvation. You know how that survival system can either interfere with or help you in your efforts to become lean, healthy, and happy. And you've become familiar with the twelve avoidable stressors that can signal that system into defensive action, causing it to store fat and reduce your energy. This knowledge will prepare you for all the principles that follow. It will prepare you to change your patterns of behavior and your attitudes in a way that will promote positive changes in your body. This knowledge is the basis for all else that follows in the upcoming chapters.

Until now, your life may have seemed out of control. Through starvation dieting, you may have been eating very little but still gaining fat with every meal. You were much like the driver of car without a steering wheel, careening down a twisty mountain road on a course to disaster. Now you may think of the knowledge you've just gained in this chapter as your steering wheel, the tool by which you can take control of the course of your life. With this knowledge you can control your destiny and safely steer your way though the twists and turns of life. You are already on your way to your destination: a lean and healthy life filled with energy, joy, and service to others.

Refer to this chapter often to reinforce your new awareness about how your body works. Remember that it is this knowledge that provides you with power—the power to take control of your body, to nurture and nourish yourself with love and food, to steer yourself toward a life of leanness, freedom, and happiness.

To complete this marvelous process of transformation, you will need strong commitment and deep motivation. This, too, you can obtain. And you can do it, in part, with the knowledge you've just gained. In chapter 2, I'll show you how to successfully motivate yourself to start and experience the joy of being lean and free.

QUESTION: *What is the thirteenth avoidable fat-storing stressor?*

ANSWER: *Too rapid an increase in calories and high-fiber foods is the thirteenth stressor. This can encourage unnecessary excess fat gain and cause gas and bloat-ing. On page 237, write down what you are eating right now on an average day. Then, very* gradually *increase the amounts of food you are eating if you have been a dieter or a meal skipper. Start by eating six small meals if your schedule will permit. You should never be miserably stuffed any more than you should be hungry after a meal. Your hunger will gradually increase as your metabolism increases. Listen to* your *body. And start out with canned and steamed vegetables and fruits and* part *whole-grain breads and cereals. Gradual change will encourage much more rapid body fat loss and reduce the stress on your body.*

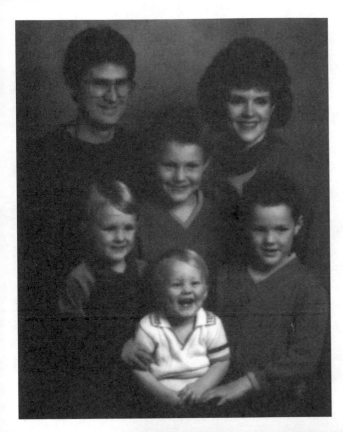

This is the last picture we had taken together before our accident.

After Nyle's passing, our family went through much physical and emotional healing. Aaron (our oldest son) was in a body cast and had a plate in his leg for six months. Now he is fully healed and has reduced his waist line to 30 inches.

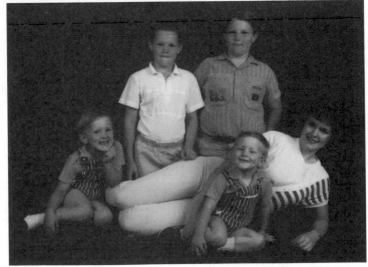

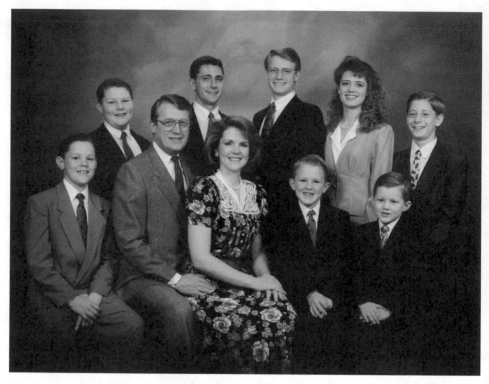

*It's exciting to join two families together, and it's also frightening at first!
We have a seven-son basketball team and one wonderful daughter.*

QUESTION: *Dana, in this chapter, I learned about the thirteen fat-storing stressors. But do I really* have *to cut out all of my wine, beer, and coffee to be successful on this program?*

ANSWER: LEAN & FREE *is an* addition, *not a* subtraction *program. Simply focus on all of the great foods you're adding to your life, and don't worry about subtracting fat-storing stressors initially. Most people notice that within just one to two weeks of following the delicious* LEAN & FREE *balanced menus, their cravings for excessive amounts of fats, sweets, artificial stimulants, and mood altering substances are GONE! Then they have the freedom to actually choose how much or how little of these stressors they want to include in their day. I'm much more moderate with desserts than I used to be, and I find amazing freedom and energy, and* no *excess body fat associated with my food choices.*

2. COMMITMENT

THE PASSION TO BE LEAN & FREE

*I*n chapter 1, you learned that the storage of fat is an inherited and natural survival function of your body. You were introduced to the twelve major stressors that can trigger your body's survival system to store excess fat. You learned that each of these fat-storing stressors is manageable, even avoidable. You also learned how low-calorie dieting and meal skipping can increase your excess fat storage more than all the other stressors combined.

Now that you have this knowledge, you have power. And you have responsibility too. Your destiny is in your hands. You understand how your body works and that you and nobody else will make the difference between your remaining overly fat or becoming lean and vibrant.

Knowledge is the first critical step in attaining a lean, healthy body—a body that is approximately 15 to 25 percent fat for a woman and 10 to 20 percent fat for a man. The second step is developing the unshakable belief that you can transform your body and your life by committing to a plan that will enable you to succeed.

When you commit to the LEAN & FREE LIFESTYLE, you are not committing to another diet. In fact, LEAN & FREE 2000 PLUS is far removed from dieting; it exists at the other end of the spectrum. To help you understand why, here's a brief comparison:

When you diet, you are looking for a quick fix, an immediate solution to a problem that may have plagued you for many years and that probably took many years to develop. In hope of that quick solution, you eat less. When you do, you lose a few pounds of water and lean muscle tissue almost immediately, and so you begin to think you've made progress. Then your body's survival system kicks in. Instead of losing weight on your 1,500 calories a day, your body adjusts, and you simply maintain your new weight, a phase often referred to as "the plateau." Your energy level also decreases, and you develop fat-storing enzymes in your diminishing muscles. Gradually, your survival system encourages your body to actually gain weight on 1,500 calories. This is called "the lose, maintain, gain diet cycle."

In response, you decrease to 1,200 calories until your survival system gradually gears down. You lose at first. Then you maintain, and eventually you gain, even if you don't give in to your increased cravings for fats and sweets. In desperation, you decrease to 900 calories, then 700, then 500. I know many people who were actually gaining weight on well under 1,000 calories before they were introduced to this program.

During this "lose, maintain, gain diet cycle," your self-esteem suffers. You think you've failed because you've not only gained all your original weight back,

DIET CYCLE

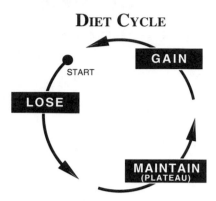

but you've also probably gained more. In fact, you may have been absolutely heroic in your resolve. It wasn't a lack of willpower that defeated you; it was one simple fact: diets do not work!—except in reverse. They can't work. And furthermore, they abuse your body; they cause physical discomfort; and they create a sense of deprivation, thus withholding from you much of the joy of life. While you're on a diet, you may be weak, hungry, and miserable.

By contrast, the LEAN & FREE LIFESTYLE does not promise a quick fix. It does promise the freedom to eat the way you were meant to eat, success through gradual and permanent changes in your body. When you abundantly provide your body with all the food and nutrients it needs, your body will naturally respond by becoming healthy, vibrant, and lean.

You didn't gain your extra fat overnight, and you cannot lose it overnight either. As you implement the LEAN & FREE LIFESTYLE, your progress may seem slower than it would in the first stages of a diet, but there is a major difference: LEAN & FREE progress is permanent.

If you find it difficult to abandon the hope of a quick solution, consider this: the time you will spend on this program is going to pass anyway. Your choice is to use that time by following the principles of this program and becoming lean and healthy, or to waste that time by continuing to try quick-fix diet plans that will eventually leave you fatter than when you started, or old, saggy, wrinkled, and skinny. It's as simple as that. The LEAN & FREE LIFESTYLE is actually the fastest fat-loss program in the world because, I believe, it is the only one that really works!

By closely following LEAN & FREE principles, you can lose fat and inches, reduce your clothing size, and actually appear to grow younger, not older as you do when you diet. Remember the woman I told you about in the introduction? She totally changed her body, dropping forty inches and several dress sizes, and yet her skin looked wonderful. Amazingly, all this occurred with only a one-pound weight loss.

But to become lean and healthy, not only do you need to start with this program, but you must also stay with it! And that takes commitment. You must believe that the principles in the LEAN & FREE LIFESTYLE are correct and will work for you.

This commitment cannot be a blind one, based on faith alone. It is built through experience and fueled by long-lasting improvements in how you feel and look. Remember, you are making a lifestyle change, and once that change is made, it is permanent. Believe me, you won't be able to tolerate the thought of going back to your old ways.

Committing to any new program and staying with that program for life requires a plan. It's not as simple a process as "read the book and go do it."

Commitment is the result of building a passion to be lean and free. That passion is a fire of emotion deep inside your heart that motivates you to work with correct principles until your survival system can create the changes that will make you lean and free. It is this fire of emotion that keeps you going, without giving up, until you have successfully reached your goal, no matter how long it takes or how far you have to go. I have learned that this kind of commitment is built through a simple five-step process.

FIVE STEP COMMITMENT PROCESS

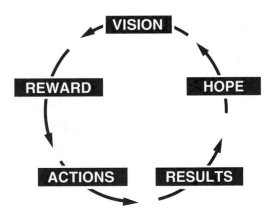

Step 1: Hope

The first step in building the fire of commitment is the development of hope. When you have hope, you believe it is possible for you to change. This sense of possibility renews spirit, revitalizes your thinking, and gives you the faith necessary to start and successfully follow a plan of action that will take you to your goal. Hope is the cornerstone of all change. When you lose hope, you lose motivation and the will to persevere. You become resigned to a life of despair, anger, and frustration.

Hope is created through knowledge ("I know how my body works, and I know what I must do to change it"). And hope is created through the inspiration gleaned from knowing that other people have successfully applied that knowledge to make dramatic changes in their lives ("If it has worked for other people, then it can work for me"). A sense of hope fuels you, supplying energy for what you must do and enabling you to overcome obstacles.

Step 2: Vision

Once you have hope, it is easier to picture yourself as a lean and free person. Without hope, it is nearly impossible to do so. This ability to picture yourself in vivid detail as lean and free from diets and excess body fat is what I call vision. The clearer you can see yourself, the more real the picture seems. And the m⌐ real it seems, the more inspiration and excitement you feel.

When you combine your desire to be lean and free with a vision of yourself as lean and free, you can create within yourself motivational forces far beyond what you may have previously imagined. These motivational forces will enable you to free the lean body within, just as Michelangelo freed his works of art from stone.

Michelangelo, the great Renaissance artist, provides an example of how compelling vision can be. Someone once asked Michelangelo the secret of his genius in sculpting from marble detailed, life-like images.

"Rather than thinking about carving a statue out of stone," he said, "I picture in my imagination the completed work, in all of its exquisite detail. I then project the picture from my mind into the stone, where it becomes entombed, imprisoned within the stone. My job as the artist is not to carve an image into the stone but to free it from the stone. And this I do with passion because I know the image is already there, alive and breathing. The process," he concluded, "is quite simple. That which I desire, I must first imagine. That which I can imagine, I create."

Step 3: Reward

With hope and vision it is now possible to imagine what your life will be like when you succeed, the rewards you'll experience when your vision becomes a reality, and your success all along the way. Reward is the third step to commitment. Imagine what it will be like when you are lean, healthy, and full of energy. Imagine wearing clothes in sizes you have only dreamed about until now. Imagine the ability to do active things without pain, strain, or embarrassment. Imagine people making positive comments about you. Imagine having glowing skin and shiny hair. Imagine the new-found self-esteem you'll feel just from looking in the mirror. Imagine becoming more attractive to others around you.

Concentrating and focusing on how much better your life will be every day as you lead your new LEAN & FREE LIFESTYLE further fuels your fire of emotion and deepens your commitment.

Step 4: Action

The fourth stage of commitment is action. Action is the steady, patient application of what you are learning in this program. You have to take action to achieve results and rewards. And every action that follows correct principles further builds hope and commitment and speeds the process of change.

Step 5: Results

Finally, the fifth stage of commitment is results. The key to this phase is being able to identify and register even the most subtle positive changes in your body and emotions. Results supply the fuel that keeps you going. When you see results, it increases your hope, solidifies your vision, and brings to reality the rewards you had previously imagined. All of these steps combined create a positive, compounding cycle of emotion that gives you the motivation and commitment, the emotional power, to patiently carry you through the natural process of becoming lean and free—to eat as you've always dreamed for life.

Once you know the five steps that build passion, motivation, and commitment, you must practice them every day.

The key to success is to take these five steps and practice them daily to build the emotion that leads to unshakable commitment.

Hope is sustained by the continual gathering of information. Your *first step* is to completely read this book. It contains valuable and accurate information about how change occurs within your body and how you can participate in that change. Then you must continue to reinforce that learning by rereading the book and regularly listening to your LEAN & FREE audio and video tapes. This keeps essential knowledge in the forefront of your mind, where it can continue to guide your actions.

This first step also includes identifying people who have succeeded on this program and studying them. You'll find inspiring success stories in the chapter entitled LEAN & FREE SUCCESS STORIES. Their success will motivate you and increase your sense of hope.

The *second step* is to create a detailed mental structure, a vision, of how your body will look and feel when you become lean and healthy. If you were lean at one time, use that image as a beginning point. If you've always been overly fat, find someone with your basic body structure (tall, short, etc.) who is lean and imagine yourself looking like that person. This can be a person you know, a picture out of a magazine, any image you can admire and relate to.

The richer and more lifelike you can make this image, the better. Imagine exactly how you'll look, in as much detail as possible. What are you wearing? Are you smiling? How does your skin look? Your hair? How do you feel when you look in the mirror? How does it feel to move gracefully, lightly, and freely? How does your stomach feel being flat and taut? How does it feel to be of service to your family and friends without carrying the encumbrances and embarrassments of excess body fat? How does it feel to eat all you want and have abundant energy? When creating these images, bring all the five senses into play: sight, sound, taste, smell, and touch.

Once you have the vision, experience it in your mind many times a day. See and feel it when you wake up, see it in your daydreams during the day, and replay it in your imagination as the last thing you do before you drift off to sleep at night. Over time, as you replay the image, you'll find that it changes, that it adapts to any new hopes, desires, or ideas you have. And, if it is an image you can realistically achieve, it can't help but inspire you.

Step three is to develop a detailed list of the rewards you'll experience as a lean, healthy, and energetic person.

List all of the positive things people will say to you when they start to notice your personal transformation. List the health rewards you'll experience.

List the rewards of emotional stability and renewed confidence.

List the rewards of being able to wear the clothes you've always wanted to wear, being able to vacation and feel good about how you look and feel, being able to eat all the good food you want, staying lean and trim in the process.

List the phenomenal rewards of remaining lean and healthy even when your eating and exercise habits veer off the track for a while, because in this program there is wonderful freedom for imperfect habits.

When you are finished, study the rewards on your list. Vividly imagine what it will be like to achieve each and every one of them, and add new rewards as they occur to you. Finally, incorporate this list of rewards into your daily vision exercises, where you imagine yourself healthy and lean.

The *fourth step* in building commitment is to follow the principles you're learning in the program. Later in this book you'll be given specific actions to follow, and the closer you adhere to them, the more successful you'll become.

The *fifth* and final step is to carefully monitor your progress. Look for signs that your vision is merging with reality. Look for signs that the rewards you have identified and imagined are beginning to materialize.

Once your imagination becomes reality, your level of motivation and commitment will be so high that you'll never dream of returning to your old patterns of living and being.

This close monitoring is critical because many of the changes you'll experience on this program are subtle and extremely important. If you've been dieting for a while and have gained several extra pounds, or if you have starved yourself skinny, it will take time to transform your body from a fat-storing warehouse into a neutral state and then to a fat-burning machine. The time varies from person to person, depending on how many of the fat-storing stressors are at work in your life and how long they've been stressing you.

Rather than establishing a deadline or trying to predict a time-frame for how long it will take to make the desired changes, it is much more effective to view the process of change in stages. By measuring your progress in terms of time, you may actually stress your body. You may impose standards that are personally unrealistic. This "time" stress may trigger your body's survival system to store excess fat, thus counteracting many of the changes you are working toward achieving. By trusting your body and being sensitive to its needs for food and nourishment, you will reap rewards beyond your wildest imagination—one day at a time, starting with the day you begin this program.

To help you measure your progress, I have listed the four stages your body will go through and the signs of success that accompany each stage.

Stage 1—Level A (Fat-Storing to Neutral)
(You are most likely in this stage if you have been a regular dieter or meal skipper.)

❑ A gradual increase in energy.
❑ A loss of cravings for sweets and fatty foods.
❑ A marked increase in your appetite for good food as your lean muscle tissue increases and your metabolism quickens.
❑ A calmness that you never felt while dieting.
❑ A possible increase in weight due to increases in body water and lean muscle tissue. (Both elements are essential for future fat loss.)
   (Examine the Body Composition Chart on page 45.)

Stage 1—Level B (Neutral to Fat-Burning)
(If you are overly fat but have never dieted and skipped meals, you are most likely in this stage.)

❑ Your body becomes weight stable. You may begin to notice a significant firming and toning of your muscles. Many people begin to experience moderate to significant loss of inches (clothes fit much looser). This is often accompanied by weight stability, weight loss, or even weight gain because newly developed muscle weighs twice as much as fat yet takes up half the space.

❑ Your muscles begin to change shape, becoming longer, leaner, and firmer.

❑ Your energy level may increase significantly as you follow the complete principles of the LEAN & FREE LIFESTYLE (which include supplying your body with adequate amounts of sleep).

❑ Many health problems such as high cholesterol, high blood pressure, diabetes, hypoglycemia, chronic fatigue, and depression may markedly improve or disappear completely.

❑ Your skin may look more youthful, glowing and supple.

❑ Wrinkles are often less pronounced as your body's percentage of water increases to a normal level, and muscles firm. (The difference is like going from "prune skin" to "plum skin".)

❑ Your hair may begin to thicken and develop a healthy sheen.

❑ Your nails may become stronger and less brittle.

Stage 2 (Fat-Burning)
❑ Marked loss of inches with moderate weight loss may be noticed. Many people experience significant weight loss.

❑ Some people drop more than a hundred pounds during this stage while others may drop as much as five sizes and stay the same weight.

❑ Peace of mind from adherence to correct health principles may become constant.

❑ A marvelous phenomenon begins to be enjoyed. Even when these people eat too much fat and sugar for a period of time, they experience no significant weight gain and quickly return to "pre-splurge" size when the ideal health habits they learn in this program are resumed.

Stage 3 (Fat-Loss Acceleration)
❑ With ideal health habits, people see consistent and regular body fat loss and drop as much as one or more sizes per month until reaching their ideal percentage of body fat.

BODY COMPOSITION CHART

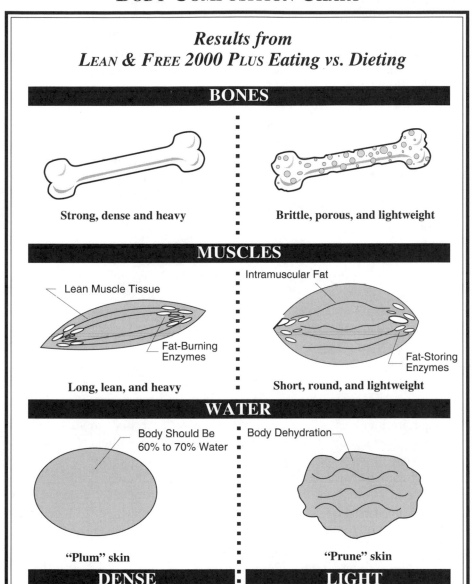

Results from
LEAN & FREE 2000 PLUS Eating vs. Dieting

BONES

Strong, dense and heavy

Brittle, porous, and lightweight

MUSCLES

Lean Muscle Tissue

Intramuscular Fat

Fat-Burning Enzymes

Fat-Storing Enzymes

Long, lean, and heavy

Short, round, and lightweight

WATER

Body Should Be 60% to 70% Water

Body Dehydration

"Plum" skin

"Prune" skin

DENSE

LIGHT

- ❏ At this point it becomes abundantly clear why dieting cannot produce permanent loss of body fat.
- ❏ This person regularly eats to comfortable satisfaction on high quality, balanced foods and experiences very high energy and consistently high mood states. They neither stuff themselves, nor go hungry.
- ❏ The metamorphosis from a fat-storing body to a fat-burning body becomes complete.
- ❏ Total freedom from excess body fat may become a reality.
- ❏ Service to others may become a joy and not a burden.
- ❏ Fear of vacations and parties becomes a thing of the past.
- ❏ Peace of mind and self-esteem may become constant companions.

THE THREE STAGES OF METABOLISM

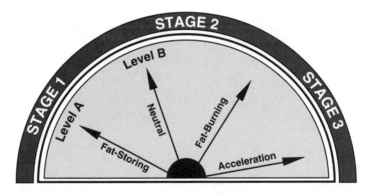

Again, it is important to emphasize the virtue of patience. Becoming naturally and permanently lean is a very different process from becoming artificially skinny. Fifty percent of people will experience stage 3 within a period of months; 25 percent will experience complete success in weeks; and the remaining 25 percent will experience complete success within one to two years. This latter group includes people who have dieted or skipped meals regularly for many years. The time it takes to achieve results depends on your own body, how many times you have dieted, and how consistently you follow the LEAN & FREE LIFESTYLE principles.

Remember, it is insignificant how long it takes to become naturally lean; that time is going to pass anyway. Your success, freedom from dieting, and happiness can begin the day you start this program, because in starting and gaining the initial knowledge that will bring you your desired results, you have already taken the most critical step. The important idea is to avoid cutting the process short or sabotaging it by attempting to find ways for quick, short-term results. Short-term results can only mean dieting, and, as you know now, diets can trigger your body's survival system to store excess fat as they did for me until after age twenty-three. Then I finally stopped dieting and ruling my life by the scales. Notice in the following chart that I did not weigh too much at age seventeen. My body composition simply needed to change.

Dana's Weight Chart

Age	Height	Daily Calories	Weekly Exercise	Weight	Body Fat %	Dress Size	Pant Size	Energy Level
14	5'8 1/2"	2500	3 days 30 min.	119	23%	8	10	Good
17	5'9 1/2"	1500	5 days 1 hr	150	34%	10	14	Lagging
19 (while dieting)	5'9 1/2"	300	6 days 2 hr	136	30%	8	12 tight	Extremely low
6 weeks later	5'9 1/2"	1200	6 days 90 min.	154	35%	10	14 tight	Low
23	5'9 1/2"	800	6 days 90 min.	204	42%	14	18 tight	Felt very weak and depressed
24	5'9 1/2"	3000 to 4000 (nursing a baby)	6 days 60 min. aerobics	145	15.5%	6	4	High-feel calm and peaceful
34	5'9 1/2"	2000 to 3500	3 days 60 min. aerobics (plus 15 mini floor exercise)	150	15%	6	4	High-feel calm and peaceful

If you have the sincere desire to change, this program is your answer. Like anything worthwhile, the LEAN & FREE LIFESTYLE requires commitment and time. By following what you've learned in this chapter, you can build that commitment. And you can sustain it through the transformative months ahead, which will lead you inevitably to the fulfillment of your dream

In this chapter I've reinforced the difference between diets and the LEAN & FREE 2000 PLUS ULTIMATE WELLNESS/WEIGHT CONTROL LIFESTYLE. You've learned the five steps of building a commitment to the program and what you need to do each day to implement those steps.

In chapter 3, I'll discuss the devastating effect of hating your body and why loving and nurturing your body is essential in your quest for health, leanness, and a lifetime of happiness.

3. NURTURING
How To Love Your Body Lean

*I*f you're carrying excess body fat or are out of shape, the last thing you want to do is stand in front of a full-length mirror wearing anything skimpier than a long winter coat. Why? Because you probably don't like what is hidden by the coat.

However, it is important to understand that the fat, out-of-shape image reflected in the mirror is not the real you. It is simply the result of years of misinformation and well-intentioned but misguided activities.

You are not overly fat because you eat too much good food or because you are genetically destined to be fat. You are overly fat because until now you haven't fully understood the natural laws that, if honored, can make you healthy and lean. One of those critical laws or principles is nurturing yourself, developing a loving relationship with your body.

If you're like many overly fat people, you probably hate your body. And if you hate your body, you actually help perpetuate its condition by creating fat-storing stress. This stress can actually reduce your energy level and subsequently your metabolic rate. The stress of self-hate often causes feelings of desperation that result in extreme eating behaviors such as total starvation or excessive consumption of fats and sweets. As we have already discussed, both of these extremes can lead to excessive fat storage. So until you transcend this stressful self-hate and learn to love your body, your own attitudes may work to sabotage your efforts toward the LEAN & FREE LIFESTYLE.

In this chapter I'll show you how to nurture your body by establishing a loving relationship with it, a relationship that will give you the opportunity to work with your body toward the goal of health, fitness, and service to others. The adversarial relationship you may now have must be transformed into one of harmony and cooperation. Your body must cease to be your enemy and must instead become your friend and your partner. This task, although it may sound impossible now, can be achieved through a simple change of attitude enhanced by specific mental exercises.

To begin with, you must identify and accept any negative feelings you might have about your body. Some people find it difficult to admit that they are actually directing hostile and destructive thoughts at their bodies. You're probably thinking, "I don't hate my body; I'm just uncomfortable with how it looks." But, if your answers to any of the following questions are yes, you are indeed sending negative messages to your body, messages that can trigger fat storage and that must be completely changed if you want to achieve your fat-loss goals.

Becoming a friend and a partner with your body is essential to your LEAN & FREE success. I began to like myself and my body all along the way.

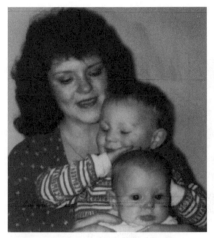

About 190 pounds and 40% body fat.

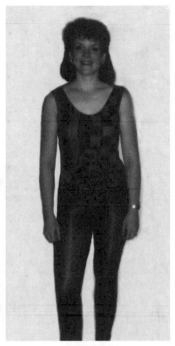

About 175 pounds.

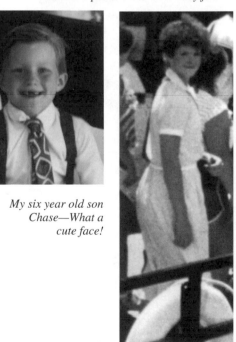

My six year old son Chase—What a cute face!

About 185 pounds.

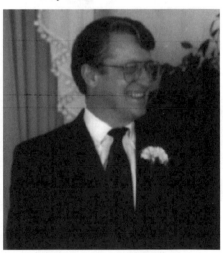

It's great becoming naturally lean, not starved skinny. While we were preparing for our 22 year old son's recent marriage, I was mistaken several times for our son's bride. Marty (my husband) got an even bigger kick out of that than I did.

49

- ❏ Are you embarrassed to be seen in public in a swimming suit?
- ❏ Do you wear clothes that hide your true shape?
- ❏ Do you feel frustrated at having to buy larger-sized clothing than you'd like?
- ❏ Do you feel envious or inferior when you see lean, healthy people?
- ❏ Do you avoid looking at yourself in mirrors?
- ❏ When you see your reflected image, do you feel frustrated, angry , or desperate?
- ❏ Do you avoid having your picture taken?
- ❏ Do you feel frustration, anger, or despair when you see yourself in a photograph or videotape?
- ❏ Do you avoid social situations because you feel ashamed of your body?
- ❏ Have you avoided or dreaded going to a class reunion because you felt ashamed of your body?
- ❏ Do you frequently make jokes about how big you are?
- ❏ Do you feel hurt when you overhear negative comments about your body or about other overly fat people?

If you answered yes to any of these questions, then you probably have animosity toward the visual appearance of your body, and that animosity needs to be resolved if you hope to become permanently lean and happy.

Hating your body is more than just an attitude. Such hate has both psychological and physiological implications.

Psychologically, hating your body creates a feeling of despair. You blame yourself for living a life of ill health and subjecting yourself to ridicule. When people make disparaging remarks about your looks, you are deflated by them and unable to rally. Even when you find out there is something you can do to change your size or shape, you are reluctant to try, thinking, "It probably wouldn't work for me anyway and I'll probably just fail all over again."

Physiologically, hating your body sends signals that it is being threatened. And you know now how your body responds to a threat, whether that threat is real or perceived. It signals your survival system to save the body by storing fat, conserving energy, slowing its ability to burn fat, and producing a desire for foods high in fat and sugar. This self-hate/fat-storing relationship becomes a vicious cycle that ultimately leads to a sense of total hopelessness.

To break this cycle you must learn to replace the hate for your body with love. That doesn't mean you must be content or satisfied with the way your body looks right now. It simply means that you must release feelings of blame or guilt for that look, develop an understanding of how your body works and why it is in its current shape, and become aware of what you need to do to nurture it back to health.

When you can look at your body in the mirror and say, "I know right now you're in pretty bad shape, but it's not your fault and its not my fault either. I have simply not known how to take care of you. Now that I know what to do, let's work together as a team to get us both in shape." When you can make such statements, you have begun the self-nurturing process of learning to love your body. When you stop resenting your body and yourself, you eliminate a major stressor that has encouraged your survival system to store excess fat.

As with most overly fat people, hating the way my body looked (especially my thighs) was a critical problem for me. Until I learned to accept and love my body as a friend, it was very difficult for me to become healthy and lean. It seemed as if all my actions and goals were met with resistance. Even when I ate well and exercised correctly, my body didn't fully respond. But when I learned how to accept and nurture myself, and to work with my body instead of against it, I began to achieve dramatic results.

One day a friend told me she had read an article on how to help children develop self-esteem and love for themselves. The article said that when children overhear positive remarks being made about them by significant people in their lives, it will dramatically improve their sense of worth. And as one would expect, overhearing negative remarks will greatly diminish that sense of self-worth to the point of being very destructive.

I realized then that my body was similar to a child. It was dependent on me for its well-being, and my attitude toward it determined whether it was healthy or unhealthy, lean or overly fat. With this realization, I developed a simple method for nurturing my body. I call it "body talk."

"Body talk" refers to a simple practice of having positive conversations with yourself about your body and imagining that your body overhears what you're saying.

Several times a day, I reinforce in my mind how fortunate I am to have a wonderful body. I remind myself that it is one of nature's most miraculous creations. As such, it is meant to be healthy, lean, and beautiful. Its natural and intended state is one of fitness, productivity, and serviceability. I talk about how forgiving and resilient my body is. I talk about the new knowledge I have about my body and about how all I have to do to transform my body into its ideal shape is apply that knowledge. As I talk to myself, I pretend that my body is eavesdropping, just like a receptive child, and absorbing the full impact of my positive comments. It's a fun exercise, and, more important, it's powerfully effective.

I also use "body talk" to respond to external circumstances and events. For instance, whenever I look in the mirror or see other healthy, lean people, or even when I see old, unflattering photographs of myself from the past, I engage in constructive inner dialogue. Rather than hurting my body with demeaning thoughts, I smother it with warm, positive, loving thoughts of gratitude for my health and my ability to serve.

This simple yet profound exercise has not only worked magic for me but can work magic for you too. I know this, because I know many others who have tried it and met with the same success I did. Talking to your body may seem odd at first, but, believe me, it has a profound effect on eliminating one of the major stressors that may trigger your body to store fat. It immediately turns self-defeating self-hate into nurturing self-love and appreciation.

The bonus of such nurturing extends far beyond the changes that will occur in your body. It will reverberate through all areas of your life, reshaping not just your outer form but also the forms hidden within. If being overly fat has caused you to hate how you look, you can do something about it. But if you can't learn to love yourself now, there is no guarantee you will love yourself even when you are lean, fit, and attractive to others. Loving yourself depends on a sense of the beauty that comes from strength, courage, and goodwill and not just from the tone of your muscles or the tautness of your skin. Yet we all know that everyone who shines with inner beauty reflects it on the outside as well. And inner beauty is the ultimate fitness, the greatest health, and the truest beauty of all.

My body is my friend and my partner.

My body is one of nature's most miraculous and
beautiful creations.

It's not my body's fault I'm overly fat. It is not my fault either.
I simply did not know what to do. Now my body and I are working
together to become healthy, energetic, and permanently lean.

I understand my body now. It is wonderfully forgiving
and resilient because now I know how to nourish it
and I listen to its hunger and satisfaction signals.

It wasn't my body's fault I was craving fats and sweets,
or my fault either. It was my survival system perceiving a famine.

My body and I are working together to become purposeful,
happy, and filled with a love for life.

I'm so grateful for my body's strength and its ability to
help me serve others.

As you nurture your body and become more serviceable
to others, you will reflect an inner beauty as well as an
outer beauty. *Inner beauty is the ultimate fitness,
the greatest health and the truest beauty of all.*

4. NOURISHMENT
How To Feed Your Starving Body

*S*o far in this book, I've introduced you to the LEAN & FREE 2000 PLUS ULTIMATE WELLNESS/WEIGHT CONTROL LIFESTYLE, discussed the circumstances that encourage your body to store fat, and suggested lifestyle and attitude enhancements that will gradually convert your body from a fat-storing warehouse to a fat-burning machine.

You've learned about the stressors that can trigger your body's survival system to store excess body fat. You've learned how knowledge, hope, and vision can keep you motivated until you attain your goal of being lean, healthy, and energetic. And you've learned why loving and nurturing your body is essential to your success.

Now it's time to learn about food, the delicious foods you are privileged to eat that nourish your body and supply you with the abundant energy to lead a productive life of service. When I refer to nourishing your body, I am referring to the ability to provide it with a plentiful supply of the foods and nutrients (vitamins and minerals) it needs to signal your survival system to burn fat and create an abundance of life-enriching energy.

I developed the LEAN & FREE LIFESTYLE program after an extensive study of nutrition and after putting what I had learned into action. I proved through my own experiences and those of thousands of other people that creating a fat-burning metabolism is accomplished not by dieting and food deprivation but by eating generous amounts of the right kinds of food.

I also learned that it was less effective to eat these foods in an impulsive, unorganized way, and far more effective to plan a complete balance of foods and a daily schedule of when to eat them. This approach relaxes and satisfies your survival system, which will in turn increase your body's fat-burning capacity. With this balance of foods I was able to create a variety of quick, tasty, desirable, and nutritious meals that not only pleased me but also my entire family. From this experience I have developed specific meal plans. These plans, which I'll detail in chapter 7, take the guesswork out of meal planning. As you follow what you're learning in this program, your survival system will begin to signal your body to naturally let go of excess body fat.

Before you can use and appreciate the meal plans in this program, it's important for you to understand why they adhere to these four principles. Let's examine each one.

Eat to Comfortably-Full Satisfaction

If you've dieted, you will most likely fear that eating to comfortably-full satisfaction will make you fat. And if you eat 2,000 calories of chocolate ice cream and nothing else, it no doubt will. But I'm recommending comfortably-full

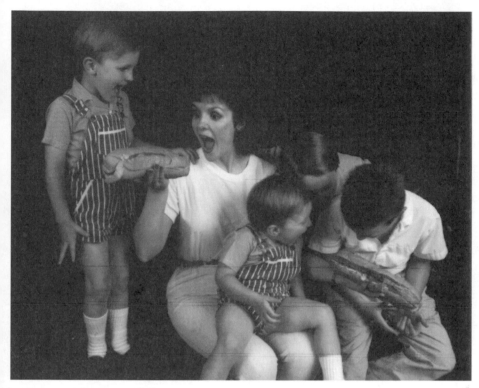

One thing my family has no problem with, is eating. We all have great appetites!

The LEAN and FREE 2000 PLUS food plans are designed to accomplish four things:

1. Provide comfortable and complete satisfaction on "high quality," balanced calories. This means you may be gradually increasing your calories if you have been a dieter or a meal-skipper. Your hunger will gradually increase as your metabolism increases, and most LEAN & FREE people, over time, require about 2,000 or more calories a day for comfortable satisfaction. However, some need more and others need less. The key is in *listening to your body.*

2. Provide an ideally moderate amount of animal protein (meat and dairy products) with total protein intake equaling 10 to 15 percent of daily calories. And encourage a fat intake of 10 to 20 percent, not to exceed 30 percent or drop below 10 percent.

3. Gradually provide an increased amount of complex carbohydrates (whole grains, legumes, vegetables, and fruits) while reducing refined carbohydrates (white flour and sugar-rich foods). Notice I didn't say you will eliminate desserts. You will still enjoy wonderful desserts following the LEAN & FREE LIFESTYLE, but *after* you have eaten to comfortable satisfaction!

4. Encourage the drinking of six to twelve eight-ounce glasses of water every day.

---

satisfaction on good nutritious food that will give you energy and prevent your body from activating your survival system to store excess fat. My experience shows that most people *gradually* increase to at least 2,000 or more high-quality calories every day once they have developed a fat-burning metabolism. Some eat less, but the important thing is that they listen to their bodies and comfortably satisfy their hunger needs by eating good, balanced foods, *often.* If they go hungry or skip meals, their survival systems may reduce their energy levels, slow their metabolisms, and increase their fat-storing capacity while heightening their cravings for excessive fats and sweets. So remember to listen to *your* body and increase calories and fiber *gradually*!

Eating to comfortably-full satisfaction may be a new experience for you if you've been a former "starver" or a "stuffer." As you begin, you may still be feeding a fat-storing body. Through dieting, lack of exercise, meal skipping, and eating unhealthy, nutrient-deficient foods that alarm your body's survival system, you have convinced your body that unless it stores fat, it may be threatened with extinction.

Eating to comfortably-full satisfaction eliminates the starvation threat. What is "comfortable satisfaction"? It is not an abstract concept. It is simply the sense of comfort that follows an adequate, well-balanced meal. It is accompanied by a feeling of overall calmness and a sense of well-being. You should not feel stuffed or uncomfortable, and you should get hungry within three to four hours after your meal.

In contrast, you can never eat exclusively fats and sweets to full satisfaction because they are nutritionally unbalanced and do not satisfy your survival system's needs. If you eat an entire gallon of chocolate ice cream, you may feel stuffed or miserably full, but you will not feel fully satisfied or completely calm.

Remember, the reason dieters have always been told to eat less or to leave the table while they're still a little hungry is because of the simple understanding that 3,500 calories equals a pound of fat. We've therefore been taught that if we want to lose one pound of fat, we must create a 3,500-calorie deficit. As you now know, creating such a deficit works at first but only at first. Then our survival system adjusts to the new lowered caloric intake. We lose energy, muscle tissue, water, and an appetite for good food, while our cravings for fats and sweets increase.

We then hit a plateau on our diet and, eventually, with our decreased metabolism, we may even gain weight. This 3,500-calorie deficit approach fails to take into account our body's remarkable ability to shift to a fat-storing mode to protect against famine or starvation. It actually goes into a state of "slow-motion metabolism."

On the other end of the calorie spectrum, people who are force-fed more than 8,000 calories may see a mere ten-pound weight gain.[1,2] Then their bodies go into states of what I call "hyper-metabolism." They produce more heat and have excess energy to spend while their bodies refuse to store any more excess fat.

So how do you decide exactly how many calories you should eat to achieve optimum health, energy, and an ideal level of body fat? You don't! You simply listen to your body, and if you aren't yet receiving clear signals of hunger and fullness, just start by eating *often* in small amounts and very gradually increase as your body tells you to do so. And if you're a *stuffer*, slow down and *enjoy* your food.

Most people eat 2,000 or more calories once they have developed a fat-burning body, but a few never get quite that high. Remember, this permanent, healthy lifestyle is about "*feelings*," not *numbers*! Listen to YOUR body–it *will* talk to you. Just give it time to trust you again.

If, when you start this program, you are used to existing on less than 1,000 calories a day, you already have a "slow-motion metabolism" that may cause you to feel fully satisfied on 1,200 calories. But allow yourself a month and you'll notice a gradual increase in your appetite as your metabolism increases. Gradually increase your caloric intake as your body signals you to do so. Increased appetite equals decreased body fat! Remember that muscles require alot of good calories to sustain them, and fat requires very few.

Since you have been told all your life that the only way you can lose weight is to eat less, you may confuse fully satisfied eating with gluttony. But they are very different. Gluttony is an "always wanting more" state. When I hear people express fear that they are being gluttonous, I ask them if they consider a sausage and egg fast-food biscuit, a cheese potato, and a taco salad with ranch dressing too much to eat in an entire day. They invariably say, "no". Then I explain that there are about 2,300 calories and more than 150 fat grams in that day's menu. Because this menu is made up of more than 60 percent fat, it takes up very little space. On the other hand, 2,300 calories of 20 percent fat food would take up two to three times as much space and provide a much greater quantity of food to eat.

People on this program are often questioned or doubted by friends when they order something like a foot-long turkey sandwich with extra veggies and no oil or mayonnaise. What the wide-eyed friend doesn't realize is that the high-fat, six-inch sandwich with onion rings and diet soda they have ordered is loaded with fat-storing stressors (through the excess fat, artificial sweeteners, and refined flour).

Eat Adequate but Not Excessive Amounts of Protein and Fat

The second recommendation of the food plan is to provide adequate amounts of protein and fat. Too much or too little of either will stress your body, threatening your health and signaling your survival system to store excess fat.

The prevailing diet wisdom is that protein builds muscle. This is true. Therefore, this wisdom suggests that more protein is better because it builds more muscle. But this is not true.

High protein levels may result in elevated cholesterol levels, loss of calcium from your bones, muscle loss, liver damage, and an increased risk of coronary disease. Low levels can deprive you of energy, damage your skin and hair, and also promote muscle loss.[4-14]

Proteins are made of small building blocks called amino acids that are required for the formation of body tissues, enzymes, and hormones.

These amino acids are also the principle materials of your cells, bones, brain, blood vessels, muscles, nerves, hair, skin, nails, intestines, and various glands. They also help deliver oxygen and nutrients to your cells through the bloodstream.

Your body manufactures all of these amino acids except nine, and those are called the "essential" amino acids. If you don't eat foods that contain all the nine essential amino acids, your body will not be able to produce the protein it requires to keep you lean and healthy. In order for your body to effectively use protein, all the essential amino acids must be present and in proper proportions. Even the temporary absence of a single essential amino acid can have adverse effects and negatively influence your body's ability to burn excess fat.

Plant proteins, the kind you get from eating vegetables and grains, are often deficient in one or more of the essential amino acids, so they're called "incomplete proteins." Animal proteins have a better balance of the essentials, so they're called "complete proteins." You might think, and logically so, that your best bet, then, is to obtain the majority of your protein from animal sources, such as meat, eggs, and dairy products. But animal proteins are also a primary source of saturated fat. So the most efficient and healthiest way to provide your necessary protein is to combine incomplete proteins (like whole grains and beans) and supplement them with moderate amounts of animal proteins, including lowfat dairy products and lean meats.

Generally, if you eat legumes along with whole grains, you've formed a partnership that provides you with the complete set of amino acids sufficient to meet your body's needs. For instance, wheat and chili beans, eaten together, supply all the essential amino acids, though each is deficient on its own. Nuts and seeds are also complete and are very high in "beneficial" fat, but be moderate with them.

Your body does not store protein. That is why you also need to eat small amounts at every meal to make certain your skin, hair, and other parts of your body are getting the help they need.

The emphasis of the LEAN & FREE eating program is on complex carbohydrates, and your protein intake is side-stage, averaging to about 10 percent of your overall caloric intake, not to exceed 15 percent. Although your percentage of protein intake may be half that of your neighbors, you'll be well within the guidelines of the National Research Council. It recommends that a twenty-five to fifty-year-old woman consume 50 to 100 grams of protein per day (or 200 to 400 calories from protein).

Since a woman following this program may be consuming 2,000 total calories a day for full satisfaction, then 10 percent of that will amount to the 200 calories or 50 grams of protein recommended. (There are 4 calories in one gram of protein.) I consume about 2,000 to 3,500 calories per day. Ten percent of 3,000 calories is 300 calories or 75 grams of protein. That math is very simple once you know the equation.

For me and many others, it was an exciting discovery to learn why eating more calories adds to, rather than subtracts from, health and balanced nutrition. And don't worry, you won't have to figure out a single protein percentage. It's all done for you.

Since your goal in the LEAN & FREE LIFESTYLE is to optimize your health while developing an optimal percentage of body fat, there is an immediate implication that fat is a "bad" word. Yet you mustn't forget that fat, too, is essential in keeping your body healthy and attractive, and it should make up approximately 10 to 20 percent of your daily food intake.

Fat helps you maintain sleek, rosy skin and shiny hair. It transports important, fat-soluble vitamins like A, D, E, and K. It also cushions and protects vital organs and helps maintain your body temperature. When fat is broken down and absorbed, the resulting particles of fat are called fatty acids. Fatty acids are important to your body because they help manufacture hormones and build cell membranes.

Both plants and animals store fat in fat cells. The primary role of fat is to provide the body with a large store of potential energy for work. Fat is perfectly designed for this assignment—it carries more than twice the energy potential per gram than either protein or carbohydrate. It is easily transported, easily stored, and readily converted into energy. And the primary reason your body will store that fat is because it isn't receiving an abundance of calories and nutrients throughout the day.

Although most fat has a bad public image, it's not fat in general that's bad for you but rather excess fat, especially excess saturated fat. Saturated fats are found mostly in meats, dairy products, coconut oil, palm oil, and palm kernel oil. High-fat meats and whole dairy products may also contain high levels of the lipid cholesterol.

Cholesterol is a white, waxy substance that animals make from fat but plants do not. It's a natural product, found in just about every tissue of the body, and it too is essential for your good health. Every day your liver produces 1,000 milligrams of cholesterol, which helps form the outer membrane of cells and aids bile formation in the liver, vitamin D synthesis, nerve-fiber strength, and the production of sex hormones. The problem with cholesterol, as with many nutrients, is that too much of it interferes with normal body functions. You don't have to eat foods containing cholesterol to be healthy; your liver can produce all it needs if you eat a moderate amount of fat. Yet if you eat the wrong fats, you may be adding too much cholesterol to your body, so much so that it collects on blood-vessel walls, narrows arteries, and causes changes in the arteries of the brain and heart that can lead to heart disease and strokes.

Unlike saturated fats, which elevate cholesterol levels, many unsaturated fats, especially monounsaturated fats, actually reduce them. For this reason, it is advisable to limit your intake of saturated fats, in particular the fats you get chiefly from meats. Instead, use more unsaturated fats from vegetables. The most advisable fats or oils to use in recipes include canola oil, olive oil, peanut oil, safflower oil, sunflower oil, corn oil, and soybean oil. Canola oil is high in linoleic acid and monounsaturated fats but does poorly when heated to higher temperatures. Look especially for oils with the label "cold pressed" or "expeller pressed." That means they have not been put through the heating process that is often used to extend shelf life but also, unfortunately, partially hydrogenates or saturates the fat in them. (Canola oil is not cold pressed but is processed in another way that prevents saturation.)

I buy safflower oil and expeller-pressed olive oil, and I keep the olive oil refrigerated to protect it from rancidity. I also purchase partially hydrogenated corn oil because it has a longer shelf-life. I include it in my food storage. Always try to buy good quality oils; their taste is superior.

These oils all contain 9 to 78 percent linoleic acid (omega-6) and 0 to 5 percent linolenic acid (also known as omega-3). These are essential fatty acids that may help to increase "good" cholesterol levels and promote a fat-burning metabolism. It is helpful to study the chart on page 62.

One of the most positive aspects of the Lean & Free Lifestyle is that it counters the extreme anti-fat movement sweeping our society and brings our perspective on fat into better balance. The fat intake in our country now averages about 40 percent of our total diets. In response, many extremists promote eliminating fat almost entirely from the diet, but this is as hazardous and unwise as eating excessive percentages of fat. Fat is an essential nutrient, and your survival system will strongly resist and defend itself against a fat deficiency. As always, it is moderation that holds the key to permanent health and leanness.

If you enjoy fat in your diet, there is even more good news about the Lean & Free Lifestyle. Let's compare this program to the guidelines of the American Heart Association. Those guidelines recommend that you limit your fat intake to 30 percent. While eating only 1,000 calories a day, you must therefore limit your fat to 300 calories, or about 33 grams of fat (9 calories per gram). But when you follow the Lean & Free guidelines, and you eat 2,000 to 3,000 calories per day, keeping your fat percentage at 20 percent, you are eating 400 to 600 calories from fat, or 44 to 67 fat grams.

FATTY ACID COMPOSITION OF
COMMON FOOD FATS

	"Bad" fats in excess	"Good" essential fats		
Oil	Saturated Fat	Linoleic Acid (Omega-6)	Linolenic Acid (Omega-3)	Monounsa-turated Fat
Safflower oil	9%	78%	1%	12%
Sunflower oil	11%	69%	0%	20%
Peanut oil	13%	33%	5%	49%
Corn oil	13%	62%	0%	25%
Olive oil	14%	9%	0%	77%
Soybean oil	15%	61%	0%	62%
Canola (Rapeseed) oil	6%	31%	1%	24%
Margarine	18%	29%	5%	48%
Chicken fat	30%	22%	1%	47%
Lard	41%	12%	0%	47%
Palm oil	51%	10%	0%	39%
Beef fat	52%	3%	1%	44%
Butterfat	66%	2%	2%	30%
Coconut oil	77%	2%	15%	6%

Sources: Canola oil: data, Procter & Gamble. All others: J.B. Reeves and F.L. Weihrauch.

What does this mean? It means you can once again say hello to moderate amounts of cheese (real cheese, not the processed variety that melts like a piece of plastic). It means hello to real butter now and then, not hydrogenated, artificial substitutes (butter is saturated by nature, not artificially saturated as substitutes are). And it means a guiltless piece of pie with ice cream on the weekends (after full meal satisfaction, of course). After all, your survival system will no longer be on fat-storing alert. It's becoming a real energy spendthrift.

Eat Plenty of Complex Carbohydrates

The third recommendation is to eat plentiful amounts of complex carbohydrates. Carbohydrates are found in all plants, and they are your body's principal source of energy. Carbohydrates are essential for the proper functioning of your central nervous system. They help in the fat-burning process, and they maintain tissue protein. You need abundant complex carbohydrates in your daily diet so that tissue-building protein isn't wasted for energy when it might be needed for muscle repair.

The two basic types of carbohydrates are *complex* and *refined*. All carbohydrates are sugars. Complex carbohydrates are made up of complex chains of sugars that form the starches in plant foods like potatoes, whole grains, pasta, bread, cereal, corn, and a variety of vegetables and legumes. When digested, these sugar chains are absorbed slowly into the bloodstream and help prevent dramatic shifts in blood sugar and energy levels. Fruits are also considered complex carbohydrates, but they are the least complex and absorb more quickly into the bloodstream. It is difficult to convert complex carbohydrates to fat that can be stored in the fat cells.

Refined carbohydrates found in cookies, soft drinks, and white and refined breads mostly contain the simple sugar called sucrose. These foods offer very little in the way of nutrients and fiber. They are broken down and absorbed quickly into your bloodstream, rapidly increasing your blood-sugar level. Increased amounts of insulin are then released by your body, and these simple carbohydrates are driven easily into your fat cells. Then your blood sugar drops, and so does your energy level. That's when you start craving sweets again.

White sugar is the least nutritious refined carbohydrate of all. Yet we each consume an average of 128 pounds of white sugar a year.

Excessive sugar may indirectly increase your serum cholesterol level, thus increasing your risk of a heart attack. It affects the pancreas and can result in diabetes. It can contribute to hypoglycemia. Perhaps most dangerous of all, sugar fills you up and supplies you with false, temporary energy that prevents you from eating foods with the proper nutrients and fiber. Sugar has been blamed for many other ills. However, based on present evidence it is only a problem in diabetics and seems to encourage obesity only if it results in excessive empty calorie consumption that displaces essential nutrients.

There is, however, a safe way to eat sweets and to include them in your new program of healthy eating and fitness. The key is to eat them for dessert after a fully balanced, satisfying meal. Then, as they combine with the more complex foods you ate during your meal, they will be more slowly absorbed into your bloodstream. As a result, it will be much more difficult for your body to store these refined carbohydrates in your fat cells, and your energy level will remain even and constant.

Another advantage to eating sweets for dessert is that you will require less of them than if you use them for snacks. For instance, one or two cookies are very satisfying after a big meal, whereas it may require one or two dozen cookies to fill you up before the meal! Welcome finally to a program not of restriction but of plenty! If you are diabetic, you will want to avoid sugar and go with highly nutritious, delicious fruit-juice-sweetened desserts. And, if you are highly resistant to fat loss like I am, you will want to be very moderate with desserts and go with "A" choice desserts 99 percent of the time.

Complex carbohydrates are far more nutritious than the refined carbohydrates. Besides the vitamins and minerals they contain, many of them are root vegetables, like carrots, beets, and potatoes. Root vegetables increase your body's reserve of nucleic acids, which may help to lower blood cholesterol levels.

Fiber is another chief advantage of complex carbohydrates over refined carbohydrates. Fiber is an indigestible substance found only in plants. It can't be categorized as a nutrient since it is not absorbed by the body, but the advantages of fiber-rich foods are many.

They play a role in diluting cancer-causing agents, and they may help reduce cholesterol levels. Fiber adds bulk to the waste products passing through your digestive system, which helps speed their elimination. Besides relieving constipation, this allows for the efficient release of toxins, helping to purify your body. It prevents the toxins from reaching your cells, where they can cause critical damage.

For most people in our country whose diets are low in bulk, the food they eat remains in the small and large intestines for about seventy-two hours. But a high-bulk diet moves through the system in eight to twelve hours. That's a difference of more than sixty hours, sixty hours during which your body is working extra hard to relieve the irritation, and sixty hours in which your body may be storing cancer-causing agents called carcinogens.

It's no wonder that a fiber-rich diet has been associated with a lower incidence of certain forms of cancer, such as cancer of the colon. In fact, 80 percent of cancer is believed to have some connection with dietary habits.

Drink Six to Twelve Glasses of Water Per Day

The final recommendation, and one of the most critical, is to drink six to twelve eight-ounce glasses of water every day. We don't often think of water as a nutrient, yet it has tremendous impact on all our body functions and a dramatic effect on the appearance of our skin and hair.

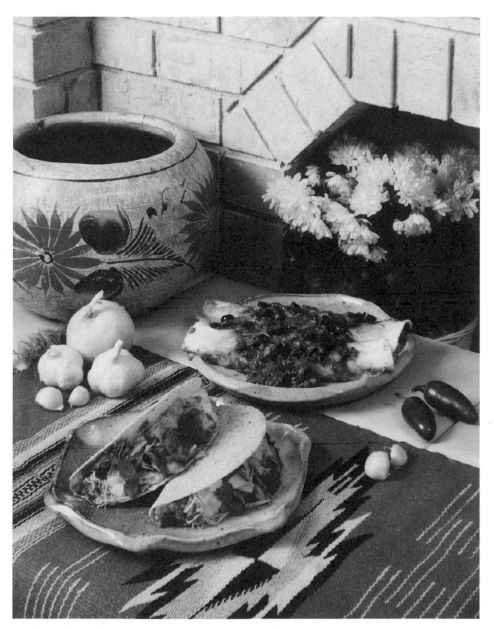

Speaking of nourishment, it's great when your meals both look and taste delicious!

Photo: Tempting Tacos p. 288
Chicken-Chili Enchiladas p. 283

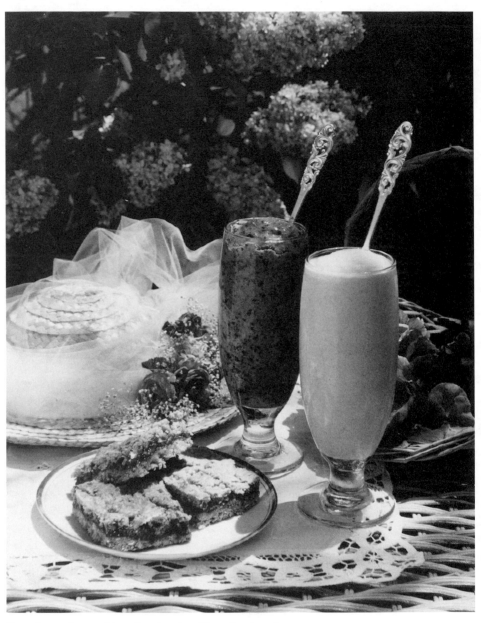

I've always thoroughly enjoyed eating. How about you?

Photo: Breakfast Shake p. 275
Instant Blueberry Ice Cream p. 278
Date Bars featured in Dana's LEAN & FREE 2000 PLUS COOKBOOK

You can live for weeks without food but only a few days without water. Water provides fluid for the circulation of blood and transfers nutrients into the cells and waste products and toxins out of the cells. It regulates your body temperature. It's the basic solvent for all the products of digestion. It works with fiber in your digestive system to help dilute toxins. And it can do wonders for your skin. This is most evident if you compare the skin of dieters with people who eat nutritious foods and include ample amounts of water in their meal plans.

Normally, water should account for 60 to 70 percent of your body weight. But if you've been dieting, chances are that your body is only 50 percent water. That is why dieters often have skin that appears dry, drawn and wrinkled, rather like that of a prune. But people who eat plenty of *high water content foods* (emphasizing complex carbohydrates), and who supply their bodies with healthy amounts of drinking water, have skin that is smooth, clear, and rosy. If the dieter has the skin of a prune, these people have the skin of a plum.

No other fluid can provide you with the pure effects of plain, clear water. Water contains no caffeine, no additives, and no refined sugars. Soft drinks often contain both caffeine and sugar, each of which can dehydrate the skin and trigger the body's fat-storing survival system. And don't be fooled by sodas with a little fruit juice added to them! Although they're a big step above artificially sweetened sodas, the few vitamins contained in the juice are hardly worth the sugar that accompanies them.

These four basic recommendations or principles are all incorporated in the LEAN & FREE SAMPLE MENUS, to which you'll soon be introduced. These menus are not only delicious and simple to prepare, but they also meet every criteria for optimal health and leanness. And you'll be eating the way you were always meant to eat—at last!

The LEAN & FREE MENUS are effective because they provide the perfect balance necessary to achieve an ideal percentage of body fat, reduce depression, reduce high cholesterol, and increase your energy level and overall sense of well-being. Remember, too much or too little of any nutrient can result in an im-balance that can trigger your body's survival system to store excess fat. But when your body recognizes that it's receiving complete caloric and nutritional satisfaction, it no longer has any need to store extra fat. The result is optimal health and permanent leanness.

Some people have asked me, "If I'm eating good, low-fat, high-fiber foods, why do I have to worry about eating balanced meals? "

The answer is simply that balance protects you against the two types of starvation that may encourage your body to store fat: (1) caloric starvation, and (2) nutritional starvation. A low-calorie diet, whether balanced or not, is a perfect example of caloric starvation. When you starve yourself in this manner, your body reacts by converting muscle into glucose for energy, storing fat to prevent what it perceives to be starvation, reducing your energy level, decreasing your metabolic or fat-burning rate, reducing your production of body heat, and developing fat-storing enzymes in your muscles. Remember, muscle burns fat, and the consumption of lean muscle tissue for energy reduces your body's ability to burn fat. And, of course, loss of muscle tissue also means a sagging, flabby body. Increased muscle tissue means a firm, shapely physique.

The other form of starvation countered by balanced eating is nutritional starvation. This occurs when a person eats sufficient calories but the calories do not include all the essential nutrients (vitamins, minerals, and fatty acids) for good health. When your body suffers from a nutritional deficiency, it not only affects your health but it also impairs your metabolism. Metabolism occurs in the cells of your body. In order for your body to effectively burn fat, the right combination of vitamins, minerals, and fatty acids needs to be present in the cells. When there is a deficiency, a higher percentage of what you eat may be stored as fat.

Both forms of starvation can result in a fat-storing body and keep you from converting to a fat-burning, healthy body, the goal of the Lean & Free Lifestyle.

Here is an example of what a balanced daily meal plan looks like:

WATER: ❑ 6 to 12 eight-ounce glasses.

VEGETABLES: ❑ large variety of 6 or more 1/2 cup servings.

GRAINS: ❑ 8 or more servings. (I usually eat a variety
of grains averaging between 8 and 12 servings.
If I include a lot of potatoes and beans in my
menu, my grain intake is slightly less.)
slice bread = 1 serving.
1 oz. whole grain cereal = 1 serving
1/2 cup cooked cereal or brown rice = 1 serving
1/2 cup pasta = 1 serving
1/2 hamburger bun = 1 serving
tortilla, roll, or muffin = 1 serving
(include corn, brown rice, oats, barley, and
millet as well as wheat)

PROTEIN: ❑ Dairy: 2+ servings–Adult, 3+ servings–Children, 4 servings–teenager, pregnant women, breast-feeding women, and postmenopausal women (unless you have a dairy allergy)
1 cup milk = 1 serving
1 cup yogurt = 1 serving
1 oz. cheese = 1 serving
1/2 cup cottage cheese = 1 serving
1/2 cup ice milk = 1 serving

                  ❑ Meat: 2 servings, 3 servings—pregnant women
3 oz. cooked lean meat = 1 serving
1 egg = 1 serving
1 tablespoon peanut butter = 1 serving
1/4 cup nuts, seeds = 1 serving
1/2 cup cooked dried peas or dried beans = 1 serving
Legumes and whole grains together equal a complete protein.

                  ❑ The average 25 to 50+ year-old or older woman requires not less than 50 grams of protein per day. The average pregnant woman requires not less than 90 grams and, while nursing, at least 62 to 65 grams. These amounts are more than adequately supplied by the LEAN & FREE serving recommendations. No additional protein gram calculation is necessary.

FRUITS: ❑ At least four servings.
1/2 cup juice = 1 serving
1 medium fruit = 1 serving
1/4 cup dried fruit = 1 serving

Eat at least one vitamin-A– and one vitamin-C– rich fruit or vegetable choice every day. See page 77 for a list of these foods.

Note: These serving sizes match the serving sizes recommended by the United States Department of Agriculture. They are standard serving sizes. I seldom measure my servings unless I'm calculating calories or fat grams on a very high-fat item. I eat generously-large helpings of complex carbohydrates and I'm moderate with animal proteins.

Fats: Ten to 20 percent of overall calories should ideally come from fat, with never less than 10 percent nor more than 30 percent. Twenty percent of 2,000 calories is 44 fat grams, 20 percent of 3,000 is 67 fat grams, and 20 percent of 4,000 calories is 88 fat grams. (Refer to the "Ideal Fat Grams for Your Calorie Intake" chart in chapter 7, page 119.)

To help you achieve a balanced eating plan, I have developed what I call the "five fingers of nutritional balance," (see page 72) which serves as the guideline for nourishment in the LEAN & FREE program. Those "five fingers" are water, vegetables, grain, protein, and fruit.

As I stated earlier, I recommend drinking six to twelve glasses of water per day. This should easily meet your body's water needs unless you are spending long hours in the hot sun or losing great quantities of water during extended physical activity.

Vegetables, grains, and fruits—the second, third, and fifth fingers of nutritional balance—are complex carbohydrates. They are rich in vitamins and proteins and contain fiber. Fruits are listed last because they are the least complex and are high in natural sugar. They are perfectly suited for dessert!

Vegetables *do not* have to be eaten raw to be nutritious. You can steam them lightly, stir-fry them in cooking spray, or microwave them for short periods of time. Don't just limit yourself to familiar and traditional vegetables. Eating carrots until you are blue in the face (actually too much carotene will turn you orange) will only bore you and is not nutritionally ideal.

Try purple cabbage cut in lacy slices, cucumber, jicama (a tasty turnip-like vegetable), broccoli, potatoes, corn, sweet potatoes, beans, and anything else that inspires you. Be patient and creative, and, in a few months–believe it or not– you'll be craving vegetables instead of chocolate bars. Your entire body chemistry will change, including your taste buds. You will even find your once-routine visit through your local grocery store's vegetable section to be an exciting, appetite-stimulating extravaganza.

Whole grains are the third finger of nutritional balance. They represent a principal source of complex carbohydrates and are rich in minerals and vitamins, particularly the B vitamins. All grains, if not refined, are high in fiber. Brown rice, corn, wheat, oats, barley, and millet all have a similar structure—a core or germ that is protein rich and a surrounding layer that's a concentrated source of vitamins and minerals.

If you haven't been eating whole grains, your digestive system may require several months of adjustment. But once you've adapted, choose 100 percent whole-grain breads, rolls, tortillas, and so on. When you're shopping, avoid enriched white flour as much as possible unless you're still adjusting and need to moderate your use of whole grains.

There are many tantalizing kinds of food to choose from in the complex carbohydrate category. Among them are whole-wheat breads (unless you are allergic to wheat), corn tortillas, whole-wheat spaghetti, artichoke pasta (found in the health-food section of most grocery stores), whole-wheat tortillas, corn bread, and whole wheat, brown rice, corn, oat, and barley cereals. Try to choose cereals based on grains other than wheat to vary your grain intake at breakfast and snacks.

Wheat plays a major role in sandwiches and rolls for both lunch and dinner. Although I consistently buy whole-wheat bread, when my children ask for refined white bread (maybe five or six times per year), I do buy it for them. I find it unwise to make any food forbidden, unless it is a critical health threat (such as alcohol or unnecessary drugs).

The fourth finger of nutritional balance is protein. Protein is essential for a healthy body. However, without sufficient complex carbohydrates and calories (as in a restrictive and poorly balanced diet), your liver must convert the protein you eat to glucose to be used for energy. This process can damage the liver and may also encourage water and muscle loss.

If you use lowfat dairy products and lean meats, make them support products rather than the focal point of your meal. Dairy products should include skim or 1 percent milk, low fat or nonfat yogurt, ice milk, and lowfat cottage cheese and cheese. If you love 2 percent milk, just be a little more moderate with your cheese intake.

Protein is also supplied by fish. Excellent fish choices include halibut, tuna in water (not oil), salmon, swordfish, orange roughy, and snapper. Include these at least twice a week, as they contain Omega 3 fatty acids that help fight "bad" (LDL) cholesterol.

White skinless turkey and chicken meat are also good protein choices. Be moderate in your use of dark meat and red meat. You might use them in soups, stews, and sauces for the flavor, but avoid using them as the feature of a meal, although you should certainly feel free to have a roast, for example, once a month. Red meat provides vitamin B_{12} and iron, but in large quantities it is associated with certain forms of cancer.

You can also obtain protein from a combination of whole grains, dried beans, and peas. Combined, they give you all the essential benefits of a complete protein. For example, meatless chili plus cornbread equals complete protein; split-pea soup plus whole-wheat bread equals complete protein. These foods are also complex carbohydrates and are very low in fat, so eat them to your heart's content!

Fruit, the fifth finger of nutritional balance, is very nutritious and high in natural sugars. It is best eaten with a meal and not on an empty stomach. Fruits are the least complex of the complex carbohydrates. They do not seem to incerease the body's ability to burn fat as much as complex vegetables, grains, and legumes. But I recommend incorporating a citrus fruit, a tomato, or a green pepper into your daily menu because each is high in vitamin C. Vitamin C helps you resist infection and improves your skin tone. However, it is water soluble, is not retained well by the body, and must be constantly replenished. Include at least three different fruits into your daily meal plan.

As the chart below indicates, eating healthy and lean is as simple to remember as 1-2-3-4-5. Just count on your fingers as a reminder!

FIVE FINGERS OF NUTRITIONAL BALANCE CHART

Working together with the five fingers of nutritional balance are vitamins and minerals. In sufficient but not excessive quantities, they may reduce stress, and stress, you'll recall, is the major cause of fat storage.

If you think you have a vitamin or mineral deficiency, follow these steps:

❑ Consult your doctor.
❑ Eat three to six or more times a day, choosing a variety of foods from the five fingers of nutritional balance. Eat to comfortable satisfaction.

❑ Exercise aerobically at least three times a week for thirty to sixty minutes to ensure maximum vitamin and mineral absorption.

Exercise is critical; studies indicate that sedentary people absorb less of the vitamins and minerals they ingest. For example, it is estimated that just 1 percent of the calcium we ingest absorbs into our bones if we do not exercise. However, if we do exercise, more than 20 percent may be absorbed. (Vitamin D is also essential for the absorption of calcium, which is why it is now a supplement to most milk. To be properly absorbed, many nutrients require being correctly combined with other nutrients. The LEAN & FREE SAMPLE MENUS provide this balance.)

If you follow the guidelines presented in this chapter, you may even be able to wear smaller-sized clothing than you ever dreamed of wearing. I never imagined myself in a size 4 pant; I thought I would need to weigh 125 pounds to wear a size 10. But today I wear a size 4 and I weigh 150 pounds. And the reason I was able to accomplish this is not because I starved myself, but because I learned to listen to my body and eat accordingly.

As you study the menu plans in my LEAN & FREE COOKBOOK SAMPLER, notice their emphasis on generous quantities of water, vegetables, whole grains, legumes, and fruits, supplemented by moderate amounts of lowfat dairy products and lean meats.

Instead of depriving yourself, you'll be eating more of the foods you crave: whole-grain breads, potatoes, pasta, chili, enchiladas, tacos, and even pizza. And you'll be eating the same amount of dairy products and meat you would have eaten if you were following the four-food-groups guideline you were introduced to as a child (although eating less animal protein and more whole-grain–legume combinations is also a very healthy option). And remember, your percentage of calories from animal protein have been greatly reduced because of your increased intake of complex carbohydrates. Examine the following program comparison chart on page 74 to see the difference between a typical diet and a LEAN & FREE 2000 PLUS menu plan.

The vitamin and mineral charts on pages 76 through 79 show why good, balanced food is so essential in your quest for optimal health, reduced physical and emotional stress, and permanent excess fat loss.

Notice how many vitamins and minerals are found in the most complex of carbohydrates, whole grains, legumes, and vegetables. Fruits, lowfat dairy products, and lean meats also contain many essential nutrients. With this knowledge, it is easier to understand why it is so difficult to feel well physically and emotionally if you're not regularly eating abundant amounts of good food.

Typical 1,000-Calorie Diet Menu	Typical 3,000-Calorie* LEAN & FREE Menu
BREAKFAST	**BREAKFAST**
Water: diet beverage *Grain:* 3/4 oz. cereal *Protein:* 1/2 c. skim milk *Fruit:* 1/2 grapefruit	*Water:* 8 oz. *Grain:* 3 French toast slices w/ 6 Tb. maple syrup *Protein:* 1 cup nonfat fruit yogurt *Fruit:* 1 large orange, sliced
SNACK: _____	**SNACK:** 8 baby carrots 12 oz. water
LUNCH	**LUNCH**
Water: diet beverage *Vegetable:* 1/2 c. broccoli *Grain:* 1 sl. diet bread & 1 t. margarine *Protein:* 1 oz. cheese and 1/2 c. skim milk *Fruit:* _____	*Water:* 8 oz. *Vegetable:* 1 sliced cucumber *Grain:* 2 slices whole grain toast w/ 2 Tb. All Fruit jam *Protein:* 1 can Campbell's Home Cookin' Chicken w/ Noodles Soup *Fruit:* 1 apple
SNACK: _____	**SNACK:** 1 cabbage chunk 8 oz. water
DINNER	**DINNER**
Water: diet beverage *Vegetable:* 1 c. green salad and 1 t. veg oil *Grain:* 1 oz. pita bread *Protein:* 3 oz. liver *Fruit:* _____	*Water:* 8 oz. *Vegetable:* 2 cups tossed salad w/ 6 Tb. fat-free dressing *Grain:* 2 carrot muffins *Protein:* 2 cups beef stroganoff *Fruit:* 1 cup peaches in juice 1 slice Minute Cherry Cheesecake ("B–" Choice)
SNACK: 1 c. plain yogurt 1 small apple	**SNACK:** 2 carrot muffins w/ 1 cup 1% milk/ sliced cucumber/ 8 oz. water

** You must adjust LEAN & FREE portion sizes to meet your current hunger and metabolic needs. Listen to **your** body!*

Isn't it nice to know that the vitamins and minerals you need are in the foods you're going to eat, right in the five fingers of nutritional balance, and not in pills or in some magic tonic? The complex issue of vitamins and minerals is actually very simple after all.

In the LEAN & FREE COOKBOOK SAMPLER, you'll discover delicious, quick low-cost menu plans to get you started on this liberating, abundant program. Included are tasty, tempting dishes that will provide you with the balanced eating program you've needed all your life. In this cookbook, you'll find special recipes designed to help you eat to full satisfaction while loving every minute of it.

This unique, balanced eating plan is based on my studies, my own experiences, and the experiences of the thousands of people who have succeeded on this program. Follow it, and you can succeed along with us!

In this chapter I've detailed the criteria for my meal plans and explained how this criteria was established. You've learned why it is important to eat to comfortably-full satisfaction on good food each day, to eat more complex carbohydrates, to reduce sugar, to balance your intake of protein and fat, and to drink at least six glasses of water every day.

In chapter 5 I'll introduce you to the next critical part of the LEAN & FREE LIFESTYLE—a breakthrough exercise system that will help you shape yourself while reducing excess body fat.

QUESTION: *What is the difference between LEAN & FREE 2000 PLUS and Weight Watchers?*

ANSWER: *Besides the obvious differences illustrated on page 74, such as the tremendous difference in the amounts of food, the normalacy of food, and the complete balance and snacks, LEAN & FREE feeds your body to be naturally and permanently energetic and lean for life. The typical 1,000-calorie menu starves your body to be artificially and oftentimes temporarily skinny. LEAN & FREE develops a fat-burning, high-energy body that looks vibrant and forgives you when you splurge. Calorie counters and scale watchers can develop a fat-storing, low-energy body that gets too skinny in some places and stays fluffy in others— a body that may gain 3 to 6 pounds every time they splurge!*

BASIC DIFFERENCES		
	Low-Calorie Diets	**LEAN & FREE 2000 PLUS**
ENERGY	Marginal to low	High
METABOLISM	Low	High
SKIN TONE	Gaunt, saggy, gray	Vibrant, supple
DISPOSITION	Irritable	Calm, peaceful
APPETITE	Low	High
CRAVINGS	High	Low
FOOD	Strict and "so-so"	Normal, delicious
AMOUNT OF FOOD	A little	A lot!
BODY	Fat-storing: *starved skinny*	Fat-burning: *Naturally Lean*

HOW DO VITAMINS INCREASE HEALTH AND PERMANENT LEANNESS ?

Vitamin (Water Soluble)	RDA (Milligrams)	Best "Lean & Free" Dietary Sources	Major Body Functions	Possible Deficiency Outcomes	Possible Toxicity (Excess) Outcomes
Vitamin B$_1$ (Thiamin)	1.5	Whole grains Dried beans & peas (legumes)	Assists in the removal of carbon dioxide	Beriberi Abnormal heart rhythms Heart failure Loss of reflexes Mental confusion	Rapid pulse Weakness Insomnia, headaches, irritability
Vitamin B$_2$	1.8	Green leafy vegetables Whole grains Milk, yogurt, cottage cheese Lean meat	Assists in food metabolism Supports vision & skin health	Reddened lips Cracks at corners of mouth Eye lesions Skin rashes	Interference with anticancer medication
Niacin	20	Whole grains Legumes Poultry Fish	Assists in food metabolism Supports health of skin, nervous system, and digestive system	Pellagra (skin and gastrointestinal lesions, nervous mental disorders)	Diarrhea Nausea Fainting Low blood pressure Flushing and burning around face, neck and hands
Vitamin B$_{12}$ (Pyridoxine)	2	Green leafy vegetables Legumes Fruits Whole grains Fish Poultry	Assists in amino acid metabolism Helps make red blood cells	Irritability Muscular twitching Convulsions Kidney stones Greasy dermatitis	Bloating Depression Fatigue Bone pain
Pantothenic Acid	5-10	Widespread in foods	Used in food metabolism	Fatigue Nausea Insomnia Impaired coordination	Frequent diarrhea and water retention
Folic Acid	0.4	Legumes Green vegetables Whole-wheat products	Used in new cell synthesis	Anemia Heartburn Diarrhea Constipation Depression Confusion Fainting Smooth, red tongue	Diarrhea Insomnia Irritability
Vitamin B$_{12}$	0.003	Fish Poultry Lean meat Eggs Lowfat dairy products	Assists in new cell synthesis Helps maintain nerve cells	Fatigue Anemia Neurological disorders Hypersensitivity of skin	None reported

How Do Vitamins Increase Health and Permanent Leanness ?

Vitamin (Water Soluble)	RDA (Milligrams)	Best "Lean & Free" Dietary Sources	Major Body Functions	Possible Deficiency Outcomes	Possible Toxicity (Excess) Outcomes
Biotin	Not established (usual diet provides 0.15-0.3)	Legumes Vegetables	Assists in fat synthesis, food and amino acid metabolism	Fatigue Depression Nausea Dermatitis Muscular pains	None reported
Choline	Not established (usual diet provides 500-900)	Whole grains Legumes	Prevents the accumulation of fat in the liver A major element of lecithin	None reported	None reported
Vitamin C (ascorbic acid)	45	Citrus fruits Tomatoes Green peppers Salad greens	Strengthens infection resistance Strengthens blood vessels Forms scar tissue Collagen syntheses (healthier skin) Iron absorption	Scurvy (degeneration of skin, teeth, blood vessels) Depression Frequent infections	Possible blood cell breakage Nausea Excessive urination Headaches Fatigue Rashes
FAT SOLUBLE					
Vitamin A (retinol)	1	Green leafy vegetables Fortified lowfat dairy products Carrots Squash Pumpkin Sweet potatoes Apricots Cantaloupe	Maintenance of proper vision and healthy skin Bone and tooth growth Reproduction Cancer prevention	Night blindness Permanent blindness Depression Impaired growth Kidney stones	Red blood cell breakage Nosebleeds Abdominal cramps Overreactivity Hair loss Bone pain Liver damage Headaches Vomiting Peeling skin
Vitamin D	0.01	Fortified lowfat dairy products Eggs Small fish (sardines)	Promotes bone growth Mineralization Increases calcium absorption	Rickets (bone deformities) Osteomalacia (softening of bones in adults) Abnormal growth Joint pain	Vomiting Diarrhea Kidney damage Irritability Weakness Nausea Mental and physical retardation
Vitamin E (tocopherol)	15	Green leafy vegetables Whole-grain products Wheat germ (whole wheat) Nuts and seeds (high in "good" fat—be moderate)	Helps the body fight infection and disease Helps prevent cell membrane damage	Anemia Red blood cell breakage Weakness Leg cramps Fibrocystic breast disease	Digestive discomfort

HOW DO VITAMINS INCREASE HEALTH AND PERMANENT LEANNESS ?

Vitamin (Fat Soluble)	RDA (Milligrams)	Best "Lean & Free" Dietary Sources	Major Body Functions	Possible Deficiency Outcomes	Possible Toxicity (Excess) Outcomes
Vitamin K	0.003	Green leafy vegetables Cabbage type vegetables Lowfat milk Fruits	Important in blood clotting	Severe bleeding Internal hemorrhages	Synthetic forms in high doses may cause jaundice

HOW DO MINERALS INCREASE HEALTH AND PERMANENT LEANNESS ?

Minerals (Water Soluble)	Amount in Adult Body (grams)	RDA (mg*)	Best "Lean & Free" Dietary Sources	Major Body Functions	Possible Deficiency Outcomes	Possible Toxicity (Excess) Outcomes
Calcium	1,500	800 to 1,500	Lowfat dairy products Dark green vegetables Legumes Small fish (with bones)	Bone & tooth formation Blood clotting Nerve transmission	Stunted growth Rickets Osteoporosis Convulsion Muscle cramps (common in calves)	None reported
Phosphorus	860	800	Lowfat dairy products Whole grains Poultry Lean meat	Bone & tooth formation Energy transfer Cells' genetic material	Weakness Demineralization of bone Calcium loss Erosion of jaw	Calcium excretion
Sulfur	300	(Provided by sulfur amino acids)	All protein containing foods	An element of active tissue compounds, cartilage, and tendon	None Known	Poor growth (Would occur only if sulfur amino acids were eaten in excess)
Potassium	180	2,500	Lowfat dairy products Fruits Vetegables Whole grains Legumes Lean meat	Acid-base balance Body water balance Nerve function Muscle contraction	Muscle weakness Paralysis Confusion Death	Muscle weakness Vomiting Death
Chlorine	74	2,000	Common salt Soy sauce	Formation of gastric juices Acid-base balance	Muscle cramps Mental apathy Confusion Growth failure in children	Vomiting
Sodium	64	2,500	Common salt Soy sauce	Body water balance Acid-base balance Nerve function	Muscle cramps Mental apathy Loss of appetite	Hypertension (high blood pressure)
Magnesium	25	350	Whole grains Green leafy vegetables	Involved in bone mineralization and protein synthesis Enzyme action Muscle contraction Maintenance of teeth	Growth failure Behavioral disturbances Weakness Spasms Hallucinations Difficulty swallowing	Diarrhea

HOW DO MINERALS INCREASE HEALTH AND PERMANENT LEANNESS ?

Minerals (Water Soluble)	Amount in Adult Body (grams)	RDA (mg*)	Best "Lean & Free" Dietary Sources	Major Body Functions	Possible Deficiency Outcomes	Possible Toxicity (Excess) Outcomes
Iron	4.5	10	Legumes Whole grains Green leafy vegetables Fruits (dried) Eggs Fish Lean meats	Part of blood Involved in food metabolism	Anemia (weakness) Reduced infection resistance Poor concentration Headaches	Liver injury Infections Bloody stools Shock
Fluorine	2.6	2	Drinking water Seafood	May be important in bone structure & teeth	Higher frequency of tooth decay Mottling of teeth	Neurological disturbances
Zinc	2	15	Whole grains Vegetables Fish Poultry Lean meat	Part of the insulin hormone Taste perception Wound healing Sperm production Fetal development Assists in digestion	Child growth Sexual failure Retardation Loss of taste Poor wound healing	Fever Nausea Vomiting Diarrhea Dizziness Muscle incoordination Anemia Accelerated atherosclerosis Kidney failure
Copper	0.1	2	Drinking water Lean meats	Assists in iron metabolism	Anemia Bone changes (rare in humans)	None reported
Iodine	0.011	0.14	Seafood Iodized salt	Component of thyroid hormones Helps regulate metabolic rate	Goiter	Depressed thyroid activity Goiter-like thyroid enlargement
Cobalt	0.0015	(Required as B_{12})	Lowfat dairy products Lean meats	Component of vitamin B_{12}	None reported	Industrial exposure may induce dermatitis and diseases of red blood cells

79

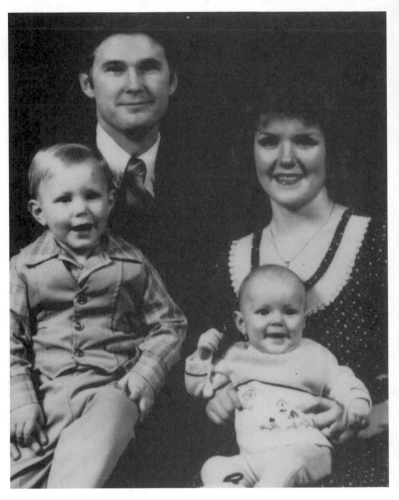

I'm a size 18 here—eating less than 1,000 calories a day (in between chocolate rampages), and I'm nursing a very hungry baby. I have little to give both physically and emotionally.

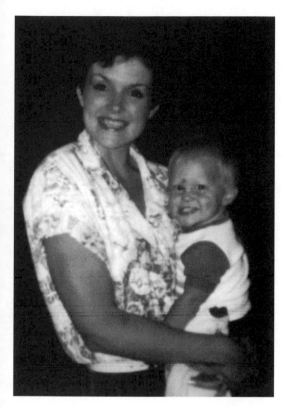

I wear a size 4 here. I'm nursing a very happy baby, and I'm eating over 3,500 calories a day. We both have a lot to give! We look like a real pair, don't we?

5. MOTION
THE SEVEN MOVEMENTS THAT CAN SET YOU FREE

*T*here is great value in simple physical movement. In fact, some evidence suggests that even backyard gardeners enjoy better health and longer lives than people of their same age who do not garden.

Except for spading, backyard gardening movements are not usually strenuous. But they do require people to move, to bend, to reach, to pull, and thus to keep their bodies flexible and functional. When you consider the other benefits of gardening as well—such as the healthy food it may produce, the exposure to fresh air and sunlight, and the sense of purpose that comes from nurturing growth, it's easy to understand why the average gardener lives longer.

Movement, or exercise, is critical to becoming healthy and lean because it stimulates your body to change from a fat-storing to a fat-burning metabolism. Exercise builds lean muscle tissue, which your body uses as its furnace to burn fat, and it produces the fat-burning enzymes that enable you to burn the food you eat for energy.

People who exercise tend to have less body fat and lower levels of cholesterol than those who don't. And they are less susceptible to heart disease, strokes, and certain forms of cancer.

As you learned in chapter 1, we have inherited the ability to store fat from our ancestors. Curiously, though, our ancestors were seldom fat. Why? Because they led a dynamic, active lifestyle that featured movement.

Our ancestors had to constantly labor for their food and survival. They pushed, pulled, reached, bent, lifted, and made moderate to rapid side-to-side movements in the course of their daily tasks. And when they needed to travel, they didn't drive cars; they had to physically exert themselves by walking, riding a horse, pushing a cart, or pulling a wagon. The machine age had not yet arrived.

With our modern lifestyle, walking to the television may be the only exercise many people experience. The grocery store, our primary source of food, is only a short drive away. We aren't required to make any effort to obtain the food sources that guarantee our survival.

But this sedentary lifestyle is not what was intended for our bodies. They are designed for activity. Activity burns extra calories; builds lean, firm muscles; stimulates circulation; and cleanses the body of impurities.

Some people have believed that optimal health could be achieved without exercise. They thought that exercise only burned calories during the workout, and that it would therefore take hours of exercise to burn off even a pound of fat. With such a theory, exercise seemed almost pointless and futile.

But modern research shows that exercise does far more than just burn calories at the time of the activity. Proper exercise creates a fat-burning metabolism that burns fat twenty-four hours a day and stimulates the body's fat-burning potential.[1,2,3]

Since most of us don't rely on movement for survival, we need to follow a simple activity program that keeps our bodies limber and healthy. In this chapter you'll learn the seven simple movements that were the basis of the activities of our ancestors, movements that, when duplicated, and when combined with eating healthy foods, can keep you as trim and fit as our early ancestors. Then I'll show you how to incorporate these movements into your daily exercise program.

It is my belief that by duplicating these seven movements through gentle, nonstrenuous exercise, you will encourage your body to burn a maximal amount of excess fat during and after each exercise session. Because of the wide range of muscle groups and movements you'll be using, you may develop more fat-burning enzymes in the muscles throughout your entire body. You may also develop a more shapely, attractive body because you will not be excluding the upper or lower body from your workout. These exercises are designed specifically to increase your energy and reduce fat. They have helped me and thousands of people I've worked with to become healthy and lean, and I feel they can be of significant help to you too.

The exercises I will recommend are not demanding or difficult. They are nonstrenuous and low-impact. Research shows that moderate, sustained, aerobic exercise is necessary to burn fat, but that strenuous exercise mainly burns sugar.[4,5,6] Moderate exercise is also safer. You should not experience shortness of breath or make yourself vulnerable to injury, because the secret to burning fat is *duration,* not intensity.

Before I explain the seven movements further, let's look at the specific benefits of exercise that make it a critical part of the LEAN & FREE 2000 PLUS ULTIMATE WELLNESS LIFESTYLE.

The rewards you'll gain from a low-impact, aerobic exercise program fall into two categories: *physical* and *emotional.*

Physically, exercise may reduce your body fat; strengthen your lungs, your heart, and other muscles throughout your body; improve circulation and coordination; help your body convert food into energy; increase your energy and stamina; reduce exhaustion; strengthen your bones; improve your appearance; and help you sleep regularly and soundly.[7-15]

As the result of a good, low-impact exercise program, you may enjoy more energy, lower blood pressure, a slower heart rate, an improved ability of the blood to dissolve clots, and less susceptibility to heart disease, stroke, and many forms of cancer. You may increase your strength, agility, flexibility, coordination, and ability to relax.[5,13,16-23]

Although some people mistakenly believe that exercise will tire them out, it can actually supply steady and consistent energy. It is the sedentary body that must work harder, because its heart and lungs are less efficient. Poor circulation deprives body tissues of oxygen and may cause muscles to deteriorate. Your body burns less energy, fat piles on, and you feel sluggish. Exercise, combined with eating to full satisfaction, reverses the cycle. It increases oxygen to all parts of the body. Oxygen is the fuel that gets you going, and it is essential for the burning of fat.

Exercise also improves your utilization and absorption of food.[13] That means it can help your digestion and also encourage your body to get the most out of the nutritious foods you are consuming.

Exercise can keep your bones strong and may help to prevent diseases like osteoporosis.[13-15] A deprivation of physical activity, as seen in bedridden patients, is associated with a dramatic loss of bone mass. Astronauts living in zero gravity show a similar loss, leading researchers to believe that the activity of muscles working against gravity is necessary for strong bones.

Emotionally, exercise can relieve depression and anxiety, clear the mind, improve self-esteem, and reduce cravings for alcohol, drugs, caffeine, tobacco, and sugar and other refined carbohydrates.[4,11,12,24] It accomplishes this partly through the way it affects the chemical processes within the brain. A low-impact aerobic exercise program stimulates the brain to release endorphins into the bloodstream. Endorphins are morphine-like chemicals that reduce pain and depression and can provide a sense of serenity, even euphoria. Since diets that are high in fat and sugar tend to promote depression, thus causing many people to eat more fats and sugars or to resort to harmful drugs and stimulants, the depression-relief offered by exercise may be one of its greatest bonuses. It can enable you to feel positive about yourself, thus increasing the motivation that can help you reach your goals. People who exercise consistently report reduced cravings for fats, sugars, and drugs and positive changes in their state of mind.[4,11,12,24]

This sense of confidence and hope is further increased by the simple fact that exercise can make you look better. It promotes firmer, smoother skin; better posture, gracefulness, and poise; lean and defined muscles; and glossier hair. The result is a more self-assured, optimistic you, one who is more attractive both to yourself and to others.

There are many other benefits to exercise; all exercisers have their own special claims as to how exercise has changed their lives. The benefits I've just listed are the most common, all verified by scientific research.[4] Even if they were the only benefits, imagine how profoundly they alone would affect your life.

Unfortunately for most of us, daily living allows few opportunities for spontaneous, natural exercise that meets the needs of an optimally healthy body. Instead we must create and plan an exercise program. Fortunately, this can be done in ways that are simple, efficient, and a lot of fun.

The primary purpose of such a program must be that it contributes to your ability to become healthy and to burn fat. That is the purpose of your exercise, and that is the only purpose. Don't take the fun out of it by imposing on yourself the same sense of competitiveness and mastery that may create stress in other areas of your life. This time, you don't need to be a super achiever—but you *do* need to persevere.

As I mentioned at the beginning of this chapter, my research has uncovered the seven basic motions that our ancestors used regularly in their daily lives and that kept them lean, fit, and healthy. They performed these movements in the course of their daily tasks, tasks that were required for survival, such as planting, growing, and harvesting their food; gathering food and hunting; and building shelters. In the LEAN & FREE exercise system, you will duplicate these movements. These movements may increase your metabolism, muscle tissue, and energy level, and, in combination with LEAN & FREE balanced eating, signal your survival system that there is no need to store excess fat. In fact, excess fat is very burdensome to keep around when you move so much.

The seven basic movements are:

**1. Walking   2. Pushing   3. Pulling
4. Reaching   5. Side-to-Side Movement
6. Bending   7. Lifting**

Of these movements, walking is the obvious focus for an exercise program because for most people it is the easiest, most readily available, and least costly. Walking requires no equipment other than comfortable clothing; well-fitting, supportive shoes; and a smooth, resilient surface to walk on. It can be practiced by yourself or with others, indoors or out, and it can be practiced at any pace or level of intensity, with very little risk of injury.

You can walk around your neighborhood, or in a shopping mall (when it's raining), or you can select a beautiful, serene setting such as a park. You can also walk in place in your own home while you watch television or listen to music or audio tapes. While indoors, I actually prefer marching in place with many varied arm movements. Those who are extremely obese need not even pick their feet up, just their heels, and gently swing their bent arms.

If you can walk at a sustained pace that raises your pulse rate into your training zone (I'll explain this fully later) for twenty minutes to an hour per day, you will receive most of the benefits exercise can provide. Those who are completely out of shape should begin with a five-to twenty-minute regimen and work themselves up to sixty minutes as it feels comfortable and natural.

It is also a good idea to vary your walking terrain as much as possible. Our ancestors walked up and down hills, over fields, through mountains, across dirt and sand, and through water. Selecting different places that provide such variety helps work different muscles, challenges your stamina and endurance, raises the intensity of your program when it becomes stagnant, and prevents boredom and tedium. Walking on a level plain for extended periods assures a constant heart rate and a consistent aerobic workout. Varying these two forms of walking is a good idea. It is important to do all you can to prevent any tedium, because you must feel challenged and interested to persevere.

If you don't have mountains or hills nearby, you can easily incorporate climbing into your exercise by using stairs instead of elevators whenever possible. You can also incorporate walking into your everyday tasks. Walk to the supermarket or at least park at the far end of the parking lot. Climb stairs in your home, if you have them. If you examine your daily routine, you may find many ways to increase your opportunities to walk and climb and thus increase your strength and fitness.

As part of your walking program, or any exercise program, remember to include some gentle stretching just after you've walked for three or four minutes and warmed up your body. Also, stretch after you've finished. This is often referred to as the "warm up" and "cool down." Both help prevent injury and stress to your body by offering your muscles a chance to flex and relax before you launch into full activity. Stretching increases your circulation, supplying warm blood to cold muscles that can easily be strained without proper preparation. Your stretches should be simple but should include the major muscles of the body, in your legs, arms, back, and neck. Toe touches (from sitting and standing positions); arm reaches; waist bends to front, back, and sides (with arms extended); and neck rolls from side to front to side are some of the most common and easiest to perform. A sixty-minute exercise program should include at least three to five minutes of stretching both before and after.

As you proceed with your LEAN & FREE exercise program, you'll find that its benefits will carry over into all your activities. You'll walk with a zest that is completely new and at a pace you can't even consider now. This "spring in your step" won't feel like exercise. It will feel like a natural expression of the abundant energy you have gained. This is the distinct advantage of a high-energy, fat-burning metabolism. Your whole existence becomes energized and accelerated because you're not only exercising correctly but you're also eating to full satisfaction. This gives you the energy you need to convince your survival system to burn excess fat.

Walking, by itself, does not incorporate all the seven movements. However, I have developed a few simple exercises that supplement your walking program and incorporate the other movements.

The pushing and pulling movements can actually be practiced while walking. Push your arms forward and pull them back in rhythm with your walking. Do this from ten to twenty times every so often as you walk. You can also duplicate these movements through wall pushes (these are like pushups done in a standing position against a wall) or by tug-of-war with a rope or elastic band.

Reaching is duplicated through a simple stretching exercise. While standing still or walking in place, reach up with your right hand and bend to your left. Then reach up with your left hand and bent to your right. Do this ten to twenty times at intervals during your workout.

To duplicate moderate side-to-side movements, start from a standing position with your hands on your hips. Step right with the right foot and then touch the left toe next to it. Then step left with the left foot and touch your right toe next to it. Develop a rhythm or listen to appropriate music. Repeat ten to twenty times at intervals during your workout.

Bending can be duplicated in a number of ways during your warm up and cool down (not during your more intense workout). Here's what I do:

❑ Put both hands on your hips and bring your right foot straight back behind you.
❑ Bend both knees slightly and press your back heel into the floor. Do the same stretch with your opposite leg.
❑ Then bend both knees slightly and stand with your feet shoulder-width apart.
❑ Bend forward, bringing your chest comfortably toward your bent knees.
❑ Lock your hands behind your back and raise your locked arms as high as you can comfortably reach behind your back. Drop your arms and slowly stand up.
❑ Gently roll your shoulders backward and forward. Bring your head forward and around to your left.
❑ Then bring your head forward and around to your right.
❑ Lifting can be done with light weights, or it can be simulated by this exercise:
❑ Lie on your floor or bed. Bend your knees, plant your feet, and lock your hands

behind your head. Put your chin and your forehead back slightly and lift your shoulders, head, and upper back off the floor. Lift from the lower back, strengthening and firming the abdominal muscles and strengthen ing the lower back. Do this slowly for one to four minutes.

By using the seven movements that helped keep our ancestors lean, your body will be stimulated to begin building lean muscle tissue, increase your metabolism, and burn excess fat.

When I exercise, I make it as interesting and stimulating a time as possible by listening to upbeat music, motivational tapes, and tapes of classic books. If you have a portable cassette player, you can do this while walking. Often I exercise (walk in place) while watching my favorite television show. It is critical to design a program that is easy, convenient, and fun. If your program doesn't meet your personal needs, you'll find it difficult to persevere.

Here are answers to some common questions about the design and maintenance of a personal exercise program:

How often should I exercise? To be most effective at reducing body fat, six days a week is ideal. But unless you are already exercising, you'll need to build up to that, starting with three days a week. Even with three days a week, many people experience substantial fat loss. Also, three days a week is a great place to maintain your loss or to coast between more dedicated fat-loss periods.

When do I exercise? Preferably in the morning. Studies show that morning exercisers meet with greater success and are more faithful to their exercise program. Seventy-five percent of the exercisers who plan their exercise for later in the day never get around to it. And of those who exercise regularly in the morning, 75 percent stay with their program permanently. Morning exercise also allows you to apply its benefits (increased energy, clearer thinking, and more stable emotions) to the daily tasks ahead of you.

My exercise has followed a Monday, Wednesday, and Friday morning schedule for ten years. To ensure that I get sufficient rest for early morning workouts, I try to be in bed by 10 P.M. I exercise only three days a week when maintaining my fitness and body-fat level. I increase to six days a week if I want to see extra fat loss. On Tuesday and Thursday, I exercise at 8:45 and on Saturdays (an exception) I exercise at 10 P.M. while watching my favorite detective show.

If you watch television for a half hour to an hour every day, it's a perfect opportunity to walk in place, do aerobic dance, or use a cross-country ski machine or exercycle while you watch.

It is important that exercise not create more stress for your body. To avoid overdoing it, learn to recognize and respond to your body's signals. Ignore "fitness" tests that confuse you into thinking you're not succeeding if you can't meet some artificial standard. And don't compete with anyone, even yourself.

How long do I exercise? For the maximum fat loss, the optimal time is one hour per day, six days a week. For health and fitness maintenance, three days a week for twenty to sixty minutes is ideal. However, you need to establish your own pace. If you can comfortably exercise for only five minutes at a time, then do it. Gradually add minutes as your coordination and stamina increase. Exercising for ten to thirty minutes twice per day can be helpful and less stressful for a person who is just beginning an exercise program and has a high percentage of body fat.

If you're already fit and have only a small percentage of fat to lose, a recent study out of the University of New Hampshire may interest you. Fit women ran on a treadmill for twenty, forty, or sixty minutes, then sat quietly for three hours while researchers monitored the rate at which they burned calories (resting metabolic rate).

Scientists found that the forty minutes did not boost metabolic rate more than twenty minutes did. However, sixty minutes doubled their calorie burning afterward! Therefore, sixty minutes of moderate aerobic exercise may be ideal for optimal fat loss, once you've gradually increased to that point.

How hard do I exercise? Your goal is to burn fat, not glucose or sugar, so you should not exercise so hard that you cannot talk. If you're out of breath and find it difficult to speak at a comfortable rate, you're overworking yourself. Your heart rate should also stay in your training range, which is 60 to 90 percent of your maximum heart rate. Your maximum heart rate is determined by subtracting your age from 220. For instance, if you are forty, your maximum heart rate is an estimated 180. Your training range or target pulse rate (60 to 90 percent of 180) is between 108 and 162 beats per minute. You can find your pulse rate by holding your index finger to your neck or wrist for six seconds. Count the beats and multiply by 10. This will give you the total beats per minute.

If you are walking, jogging, or dancing, don't focus on how long you exercise or on how much distance you cover. Time or distance goals create stress. Focus on other issues, and the time will seem to simply disappear. When I exercise, I like to combine the building of my body with the building of my mind. I listen to educational audiocassettes. As I mentioned, I also watch my favorite TV shows. This takes my mind off the time.

If walking is not vigorous enough for you, consider low-impact aerobics or cross-country skiing. They work the entire body—upper and lower—and stimulate much more efficient fat loss in many people.

The final question is *what kind* of exercise should I do and which is the most effective? While walking is the most convenient and universal exercise, there are eight effective alternatives you may prefer.

1. Treadmills. These offer varying degrees of walking intensity, and they can simulate different terrain. They leave out the movements of pushing, pulling, reaching, side-to-side movement, bending, and lifting, but these can be added after your walk. Jogging increases the efficiency of fat loss for some people, but it also greatly increases their risk of injury. While you walk, listen to exhilarating music or walk- march in place and swing your arms while you watch TV. Have fun with it.

2. Cross-country skiing (or simulated movements). This exercise provides a variation of walking, as well as pushing and pulling movements. While it does not encompass all seven movements, it is a proven method for developing fat-burning muscles and increasing cardiovascular fitness. It is also a non-impact exercise and may significantly decrease injury risk. Cross-country skiing is highly effective for encouraging excess fat loss for those whose bodies seem resistant to change. For many people on a time schedule, twenty to thirty minutes on a Nordic Track seems to be at least as effective for fat loss as a sixty-minute walk.

3. Cycling (or exercycling). Cycling, when the upper body movements are included, includes pushing (legs and arms) and pulling (legs and arms) if you use stirrups. It provides cardiovascular conditioning but is generally not as effective for fat loss as brisk walking, jogging, aerobic dance, or cross-country skiing.

4. Rowing machines. Pushing, pulling, bending, and reaching are all included in a workout on a rowing machine. These machines can be effective fat-loss tools for some people, but others find them too strenuous for the lower back. They can also produce muscle fatigue before the heart rate rises to its aerobic zone.

5. HealthRider. A HealthRider is an interesting cross between an exercycle and a rowing machine. It very effectively works upper and lower leg muscles, buttocks muscles, arms, shoulders, back, and abdominals muscles. It provides a workout that is very gentle, yet strengthening to the back, legs, feet, and entire body. It can be adjusted to all levels of fitness from very-low to high. It is an excellent cross-training machine encouraging the production of fat-burning enzymes throughout the entire body. I even recommend this machine to arthritic sufferers.

6. Stair-stepping or stair-climbing machines. Stair-stepping machines simulate stair-walking. The benefits are mostly to the lower body. It can be a good fat-loss exercise but not the best because it excludes the upper body. And it can be too strenuous for some people, putting them into an anaerobic or sugar-burning state.

7. Swimming. Swimming and walking in hip-deep water is an excellent exercise for cardiovascular fitness and stress reduction. However, it is not extremely effective for fat loss because fat floats, and the body is buoyant in the water. Some arthritis sufferers see increases in good health and decreases in excess body fat from their water exercise and good eating habits.

8. Aerobic dance. This is my exercise of choice along with my HealthRider and my Nordic Track. During my low-impact aerobic dance, I use all seven survival movements, making it highly effective for fat loss.Walking, pushing, pulling, reaching, and moderate side-to-side movement are all included. Bending is incorporated into the flexibility portion. In my aerobic dance video programs, I use all the elements of motion by including body weight "lifting" as part of the post-exercise, cool-down period. These movements help to markedly increase metabolism and create fat-burning enzymes throughout all the muscle groups of the body.

If walking doesn't suit you or doesn't seem to effectively encourage your body to drop excess fat, my next choice for a fat-loss exercise would clearly be aerobic dance. Aerobic dance exercises the entire body, not just the lower or upper torso. For both men and women, such a workout may result in substantial metabolic increases.

Whatever program you choose, there are some final important points to remember for safety and effective results:

Never exercise for even one minute without proper equipment. Generally, the only equipment you'll need is a pair of comfortable, well-fitting shoes designed for the particular exercise. If you walk just one mile, during that time the twenty-six tiny bones in each foot are subject to the full impact of your body weight at least 2,000 times. Visit a sports store that has a knowledgeable shoe sales staff and have them recommend a shoe for the type of activity you have chosen. Then make sure those shoes fit properly.

Always remember that each exercise requires a shoe built for that exercise. For example, an aerobic dance shoe requires good lateral support to prevent ankle sprains. I know. I have suffered two severe ankle sprains from falling off the rear platforms of jogging shoes while dancing.

Breathable, supportive, comfortable clothing such as leotards, support tights, good bras, and layered sweat clothing is also recommended for exercise. Rubber clothing should never be worn. Rubber clothing promotes excessive perspiration, which can result in dehydration. Rubber clothing can be dangerous, increasing the risk of heat exhaustion, which can lead to heart attack and stroke.

Suspended wooden floors, rubberized track surfaces, or athletic tiles are the best surfaces on which to exercise. Avoid bare cement, carpeted cement, and asphalt. Ten minutes of exercise on hard surfaces such as these can create a full week of lower back pain for me.

Be moderate in your approach. Don't over-exercise one day to compensate for not exercising the previous day. You'll make up for it all right—possibly with a week in bed, maybe even in traction. Remember, hard exercise is anaerobic, burns mainly glucose, and may not result in a lean metabolism. (Refer to the following charts.)

What Are the Differences between Aerobic and Anaerobic Exercises?

Aerobic	Anaerobic
1. Continuous (nonstop)	1. Start and stop
2. Rhythmic	2. May or may not be rhythmic
3. Extended duration	3. May or may not be lengthy
4. Uses entire body at same time	4. Generally uses only portions of the body
5. Burns mainly fat	5. Burns mainly sugar
6. Talk is reasonably comfortable	6. Usually feel out of breath or not taxed at all
7. Feel energized	7. May feel fatigued
8. Helps create a fat-burning metabolism afterward	8. Does not effectively create a fat-burning body
9. Creates fat-burning enzymes in the muscles	9. Does not effectively create fat-burning enzymes

Aerobic Exercises	Anaerobic Exercises
1. Brisk walking (moderate jogging)	1. Tennis
2. Cross-country skiing	2. Basketball
3. Cycling (with arm work)	3. Racquetball
4. Stair stepping (with arm work)	4. Handball
5. Rowing	5. Soccer
6. Swimming/walking in water (marginally effective)	6. Baseball
7. Low-impact aerobic dance	7. Lawn mowing and snow shoveling
	8. Golf
	9. Bowling
	10. Weight lifting and floor exercise
	11. House cleaning
	12. Roller skating

You want steady, comfortable aerobic exercise that pushes your pulse rate into your training range (60 to 90 percent of maximum for your age). The following chart shows you where your pulse should be.

PULSE RATE CHART

AGE	Average Maximum HEART RATE (Beats per Minute)	60 to 90% Target Zone (Beats per 6 sec.)	60 to 90% Target Zone (Beats per 60 sec.)
10	(220–10 = 210)	13—19	126—189
20	(220–20 = 200)	12—18	120—180
30	190	11—17	114—171
40	180	11—16	108—162
50	170	10—15	102—153
60	160	10—14	96—144
70	150	9—14	90—135
80	140	8—13	84—126
90	130	8—12	78—117
100	120	7—11	72—108

Use the "talk test." If you can comfortably (breath) hold a conversation (breath), this is a better estimate (breath) of your fat-burning level (breath) than your estimated training zone (breath). If you (pant-pant) talk (pant-pant) like (pant-pant) this (pant-pant), you're burning mainly glucose.

A little stiffness or soreness is natural. A lot is not and may result in injury. If you do suffer an injury, immediately apply ice to it to reduce swelling. Then see your doctor and ask him or her about the "ice-heat-ice-heat-ice" recovery approach.

Exercise increases your hunger for healthy foods. Your body requires more complex carbohydrate calories when you exercise aerobically. In one study, three control groups were required to run on a treadmill at 70 percent of their maximum heartbeat until exhaustion. Two of the groups had received a 70-percent increase in carbohydrate intake. The other group had received an increase in fat and protein with a calorie value equal to that given the carbohydrate groups.

The carbohydrate groups increased their running times to exhaustion by up to 26 percent. The fat and protein group experienced no significant increase[25]. So, get excited if your exercise makes you hungrier. Your new lean muscle tissue requires more high-quality calories to sustain itself, unlike low-metabolic fat. If you're trying to lose excess fat, you need to get your body out of its fat-storing, starvation mode and into a fat-burning mode. Just make sure you drink water and eat vegetables, grain, protein, and fruit to comfortable satisfaction. Some days, you'll feel extremely hungry, and other days you won't. Don't *starve* or *stuff*—just listen to your body!

Moderate exercise programs encourage your body to burn fat all day. As I said earlier, a moderate exercise program doesn't just burn calories while you're working out—it alters your body so that it will burn fat and calories twenty-four hours a day, seven days a week. In lean people, many of these fat calories are burned at rest. But this full-time fat-burning process is triggered only by exercise programs that are moderate. The results will be different and less effective if your program is too intense. If it's not intense enough, you may not see effective fat loss either.

If you dance extremely vigorously for one hour, burning 435 calories, feeling light-headed and even nauseous, you may burn only 10 percent fat. The rest of your energy may come from the cannibalization of muscle tissue in your body. And your body may not continue to burn a substantial amount of fat or glucose; the "burning" will quickly decrease after the workout is completed.

However, if you dance moderately, burning 271 calories in an hour, working up a good sweat and feeling reasonably energetic the entire time, you may have burned up to 60 percent of your calories in the form of fat. You may also have developed fat-burning enzymes that continue to increase your fat-burning capabilities for one to two days after the exercise session.

Exercise will make you feel good. When you exercise, endorphins are released into your bloodstream, elevating your mood and clearing your thoughts. In fact, that emotional well-being is one of the first recognizable and most delightful benefits of exercise—if you don't overdo it!

I call exercise the "dessert" of my day. It is the only dessert I ever indulge in before a complete meal.

On pages 85 and 86 you'll find five weekly exercise schedules that range from an "A+ fat-burning" schedule to a "death-wish F" schedule. Each schedule is like a report card. Look at them closely to determine which applies to you now. Then gradually work your way from where you are to an A or a B schedule.

Proper sleep is essential to effective fat burning. A critical element of the "A+ fat-burning" exercise schedule is sufficient rest. Seven to eight hours of sleep a night is generally recommended for adults; children and teenagers need more. Naps are acceptable and may provide refreshment, but long naps can interfere with normal sleep patterns.

Six Percent of Waking Time

A+ "Fat-burning" Exercise Schedule					
(after you have built up to this level)					
Monday	Tuesday	Wednesday	Thursday	Friday	Saturday
60 min. low-impact aerobic dance (includes warm-up and cool-down)	60 min. "moderate" Nordic Track (includes warm-up and cool-down)	60 min. low-impact aerobic dance (includes warm-up and cool-down)	60 min. "moderate" Nordic Track (watch favorite TV show)	60 min. low-impact aerobic dance (includes warm-up and cool-down)	60 min. "moderate" Nordic Track
15 min. weight resistance (floor exercise)		15 min. weight resistance (floor exercise)		15 min. weight resistance (floor exercise)	
Keep abdominal muscles tight throughout the day.					

One Percent of Waking Time

B "Coasting" Exercise Schedule					
Monday	Tuesday	Wednesday	Thursday	Friday	Saturday
30 min. brisk walk (includes warm-up and cool-down)		30 min. brisk walk (includes warm-up and cool-down)		30 min. brisk walk (includes warm-up and cool-down)	
Keep abdominal muscles tight throughout the day.					

Your body is not technically at rest during sleep; it is actually working. Both your body and your mind are regenerating themselves. I know that if I get less than seven hours of sleep a night regularly, or less than six hours a night plus a one-hour afternoon nap, I can inevitably predict the arrival of a cold or sore throat. However, when I sleep nine hours, moderate my exercise routine, and continue eating to full satisfaction, I can avoid a cold or recuperate from one in about a week. Before I developed this program, it used to take me almost six weeks to clear up a simple cough.

If, after reading this chapter, you are not convinced that you should exercise regularly and you wonder if you should continue dieting or skipping meals, I have one word of advice for you: don't!

Recent studies indicate that even if you do no exercise at all, you will be leaner if you eat to comfortably-full satisfaction on good, balanced calories than if you diet.

"C" Exercise Schedule					
Monday	Tuesday	Wednesday	Thursday	Friday	Saturday
1 hour lawn mowing		1 hour playing basketball		1 hour weeding garden	

"D" Exercise Schedule					
Monday	Tuesday	Wednesday	Thursday	Friday	Saturday
3 hours videos (chew popcorn vigorously)			Walk to 7-11 for a Slurpee		Bike ride down to the local drive-in for a burger and fries

"F " Exercise Schedule					
Monday	Tuesday	Wednesday	Thursday	Friday	Saturday
3 hours videos (chew caramels and chocolates vigorously)			Walk to TV room to pick up remote control		Drive to local store for more videos and diet cola

This is because your survival system is not being signaled to store excess body fat by a perceived caloric or nutritional famine. Of course, you will never experience the optimal health, leanness, and emotional stability that you will if you combine nutritious eating with moderate exercise.

Now let's review what you've learned in this chapter.

First you learned if you are consistently eating to comfortable satisfaction on balanced calories each day, a regular, nonstrenuous exercise program burns fat and calories not just during the time you are exercising but also for up to twenty-four hours after the exercise session.

Then you learned the special benefits of exercise when it is used in conjunction with the balanced LEAN & FREE eating system.

Then I introduced you to the seven movements that kept our ancestors lean and healthy, and I suggested exciting, effective ways to duplicate them.

And, finally, since variety helps you stay on any exercise program, I introduced you to eight forms of low-impact, aerobic exercise that best duplicate most or all of the seven movements used by our ancestors. These will help you customize your own exercise routine so that you can optimize your body's fat-loss capabilities.

Eating good food and following a low-impact, aerobic exercise program can completely change your life and dramatically increase your energy level. In chapter 6, we'll explore the ways you can channel and use your new energy to increase your sense of purpose and lead a more productive, fulfilling, and joyful life.

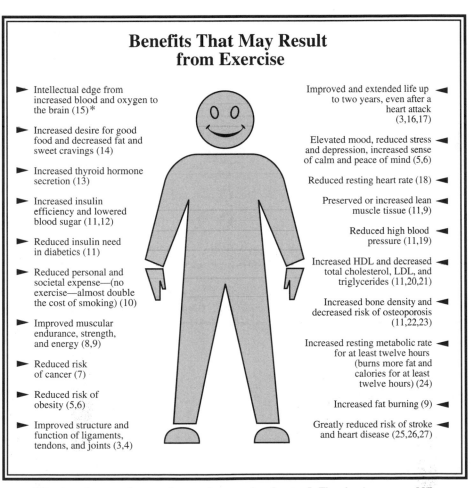

Benefits That May Result from Exercise

► Intellectual edge from increased blood and oxygen to the brain (15)*

► Increased desire for good food and decreased fat and sweet cravings (14)

► Increased thyroid hormone secretion (13)

► Increased insulin efficiency and lowered blood sugar (11,12)

► Reduced insulin need in diabetics (11)

► Reduced personal and societal expense—(no exercise—almost double the cost of smoking) (10)

► Improved muscular endurance, strength, and energy (8,9)

► Reduced risk of cancer (7)

► Reduced risk of obesity (5,6)

► Improved structure and function of ligaments, tendons, and joints (3,4)

Improved and extended life up to two years, even after a heart attack (3,16,17) ◄

Elevated mood, reduced stress and depression, increased sense of calm and peace of mind (5,6) ◄

Reduced resting heart rate (18) ◄

Preserved or increased lean muscle tissue (11,9) ◄

Reduced high blood pressure (11,19) ◄

Increased HDL and decreased total cholesterol, LDL, and triglycerides (11,20,21) ◄

Increased bone density and decreased risk of osteoporosis (11,22,23) ◄

Increased resting metabolic rate for at least twelve hours (burns more fat and calories for at least twelve hours) (24) ◄

Increased fat burning (9) ◄

Greatly reduced risk of stroke and heart disease (25,26,27) ◄

Numbers in parentheses refer to references for chapter 5. They begin on page 227.

Low-Calorie Dieting May:

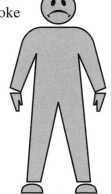

1. decrease resting and working metabolism (calorie burning) [1,16,17,18]
2. decrease bone density
3. increase blood pressure,[1,5] blood cholesterol levels, and risk of heart disease [10,12,13] and stroke
4. decrease lean muscle tissue [5,19]
5. increase depression and moodiness [14]
6. shorten life [9-13]
7. increase fat and sweet cravings and food preoccupation [5]
8. encourage abrupt increases and decreases in blood sugar levels [14]
9. decrease muscular endurance, strength, and energy and increase injury risk [14,19,21]
10. greatly increase risk of obesity [2,3,4,23,25]

(Footnotes: "The Devastation of Dieting.")

QUESTION: *What's the difference between LEAN & FREE 2000 PLUS and other high-fiber, lowfat programs that say "eat lots of high-volume, lowfat foods.*
ANSWER: *My definition of dieting is "not eating as much as I want," or "not eating the kinds of food I love to eat." So, as a fat twenty-three-year-old mother of two, it was very disheartening for me to read that everything I put in my mouth should be under 20 percent fat, that I shouldn't eat desserts with sugar ever again, and that I should completely avoid meats and dairy products, which is practically what you have to do anyway if you don't ever eat foods over 20 percent fat!*

Tell me to eat truckloads of beans, tubs full of brown rice, and ninety baked potatoes, and I'd simply rather not eat at all! It's not that I don't like beans, rice, and potatoes—it's just that I love frozen yogurt, cheese enchiladas, pizza, and beef stroganoff, and too much of anything gets awfully old after a while.

So digest the nourishment chapter and the menus and recipes extremely well! Learn to keep your whole day under 20 percent fat, not every food. Eat like a real person. You deserve normal food–fast food–economical food. This is family food. This is delicious, real food, and LEAN & FREE really works! According to my diet definition, this is the only program out there that is truly not a diet. It's freedom to eat at last!

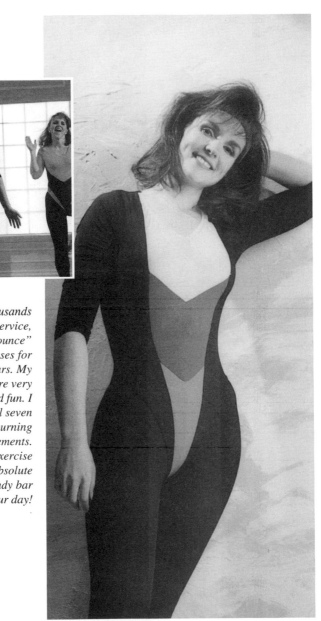

I've taught thousands of community-service, "low-bounce" aerobics classes for eleven years. My aerobics are very unique and fun. I incorporate all seven of the fat-burning survival movements. This type of exercise can be the absolute dessert or candy bar of your day!

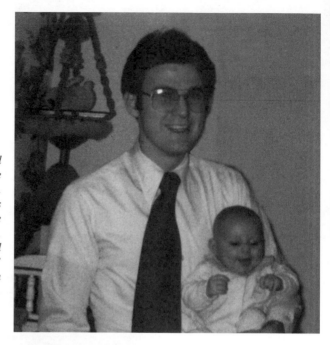

Nyle's life revolved around lightening the loads of other people. After he started living this program with me, he commented one morning, "I didn't know you could feel this good in this life." Nyle passed away after a car accident at age 33.

Living the LEAN & FREE LIFESTYLE does not necessarily give us claim to a longer life. However, we can certainly enjoy and cherish the time we have here a great deal more.

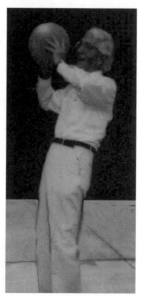

My grandfather, Dan Riley, had a massive heart attack at age 63. He barely survived. He then began to eat well and exercise 20 minutes six days a week. He is now 92 and the picture of health. I'm named after Grandpa Dan Riley, and so is my son Riley Dan. Grandpa's entire life is focused on service to others. He's one of my greatest mentors.

6. SERVICE
YOUR LEAN AND FREE FOCUS

*T*he LEAN & FREE 2000 PLUS ULTIMATE WELLNESS/WEIGHT CONTROL LIFESTYLE is designed to change your life in many ways. It is designed to resculpt your body so that it is lean and attractive, fit and healthy. It has been developed to help you generate more confidence and a sense of empowerment over yourself and your future. It is also designed to encourage more physical vitality and energy so that you can broaden your experiences and take a more fulfilling and active role in life.

This renewed energy must be channeled and directed toward a goal or activity that offers you a full expression of yourself. Without such purpose, this energy is wasted and may even be misdirected. More important, without such purpose your survival system will detect no need for increased energy, and it may begin to decrease its production of energy by storing fat instead of burning it.

It is we ourselves, through our thoughts and actions, who telegraph to our bodies a message of whether we have an important life purpose or not. And that purpose may take many forms: a family, a career, a project, a hobby, a course of study, and so on.

The stronger and more compelling the purpose and the more it aligns with our own highest standards, the stronger is the message to our survival system that we require energy. In my experience and the experience of many others, there is one purpose that seems strongest and most compelling of all, and that is the purpose of service to others. This one purpose, because it transcends our own egotism and selfish desires and because it unites us with humanity and with specific individuals, seems to elicit the most profound response and changes within our physical structure. I can cite many examples of this experience, but the following is among my favorites.

I know of a woman who was overweight, chronically ill, depressed, and lonely. She tried everything she could think of to improve her life but without success. Finally, as a last resort, she consulted a psychiatrist .

The psychiatrist told her that she was so absorbed by her problems that she could focus only on herself, thus alienating most of the people she met. And he wrote out a simple prescription. It said: "Find a children's hospital in your area and volunteer to read stories to sick children for one hour, two days a week."

The woman was insulted by this "prescription." She called the doctor a quack and demanded her money back. But he stuck to his prescription and said, "If you follow this advice, many of your problems will go away."

His confidence and insistence affected her. She became thoughtful and spent a week reconsidering the "prescription." Finally, she decided she had nothing to lose. So she located a children's hospital and began reading stories to the children.

YOUR LEAN AND FREE FOCUS

It is the purpose of the LEAN & FREE LIFESTYLE to:

❑ increase your happiness and peace of mind.
❑ greatly increase your physical energy.
❑ redesign your body so that it is,
   fit and healthy, lean and attractive.
❑ help you generate more confidence and a sense of
   empowerment over yourself and your future.
❑ free you from the bondage and misery of low-
   calorie dieting and meal skipping forever!

Your renewed energy must be channeled and directed toward a goal or activity that offers you full expression of yourself. Without such purpose, the energy is wasted, and your survival system may detect no need to increase your energy and may store excess fat instead of burn it.

There is one purpose that seems strongest and most compelling of all, and that is the purpose of service to others.

It transcends our own egotism and selfish desires, and because it unites us with humanity and with specific individuals, it seems to elicit the most profound response and change within our physical and emotional structure.

Soon, a miraculous transformation occurred. The children responded enthusiastically to her; they began to look forward to her visits and the stories she read. Eventually, they had clearly developed a real affection for her. And in turn, for the first time in her life, she felt needed and loved. More important, she developed the capacity to give love.

Soon she began to regain her self-respect and her self-esteem. Her depression lifted, her illnesses subsided, and her energy increased. She escaped, even resolved her own problems by serving others. This capacity to serve impassioned her life and defined a life's purpose stronger than any she'd experienced before. Now she values life. Today she has lost her excess body fat and is a happy, healthy, and productive person.

Without a strong, clear purpose in life, as this woman has, it is difficult, and perhaps even impossible, to make the changes you need to be healthy and lean. This is because within you is the understanding that there is no point to developing abundant energy if there is no place to direct it or no adequate use for it.

By teaching you to nurture your body, to nourish it with the right foods, and to strengthen it with exercise, the LEAN & FREE LIFESTYLE creates energy—lots of energy, perhaps more than you've ever had before. And, while that energy won't in itself make you a happy person, it will certainly provide you with the means to become one. It is your responsibility, and your special opportunity, to guarantee that your life provides experiences worthy of the energy you have worked so hard to develop and maintain.

For the overly fat person, happiness is ever elusive. While you're in a life-and-death struggle with your own body, it's impossible to find complete contentment or joy. You hate what you look like. You hate how you feel. Movement is difficult and awkward. You're easily tired. You feel unattractive, and you lack confidence. And you are constantly feeling dissatisfied and deprived by dieting or eating meals and snacks that don't meet your needs.

Once that begins to change, once you become healthier and leaner and more energetic, you will be looking for ways to use and express the new you. You will find new activities and goals, and as you involve yourself more and more in these experiences, your energy will increase again.

Having a purpose will continually inspire and motivate you. It creates a balance between your mind, your body, and your actions that makes you healthy and happy in the deepest sense. In the first phase of this transformation will come the freedom and relief of realizing you no longer have to devote your time and thoughts to your weight or your health. In the next phase will come the pleasure of nurturing yourself and your own pursuits and interests. And in the final and consummate phase will come the joy of finding you have time and energy and can reap the highest rewards of all from giving to and serving others.

For many people, identifying a life's purpose is a difficult task. We have so many skills and interests and so many choices. How and what do we choose? When people ask me this, I offer a simple guideline: "What kind of legacy do you want to leave behind when you depart this life? And what can you contribute to make this a better place than it was when you arrived?"

The answer to these questions is individual. Although we all long for true happiness, we all have different ideals and different priorities, and we define that happiness in various ways. For me and many others I've known, the most lasting happiness is achieved through acts that benefit others. Often, these opportunities occur through marriage, family, and service to the community. It usually isn't necessary to look too far; those to whom you can offer the most help are often within your own circle of acquaintances and family members.

To many people, attaining happiness is like chasing a shadow. It is elusive, impossible to catch or contain. Even if they do catch it, it disappears again, and they begin the chase all over. This is the pattern when we seek happiness through transitory or self-serving means or goals. It is my belief that until we free ourselves from a "what's in it for me" attitude, we will never attain a happiness that is deep and lasting.

A philosopher once wrote, "Ceasing to give, we cease to have. Such is the law of love." If we sincerely want something to be our own, in this case happiness and contentment, that law requires that we first give it away, and to do that we must become actively involved in service.

Service can begin with our families and spread to our neighbors, our community, our churches or other organizations, our country, and our world. The desire to serve is a natural extension of the the LEAN & FREE LIFESTYLE because its principles free you to think beyond yourself. By meeting your physical needs, it allows you to take the energy that was focused on yourself and use it to serve others. It also increases your energy so that you have greater resources for serving.

One need look no further than the popular homily "charity begins at home" to know how to begin a life of service. Service to your family creates a foundation from which all other forms of service can extend. And there are few social structures so badly in need of an influx of love and service as the American family of today.

The family is a natural focal point for a life of service, because if you love your family, you willingly and spontaneously take opportunities to serve them. Love itself becomes the motivating force. This type of love is not passive or detached. It is love expressed through action—and that is the meaning of service. It is the active expression of love; it is the highest expression of love.

It doesn't require a sociologist, a psychologist, or an educator to know that developing more love and service within the family unit is the key to many of our current social problems. The neglect of the young (either physical or emotional) and the alienation of the old are among our two greatest crises. Unfortunately, too many families in this country are preoccupied with an intense struggle just to survive, either economically or on other levels. And, since the survival drive, as we learned when studying fat storage, triggers the body's defense mechanisms, it can interfere with other productive processes. It is much more difficult to be loving when you are under siege!

To demonstrate this, I will tell you about another woman, suffering from excess fat, who was deeply involved in her own problems and grief and unable to live a productive life. As a child in World War II, she had lost her entire family in the German concentration camps. She spent the following fifty years absorbed by this loss and by guilt over her own survival. Her body felt threatened by this guilt and worked hard to store fat and protect itself. But late in life she returned to school and obtained a degree in psychology. Although her studies were an attempt to understand her own emotional problems, she was required to do field work and found herself counseling others who had experienced loss and grief. Eventually she shifted her focus to her clients. They benefited greatly from her insight, and she began to realize that she had a purpose. From this purpose came a strong will to live, to help and serve others in grief. And although she was over two hundred pounds when she began her schooling, she is now slim and fit—without even trying!

This experience is one example of how, by refocusing on serving others rather than allowing ourselves to be absorbed by personal problems and losses, we are able to renew ourselves and create a fresh life based on an infusion of love and caring. There are many other examples. In fact, perhaps the best way to envision and plan a life of service is to search first for role models—people who have impressed us with their own commitment to service. This is one way I myself learned the true meaning of service.

I was touched and inspired by the way friends and neighbors opened their hearts to me and my injured boys after my first husband's death. They brought us meals, wrote us thoughtful notes, and visited us. And we were not the only beneficiaries of their love. Helping us made them feel positive about themselves and reinforced their own sense of purpose in life.

My current husband had the same experience when his first wife was suffering from cancer. During her final two years, neighbors and friends brought dinner in every single night and provided the type of emotional support that only genuine love and service can supply. This is the kind of service you too can provide to friends and acquaintances, but it is only one example.

At this point you may still not have a clear idea of how you might want to serve others. And since you are still struggling with fat loss, you may not feel you have the energy required. But you can't afford not to start. Service alone, with pure intent, will increase your energy, strengthen your sense of purpose, and steadily increase both your desire and your resources for serving even more. And if you have a plan for the use of that energy, it will further motivate you in your efforts to become healthy and lean. So it is now, not later, that you must begin to set goals. If you follow LEAN & FREE principles, you will begin developing the energy to attain those goals today.

Your goals for serving others may apply to an area where you currently have little knowledge or experience. But, as you're learning through this program, knowledge can be acquired. And knowledge is power. I know of a woman who exemplifies this most fully.

This woman was very depressed and led a life she considered boring. Then one day, in the course of a conversation with a friend, the subject of ants somehow came up. The friend asked her, "What do you know about ants?" And she replied, "Not much." So he suggested she read up on the topic.

Figuring she had nothing better to do, she began reading about ants, and she found, to her surprise, that she was fascinated with them. She became an expert on the topic. Intrigued by this, her friend began to suggest other subjects she might pursue. Each time the woman would study and research the topic and become an expert. This study greatly enhanced her life and the happiness she enjoyed.

If you are unsure of how you might use the extra energy that a lean and healthy life will bring you, it is good advice to choose something of particular interest to you and read extensively about it. The research will trigger ideas, perhaps inspire you with a plan, and help you determine important goals and a course of action.

Beyond your family and your own interests, the community and your church are always sources of much needed service. You can even choose a career with service opportunities. Many people fulfill their desire to serve by working in fields such as teaching, medicine, government, psychology, and many other areas. Volunteer positions are numerous, ranging from Scoutmasters to Peace Corps workers.

Many people who are extremely talented actually choose less lucrative careers because of their desire to serve their fellow beings. They are the unsung heroes of our society. This is not to say that you need to change professions once you have energy to channel toward service. There are many volunteer opportunities for service, and every community needs extra help.

There is another aspect of service, another opportunity that some people find particularly difficult to understand and accept. And that is the opportunity to allow others to serve you. To many people, the acceptance of help is a threat to their independence, competence, or pride. Others simply feel uncomfortable knowing

WHO SHOULD WE SERVE?

Family • Friends • Neighbors • Church
Community • State • Nation • World

There have never been so many neglected children, elderly parents and neighbors; and all this in a time where"saving the world" and "loving all humanity" are such fashionable statements.

"Charity begins at home."

that people are expending time and energy on their needs, and they're afraid to inconvenience friends or family. Yet the surest and greatest growth potential we have as human beings is to serve others. To deprive others of that opportunity for growth is far more grievous than our fear of inconveniencing them.

My eighty-seven-year-old grandmother recently said to me, "You know, my eyes are going, and now my legs are starting to go. I just don't want to be here if I can't help people. That's what my whole life has been about. And I don't want other people to have to take care of me."

As unselfish as this comment was, it was also in a sense a contradiction. While admitting that serving others was her greatest joy in life, she was unintentionally depriving others, particularly those who had benefited the most from her generosity, to share in the same joy by allowing them to be of service to her. It is as important that we accept help as it is that we offer it. Yet my grandmother is a masterful example of a life dedicated to service, and I'd much rather be on her side than on the side of someone who constantly needs a handout and expects people to bow to his or her every beck and call.

It's also important to remember that you are never too old to be of service. I have an aunt, who recently passed away at age 107, who took in a family of seven (the youngest was four years old) when she was eighty and raised them to adulthood. The last two years of her life, she had to allow others to help her "just a little." And all of those who helped her benefited from the experience even more than she did.

Spiritual leaders have taught us through the centuries that losing yourself in the service of others is the only way to find your true self. Those who base their lives on service are among the happiest and most fulfilled people on earth. By aligning themselves with causes and projects of goodwill, they gain a certain youthfulness and vitality that can actually contribute to their longevity. Thinking beyond yourself has a life-sustaining power that can keep you healthy and active far into your later years.

In a Harvard University study, ninety-one elderly patients in a nursing home were divided into two groups, and each was given a small house plant. The patients in the first group were told that the nursing-home staff would care for their plant; the patients had no responsibility for the plants whatsoever. The second group was fully responsible for keeping the plants alive.

Eighteen months later the two groups were evaluated. The patients who had been given the responsibility for their plants were more alert, more involved in activities, and more socially responsive to their staff and visitors. The patients who were given no responsibility for their plants showed no physical or emotional improvement, and their death rate was twice as high.

You may wonder how taking care of something as simple as a house plant can make such a difference—in some cases the difference between life and death. It's simply because the patients who had responsibility for their plants felt needed. A plant may not seem like a powerful reason to live, but it made all the difference to some of these elderly people.

When you're battling the problem of excess body fat caused by dieting, you are totally in the fat-storing, survival mode and completely focused on yourself. But once you begin to eat to comfortably-full satisfaction on balanced, high-quality calories, and you eat three to six times a day, you'll have energy to burn. Helping those around you is the greatest and most fulfilling way to use your newfound energy.

After seeing how this program has worked for me and others, one of the most exciting, energizing things I do now is introduce these principles to people and help them become lean, free, and happy too.

In this chapter, I've discussed the beautiful new opportunities that can enrich your life when you become successful on this program. As you gradually become lean and free, you will have the energy to help others, starting with your family and extending to your community. As you feel and look better, your self-esteem and self-confidence will dramatically improve. And when you begin helping others, your self-esteem and self-confidence will take another significant jump to a state of happiness you may never have been able to envision before.

Right now, you may be too concerned about your own problems and your excess body fat to see the broader, more hopeful picture. And that's normal. But soon, as your energy increases, your desire to serve will increase too. At that point, you will have experienced the ultimate goal and the greatest success this program can offer.

If you have specific ideas about what you'd like to do when you become lean and healthy, I recommend that you focus on them now. Take action on them, starting today. They'll provide you with inspiration and motivation all through your process of change. Begin reading about subjects that are of interest to you. Find an area in which you can contribute, an area that excites you and inspires you to become lean, healthy, and, most important of all, happy and full of love. This process will signal your survival system to direct your energy into these new fulfilling activities rather than into excess fat storage.

This chapter completes the information section of this book. In the final two chapters I'll give you a plan, an exciting *plan*, that details the specific *actions* you must take to get started on your journey toward a life of fitness, health, and freedom.

QUESTION: *So, I'm supposed to be free to focus my* energy *outside myself and serve other people. Well then, why not just* "listen to my body" *and eat whatever I feel like eating and not worry about this water, veggie, grain, protein, fruit stuff?*
ANSWER: *You hit on the key to your question – energy. Without energy you don't have the freedom to live outside of yourself and enjoy service to others and purpose in life. Freedom comes from following natural, basic laws, not from "doing whatever we feel like doing." The freedom to drive a car is very short-lived if we don't obey traffic laws. The freedom to fly a plane collapses quickly if we've never had flying lessons. Our bodies are much more complex than an airplane or* any *machine known to man. So study how your body works. Learn to fly it into health, fat loss, and beautiful freedom—not plunge it into obesity, sickness, and despair. Then you'll enjoy the freedom and energy to really live, love yourself and others, and cherish every day!*

And remember that service is more "of the heart*" than "of the* hands*". Service that you hate to give, doesn't count because service should bring happiness both to you and to those you serve. So serve yourself by taking care of* your *most basic needs. Then you'll have the energy to reach out to others. A smile, a kind word, and a listening ear are three of the greatest services you can give.*

7. PLANNING
HOW TO DEVELOP
YOUR BLUEPRINT FOR SUCCESS

As we begin chapter 7 of the LEAN & FREE 2000 PLUS ULTIMATE WELLNESS/ WEIGHT CONTROL LIFESTYLE, congratulations are in order. You've been working hard to understand and absorb knowledge and information that may be new to you. You've learned about the stressors that encourage your body to store fat and how to avoid them; you know the importance of, and the means for, developing a lasting commitment to change; you know why you must work to love and nurture your body; you understand the importance of a balanced approach to eating; you've learned the value of movement; and you're becoming aware of the pivotal role in your life of service to others. Finally, you know that the ultimate reward of this program is freedom and fulfillment.

Your learning is in place. The foundation of knowledge has been firmly established. And now, you need a plan—a blueprint you can follow to transform this knowledge into action. In this chapter I will provide you with that blueprint.

All successful plans can be divided into sub-plans. Even the greatest of plans must be followed one step at a time, one day at a time. The focus of your LEAN AND FREE plan will be what I call your Daily Success Planner. It's an instrument for reducing what may seem like an enormous task to a viable, attainable series of smaller tasks. It will help you achieve total success by first achieving partial success. On page 111, you'll find a blank copy of the Planner and an example of a completed Planner on page 112. Then you will find a blank copy of the Daily Success Menu on page 113 and a filled in copy of a Daily Success Menu on page 114. You may want to use these to plan your menus, or simply follow the fast, delicious, already prepared LEAN & FREE menus. There is another blank copy of both the Daily Success Planner and the Menu Planner on pages 237 and 238 and there are more copies at the end of this book.

The Daily Success Planner* is designed to keep you continually focused on following the principles you're learning in this program. It is a microcosm of the entire program, because each day it allows you to assess your progress with each of the program's essential steps. Your LEAN & FREE plan must include the six elements, as shown on page 115. Through a simple 100-point scoring system, you'll be able to see how well you are meeting the requirements for optimal health and permanent fat loss.

*The planner I'm introducing to you in this chapter is an excellent learning tool. It takes about fifteen minutes a day to complete. I call it the **Left-Brain Planner**. Complete it at least once a week. For my Perfectly Simple **Right-Brain Planner** that takes about 20 seconds a day to complete, refer to page 244. Make certain to complete the Right-Brain Planner every day. It will tremendously speed your progress towards being lean, healthy, and happy for life!

LEAN&FREE 2000 PLUS™

THE LEFT-BRAIN PLANNER

NAME: _____ DATE: _____

```
1. KNOWLEDGE
2. COMMITMENT
3. NURTURING
4. NOURISHMENT
5. MOTION
6. SERVICE
7.            8.
PLAN       ACTION
```

PLAN — Points / 5___

Breakfast	
Lunch	
Dinner	
Snacks	
Exercise	
Failure Avoidance	Today, I foresee and resolve any problem that could cause me to fail.*

KNOWLEDGE 5___ — Knowledge: Today I studied or reinforced LEAN&FREE principles. This knowledge empowers my success.*

COMMITMENT 5___ — Commitment: Today I am realizing and enjoying signs of success and feel a passion to be LEAN&FREE.*

NURTURING 5___ — Nurturing: I am practicing positive body talk. I am a friend and partner with my body.*

NOURISHMENT

			FG/Cal
5___	Comfortable Satisfaction	**BREAKFAST**	
1___	Water		XXXXX
1___	Grain		
1___	Protein		
1___	Fruit		
2___	Water & Snack		
5___	Comfortable Satisfaction	**LUNCH**	XXXXX
1___	Water		XXXXX
1___	Vegetable		
1___	Grain		
1___	Protein		
1___	Fruit		
2___	Water & Snack		
5___	Comfortable Satisfaction	**DINNER**	XXXXX
1___	Water		XXXXX
1___	Vegetable		
1___	Grain		
1___	Protein		
1___	Fruit		
2___	Water & Snack		
5___	Fat Grams	Score 5 points if fat grams are about 20% of total calories. (Record calories once a week.)	

Total FG/Cal ►

10___	Stressors*	Score 10 points for avoiding ALL of the following fat-storing stressors—0 points otherwise.
	A.	Alcohol, unnecessary drugs (smoking & caffeine), and artificial sweeteners.
	B.	Excessive amounts of refined flour, sugar, and salt.
	C.	Desserts and sweets, except after comfortable satisfaction on W.V.G.P.F.
	D.	Extreme anger with self or others.

MOTION

TYPE (Non-stop aerobic)	MINUTES (Goal 30 - 60)	PULSE (110 - 180 per minute)

15___ Exercise / 5___ Adequate sleep — Score 15 points for meeting your exercise goal and recording your exercise pulse*. Score 5 points for receiving adequate sleep. (Hours slept:_____)

SERVICE 10___ — Personal Service: Today, I used my increased health and energy in service to myself and others.*

ACTION — Do It Now! Action enables you to feel LEAN&FREE success daily and get on with living a happy, fulfilled life. Take it just ONE DAY at a time. Get Excited! Go for it!

DAILY SCORE — 100 Total — Scoring:
"A" Day = 90 to 100 pts. = Superior day for physical and mental health.
"B" Day = 80 TO 89 pts. = Very good "coasting" day.
"A" Week = 630 to 700 pts.
"B" Week = 560 to 629 pts.

You may want to record your feelings and observations in your Journal Entry on the back.

© Dana Thornock 1994   *At the end of this book, you'll find Success Planners with "Journal Entry" backs.*

111

LEAN&FREE 2000 PLUS™

THE LEFT-BRAIN PLANNER

NAME: _Dana_ DATE: _8-20_

1. KNOWLEDGE
2. COMMITMENT
3. NURTURING
4. NOURISHMENT
5. MOTION
6. SERVICE
7. PLAN 8. ACTION

PLAN			
	Breakfast	Kellogg's Just Right Cereal, 1 % milk	
	Lunch	Tossed Salad, Muffins, Chilli Potato, Canteloupe	
Points	Dinner	Pizza Wheels, Instant Peach Ice Cream	
5	Snacks	Veggies, Fruits, Cereal	
	Exercise	1 hour low-impact aerobic dance	
	Failure Avoidance	Today, I foresee and resolve any problem that could cause me to fail.*	

KNOWLEDGE	5	Knowledge	Today I studied or reinforced LEAN&FREE. principles. This knowledge empowers my success.*
COMMITMENT	5	Commitment	Today I am realizing and enjoying signs of success and feel a passion to be LEAN&FREE ..*
NURTURING	5	Nurturing	I am practicing positive body talk. I am a friend and partner with my body.*

NOURISHMENT

			FG/Cal
5	Comfortable Satisfaction	**BREAKFAST**	XXXXX
1	Water	8 oz.	XXXXX
1	Grain	1 ½ c. Just Right Cereal	0-280
1	Protein	1 c. 1 % milk	3-102
1	Fruit	(in cereal)	
2	Water & Snack	12 oz. / carrots, 1½ c. Crispix Cereal, 1 c. 1 % milk / 1 banana	3-393
5	Comfortable Satisfaction	**LUNCH**	XXXXX
1	Water	12 oz.	XXXXX
1	Vegetable	2 c. tossed salad with 4 Tb. nonfat dressing	2-200
1	Grain	2 blueberry muffins	2-140
1	Protein	lg. chilli potato	6-510
1	Fruit	1 c. canteloupe chunks	t-36
2 -1	Water & Snack	12 oz.	
5	Comfortable Satisfaction	**DINNER**	XXXXX
1	Water	8 oz.	XXXXX
1	Vegetable	4 Pizza Wheels (Cheese, Veggie, Can. Bacon + Pineapple, Pepperoni)	44-1107
1	Grain	pizza buns	
1	Protein	(meat + cheese)	
1	Fruit	1½ c. Instant Peach Ice Cream	1-191
2	Water & Snack	12 oz. / 1 Veggie Pizza Wheel	9-248
5	Fat Grams	Score 5 points if fat grams are about 20% of total calories. (Record calories once a week.) Total FG/Cal ►	70-3207

| 10 | Stressors* A. B. C. D. | Score 10 points for avoiding ALL of the following fat-storing stressors—0 points otherwise. Alcohol, unnecessary drugs (smoking & caffeine), and artificial sweeteners. Excessive amounts of refined flour, sugar, and salt. Desserts and sweets, except after comfortable satisfaction on W.V.G.P.F. Extreme anger with self or others. |

70 F.G. x 9 cal. = 630 Fat Cal.
630 ÷ 3207 = 20 % Fat

MOTION

TYPE (Non-stop aerobic)	MINUTES (Goal 30 - 60)	PULSE (110 - 180 per minute)
Low-Impact Aerobic Dance	60	160

| 15 | Exercise | Score 15 points for meeting your exercise goal and recording your exercise |
| 5 | Adequate sleep | pulse*. Score 5 points for receiving adequate sleep. (Hours slept: _8_) |

SERVICE

| 10 | Personal Service | Today, I used my increased health and energy in service to myself and others.* |

ACTION

| | Do It Now! | Action enables you to feel LEAN&FREE success daily and get on with living a happy, fulfilled life. Take it just ONE DAY at a time. Get Excited! Go for it! |

DAILY SCORE

99 / 100 Total

| Scoring | "A" Day = 90 to 100 pts. = Superior day for physical and mental health. "B" Day = 80 TO 89 pts. = Very good "coasting" day. "A" Week = 630 to 700 pts. "B" Week = 560 to 629 pts. |

* You may want to record your feelings and observations in your Journal Entry on the back.

At the end of this book, you'll find Success Planners with "Journal Entry" backs. © Dana Thornock 1994

112

LEAN&FREE 2000 PLUS™

DAILY SUCCESS MENU

Date:____

FG/CAL

Breakfast

Water
Grain

Protein

Fruit

Snack

Water
Veggie+

Lunch

Water
Vegetable

Grain

Protein

Fruit

Snack

Water
Veggie+

Dinner

Water
Vegetable

Grain
Protein

Fruit

Snack

Water
Veggie+

DAY'S TOTAL ▶

Calories: _____
Fat Grams: _____
Percent Fat: _____

At the back of this book, you'll find more Daily Success Menu sheets.

FG/CAL

Breakfast

Water	8 oz.
Grain	Kellogg's Just Right Cereal
Protein	1 % milk
Fruit	(in cereal)

Snack

| Water | 12 oz. / carrots, cereal, 1% |
| Veggie+ | milk, banana |

Lunch

Water	12 oz.
Vegetable	tossed salad + nonfat dressing
Grain	blueberry muffins
Protein	chilli potato
Fruit	canteloupe

Snack

| Water | 12 oz. |
| Veggie+ | |

Dinner

Water	8 oz.
Vegetable	Pizza Wheels
Grain	pizza buns
Protein	(meat + cheese)
Fruit	Instant Peach Ice Cream

Snack

| Water | 12 oz. |
| Veggie+ | Pizza Wheels |

{Adjust calories + fat grams to the amount of food you eat for comfortably full satisfaction.}

DAY'S TOTAL ▶

Calories: _____
Fat Grams: _____
Percent Fat: _____

At the back of this book, you'll find more Daily Success Menu sheets.

© Dana Thornock 1994

If you take a look at the Planner, you'll see that at the top is a daily menu and an exercise schedule. Every morning or evening preceding your day, you'll write down what you'll eat for breakfast, lunch, dinner, and snacks and what type of exercise you are going to do that day. You'll notice that at the bottom of this first section are two lines that read, "Today I foresee and resolve any problem that could cause me to fail." Quickly scan your day for roadblocks such as parties, guests, an extremely busy schedule, and so on. Then plan ways to overcome those roadblocks.

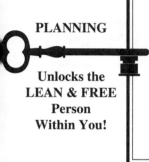

PLANNING

**Unlocks the
LEAN & FREE
Person
Within You!**

1. KNOWLEDGE of how your body works.
2. COMMITMENT to be lean and free.
3. NURTURING and loving your body lean.
4. NOURISHING your starving body.
5. MOTION and the magic in the seven survival movements.
6. SERVICE—your LEAN & FREE focus.

In this example, for breakfast I'm planning to have Kellogg's Just Right cereal with 1% milk, topped with strawberries.

For lunch I'll have a chili potato, green salad, a blueberry muffin, and cantaloupe.

For dinner I'll have four pizza wheels with cheese, vegetables, Canadian bacon, pineapple, mushroom, and pepperoni. For dessert I'll have 1 1/2 cups of Instant Peach Ice Cream.

My snacks will include 1 1/2 cups of Kellogg's Crispix cereal, 1 1/2 cups 1% milk, 1 banana, and 1 vegetable pizza wheel.

I also forsee and resolve any problems that could cause me to fail, such as parties, a busy time schedule, and so on. Give yourself five points for completing this planning section.

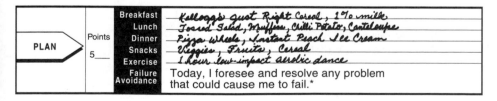

Let's move now to section two of your planner—the "knowledge" section. Score five points for studying or reinforcing LEAN & FREE principles. This includes reviewing this book, listening to LEAN & FREE audiocassette tapes, and simply thinking through the program.

The two purposes of the Daily Success Planner are to increase your knowledge and self-awareness and to evaluate your adherence to the principles of this program. Every time you record a feeling or thought or describe what you've eaten or how much you've exercised, you add to your understanding of how your body works. This understanding or knowledge leads to hope, and hope leads to the belief that you can accomplish your goals. Every day you'll accumulate more knowledge about yourself and the program, and you'll thereby be freeing yourself to more closely follow the correct principles that result in a healthy, lean body.

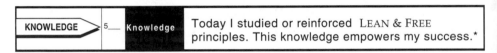

The third section of your planner is "commitment." When you are noticing and enjoying signs of success and feel a passion to be lean and free, score five points. Clearly envision yourself as a lean, happy, service-oriented person. Record your thoughts on the back of your planner in the journal section. Example: "Today I envision myself as a lean, energetic person who is of great worth to myself and others. I feel a sense of lightness and freedom."

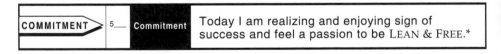

"Nurturing" is the fourth section of your planner. You learned in chapter 3 that it's essential to nurture your body if you want to become the lean, high-energy person you envision. And you learned how positive body-talk can contribute to a positive and productive relationship between you and your body. If you are a friend and partner with your body and are practicing positive body talk on this day, score five points. If you did not, or if you were critical of your body, give yourself no score. Examples of body talk statements you should be recording in your journal entry on the back include:

❑ I love my body. It is wonderful and forgiving, and it is becoming leaner, healthier, and more energetic.

❑ My body and I move freely and easily together.

❑ My body and I have control over sweets.

❑ My body has the potential to be healthy, lean, and beautiful. All I have to do is give it the opportunity to express itself. I will do this by following the principles of the LEAN & FREE LIFESTYLE.

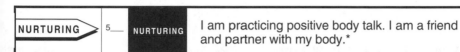

| NURTURING | 5___ | NURTURING | I am practicing positive body talk. I am a friend and partner with my body.* |

Remember, no matter what people have told you, it is not your destiny to be fat or even "pleasantly" plump. It's not your fault or your body's fault that you are overly fat. You became fat because you were inadvertently triggering your body's survival system to store excess fat. Now you realize there is no reason to hate or resent your body. You can simply love it into leanness.

"Nourishment" is the fifth section of the planner.

				FG/Cal
	5___	Comfortable Satisfaction	**BREAKFAST**	XXXXX
	1___	Water	8 oz.	XXXXX
	1___	Grain	1 ½ c. Just Right Cereal	0-280
	1___	Protein	1 c. 1% milk	3-102
	1___	Fruit	(in cereal)	
	2___	Water & Snack	12 oz. / carrots, 1 ½ c. Crispix Cereal, 1 c. 1% milk / 1 banana	3-393
	5___	Comfortable Satisfaction	**LUNCH**	XXXXX
	1___	Water	12 oz.	XXXXX
	1___	Vegetable	2 c. tossed salad with 4 Tb. nonfat dressing	2-200
NOURISHMENT	1___	Grain	2 blueberry muffins	2-140
	1___	Protein	lg. chilli potato	6-510
	1___	Fruit	1 c. cantelope chunks	1-36
	2___	Water & Snack	12 oz.	
	5___	Comfortable Satisfaction	**DINNER**	XXXXX
	1___	Water	8 oz.	XXXXX
	1___	Vegetable	4 Pizza Wheels (Cheese, Veggie, Can. Bacon + Pineapple, Pepperoni)	44-1107
	1___	Grain	pizza buns	
	1___	Protein	(meat & cheese)	
	1___	Fruit	1 ½ c. Instant Peach Ice Cream	2-191
	2___	Water & Snack	12 oz. / 1 Veggie Pizza Wheel	9-248
	5___	Fat Grams	Score 5 points if fat grams are about 20% of total calories. (Record calories once a week.) Total FG/Cal ▶	70-3261
	10___	Stressors* A. B. C. D.	Score 10 points for avoiding ALL of the following fat-storing stressors– 0 points otherwise. Alcohol, unnecessary drugs (smoking & caffeine), & artificial sweeteners. Excessive amounts of refined flour, sugar, and salt. Desserts and sweets, except after comfortable satisfaction on W.V.G.P.F. Extreme anger with self or others.	

Spaces are provided to record what you ate in each of the five recommended food categories at breakfast, lunch, and dinner, and for snacks. You'll also find a place to write down the fat grams and the calories contained in those foods. Information is provided on the next page concerning how to determine the number of fat grams you should ideally eat proportionate to the number of calories you eat to achieve comfortable satisfaction for you. You'll want to very *gradually increase* your calories if you were a dieter or a meal skipper prior to beginning LEAN & FREE. It is imperative that you write down at least three or four days of your average food intake before you begin this program, so you'll know how many calories and fat grams are consuming before you start. Increasing calories too rapidly can result in unnecessary body fat increases. Gradually eat more as your energy level, muscle tissue, metabolism and appetite increase. And remember that it's normal for your hunger to vary from day to day. Just listen to your body and follow its signals. Start by eating five or six little meals each day.

You'll be recording calories so you can adjust your fat intake to approximately 10 to 20 percent of your total calories—10 to 15 percent is ideal for individuals whose bodies are highly resistant to fat loss—like mine.

Look at the planner, and you'll see that the total score possible in the "nourishment" section is 50 points.

Score one point each for consuming water, vegetables, grain, protein, and fruit for each meal. If you are ill or are participating in a rare fast for medical or religious reasons, give yourself full credit. You'll notice that vegetables are left out at breakfast because they don't easily fit into your typical breakfast (unless you have a vegetable omelet).

Score five points for reaching comfortable satisfaction at each meal, which includes water, vegetables, grain, protein, and fruit. If you're missing one of these groups, score four points for comfortable satisfaction (except at breakfast); even if you're completely full. The following chart shows you how to score this section.

COMFORTABLY-FULL SATISFACTION CHART

Ideal	**5**	Comfortably satisfied on the five fingers of balance. (Sense of well-being—not hungry or stuffed.)
	4	Completely full on improper balance.
	3	Hungry.
	2	Very hungry.
	1	Famished to the point of weakness. You may be experiencing no hunger signals at this level.

IDEAL FAT GRAMS FOR YOUR CALORIE INTAKE

Calories	Fat Grams (10 to 20% = "A" Fat Loss Day)	Fat Grams (30% = "B" Coasting Day)
1600 to 2000	**18 to 44**	57 to 67
2001 to 2300	**22 to 51**	67 to 77
2301 to 2600	**26 to 58**	77 to 87
2601 to 2900	**29 to 64**	87 to 97
2901 to 3200	**32 to 71**	97 to 107
3201 to 3500	**36 to 78**	107 to 117
3501 to 3800	**39 to 84**	117 to 127
3801 to 4100	**42 to 91**	127 to 137
4101 to 4400	**46 to 98**	137 to 147
4401 to 4700	**49 to 104**	147 to 157

Just coming off a diet and gradually increasing calories as your hunger directs, you would have the following calorie/fat gram ratio.

1000 to 1300	**11 to 29**	37 to 47
1301 to 1600	**14 to 36**	47 to 57

SPECIAL NOTE CONCERNING CALORIC INCREASES:

These Calorie recommendations are simply suggestions. Some women have eaten less than 1000 calories faithfully for many years and fall into the "extreme chronic dieter" catogory.

These women need to listen "very" closely to their bodies and neither stuff themselves nor go hungry. Both extremes can encourage excessive body fat gain. They may want to increase their calories as gradually as 50 calories per month once they have reached 1200 calories. (Example: November = 1200 daily calories; December = 1250...) These women may ultimately find comfortable satisfaction between 1600 and 2500 calories. Chronic dieters may also experience more optimal fat loss when they eat six relatively small meals per day and keep their fat intake between approximately 10 and 15 percent of their total caloric intake.

FOR OPTIMAL HEALTH AND FAT LOSS — LISTEN TO YOUR BODY! YOU'RE AIMING FOR AN ENERGETIC "FEELING", NOT A CALORIE NUMBER.

Snacks between meals are scored this way: score one point for drinking water and one point for a nourishing snack between breakfast and lunch; between lunch and dinner; and between dinner and bedtime. Eat a vegetable if you aren't hungry and a vegetable as well as any other nourishing foods if you are hungry. (Leftovers make great snacks.) If you can't or don't snack on a particular day, you will lose only three points, and 90 to 100 points equals a great "A" day for fat loss. However, nourishing snacks help to increase your metabolism and encourage more rapid fat loss.

Score five points if you kept your fat grams in the 10 to 20 percent range for the day. Score no points if you are in the 22 to 30 percent range or below 9 percent. And score minus ten points if you are above 30 percent, as this is not a healthy range and can encourage heart disease, obesity, and cancer.

Score ten points each day for avoiding the following fat-storing stressors: alcohol and unnecessary drugs, including tobacco; artificial sweeteners and caffeine; excessive amounts of refined flour, sugar, and salt; and dessert or sweets consumed when you were not fully satisfied first by water, vegetables, grains, protein, and fruit. (And leave the sweets out if you are highly resistant to fat loss, or suffer with diabetes or hypoglycemia.)

I calculate my calories only once a week. Then I determine my percentage of calories derived from fat. To do this I multiply my fat gram total by nine, because there are nine calories in one gram of fat. Then I divide that number by the total number of calories that day.

Example: 585 calories from fat (65 fat grams times nine) divided by 3,349 total calories equals 17 percent of total daily calories from fat. Remember, good fats are essential for optimal health and leanness. If you eat too little fat, (less than 10 percent on a regular basis) you may never feel satisfied, you may crave fats and sweets, and you may weaken your immune system, thus signaling your survival system to store fat.

A fun way to further simplify fat gram figuring is to round nine calories in one gram of fat up to ten. Because we don't count traces at all, this is quite accurate. Example: Let's say you eat about 2,000 calories each day and you would like to keep your fat grams between 10 and 20 percent of your overall calories. Ten percent of 2,000 is 200. Twenty percent of 2,000 is 400. Divide 200 by 10 and you have 20 grams. Divide 400 by 10 and you have 40 fat grams. Therefore, 20 to 40 fat grams equals approximately 10 to 20 percent of your overall calories if you are eating about 2,000 calories each day. How easy! (If you aren't figuring calories, 20 to 40 fat grams is a good range to aim for.)

MOTION			TYPE (Non-stop aerobic)	MINUTES (Goal 30 - 60)	PULSE (110 - 180 per minute)
			Low-Impact Aerobic Dance	60	160
	15__	Exercise	Score 15 points for meeting your exercise goal and recording your exercise pulse*		
	5__	Adequate sleep	Score 5 points for receiving adequate sleep. (Hours slept: _8___)		

Next on your Planner is "exercise." Describe the type of exercise you did, the number of minutes you exercised, and the pulse rate you attained. Score fifteen points if you met your exercise goal recorded at the top of your Planner and if you achieved your target pulse rate.

In this completed example, I recorded one hour of low-impact aerobic dance.

120

That included a four-minute warm-up and a four minute cool-down. My peak exercise pulse was 160, or 85 percent of my maximum rate. Remember, your maximum rate is based on 220 minus your age. In my case it's 185 (220-35). Eighty -five percent of 185 is actually 157. I scored fifteen points for meeting my goal. If I had exercised only thirty minutes, I would have scored eight points. However, if my goal had been thirty minutes, then I would have received the full fifteen points.

If your pulse rate is in your training range (60 to 90 percent of maximum for your age) and you set and met a realistic goal, give yourself the full score. Refer to the pulse rate chart on page 83, or take the "talk test." If you are seriously overly fat, your beginning time goal may be only five minutes two or three times during the day. The ultimate goal, however, is to increase your exercise period to an hour six days a week when you want to see optimal fat loss, and thirty minutes three days a week for coasting.

I choose one day a week to give myself a full exercise point credit for no exercise. It's healthier and more efficient to give your body a rest. Professionals and athletes have noted that they progress more rapidly if they exercise six days a week than if they exercise seven. Give yourself credit also if you're too ill to exercise. If you're only slightly ill, exercise more moderately. Any exercise will elevate your mood, increase your circulation, and perhaps even aid in a more rapid recovery by strengthening your immune system. If you choose to exercise only three days a week, your overall weekly score can still be in the solid "B" range.

Score another five points if you received adequate sleep that day (seven to eight hours). If I consistently receive less than seven hours of sleep daily, I feel weak and tired and become more susceptible to injury and illness. Adequate sleep is essential for muscle repair, optimal fat loss, and an overall sense of well-being. When you receive too little sleep, this can seriously stress your body and signal your survival system to slow your metabolism and store more fat.

The section following exercise is "service." As I've tried to explain, service is invaluable in your quest for success and happiness. In your journal section, write down anything you were able to do for others and how it made you feel. If you performed service for other people (with a happy attitude), score ten points. These ten points are the icing on your "cake" of daily health and joy.

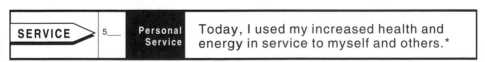

| SERVICE | 5___ | Personal Service | Today, I used my increased health and energy in service to myself and others.* |

And finally, the action section reminds you to simply take it *one day at a time.* Start by eating breakfast and *do it today.* Your goal, after adding up the pluses and minuses, is to score between ninety and one hundred points each day.

Ninety points or more is an (A) "Acclaim" day—days that, when accumulated, result in excess fat loss and happiness on a permanent and continual basis.

Eighty to eighty-nine points is a (B) "Bounteous" day. This is a great place to "cruise" for a while and enjoy your newfound freedom and excellent health. But don't expect fat loss here (although many men do see some see fat loss in this range).

Sixty to seventy-nine points (C) is a "Cholesterol" day. You can expect a reduced energy level, some depression, excess fat gain, and high cholesterol levels associated with this type of lifestyle. This is the range where your survival system kicks your body out of neutral, and you begin to develop a fat-storing metabolism.

Forty to fifty-nine points (D) is a "Diet" day. In this range your body is in an unhealthy state and becomes a very efficient fat-storing warehouse. With "D" habits, you develop many fat-storing enzymes and destroy fat-burning enzymes.

Less than forty points is an (F) "Fatal Famine" day." The types of habits that make up such days can shorten your life. It's as simple as that.

On the next five pages, you'll see plans that illustrate the scores and success grades I've just listed. The first two, the "A" and "B," are examples of my own actual success plans. You'll notice on my "A" day that I have listed only about 2,000 calories worth of food so as not too overwhelm you if you're a dieter. I actually range between 2,500 and 4,000 calories each day–quite a variation. I simply listen to my body. I eat larger portions of the same foods. It is essential that you *adjust* the portion sizes to meet your individual needs to avoid excess fat gain. I didn't start out at 3,000 calories or I would have gained alot more than seven pounds.

The "B" day was recorded during a family vacation. Flexibility is not only allowed, but it is imperative if you plan to "live" in the real world. Let these plans work with and for you, not against you. The last three "success" plans ("C, "D," and "F") are almost exact replicas of what I've seen from students in the numerous classes I've taught. Remember, you can create a fat-burning body through " A" and "B" abundance, and a fat-storing body through "C," "D," and "F" dieting and negligence.

FAT-BURNING BODY = "A" ABUNDANCE
Daily score: 90 to 100 points
on a regular basis

COASTING HABITS = "B" score: 80 to 89 points
Allows you to see little or no fat gain
when you have a "fat-burning" body

FAT-STORING BODY = "C," "D," and "F" DIETING
AND NEGLIGENCE
Daily score: Below 80 points
on a regular basis

A = "Acclaim" Day

LEAN&FREE 2000 PLUS™
GRAB 'N' GO
DAILY SUCCESS MENU — A DAY

			FG/CAL
Breakfast	**Water**	12 oz.	
	Grain	1 1/2 cups Kellogg's Just Right Cereal	2/280
	Protein	1 1/2 cups skim milk	t/129
Full Satis. 5+	**Fruit**	(in cereal)	
Snack	**Water &**	8 oz./ 6 baby carrots	0/35
Lunch	**Water**	8 oz.	
	Vegetable	1/2 foot long Subway Seafood Sandwich w/ extra veggies and no dressings	7/343
	Grain	(whole grain bun)	
Full Satis. 5	**Protein**	(seafood and cheese)	
	Fruit	1 large orange (from home)	t/62
Snack	**Water &**	8 oz./ 1/2 leftover footlong sandwich	7/343
Dinner	**Water**	8 oz.	
	Vegetable	1 cup Quick, Delicious Beef Stew* p. 256	8/302
	Grain	1 slice whole grain bread with 1 Tb. All Fruit Jam* p. 286	t/158
Full Satis. 5	**Protein**	(in beef stew)	
	Fruit	1 apple	t/81
Snack	**Water &**	8 oz./ 1 cup leftover stew	8/302

32 fat grams x 9 calories = 288 calories from fat 288÷2,035 = 14% fat	**DAY'S TOTAL ►**	Calories: 2,035* Fat Grams: 32 Percent Fat: 14

*You must adjust calories and portion sizes to your individual hunger and energy needs.

LEAN&FREE 2000 PLUS™

DAILY COASTING MENU — B DAY

			FG/CAL
Breakfast	**Water**	12 oz.	
	Grain	10 Kellogg's Frosted Mini Wheats (sugar 6 grams)	0-250
Full Satis. 5	**Protein**	1 1/2 cups 2% milk	8-182
	Fruit	1 large banana, sliced	tr-150
Snack	**Water &**	8 oz.	
		vegetables / 3 large Banana Muffins	3-451
Lunch	**Water**	12 oz.	
	Vegetable	(extra lettuce, tomatoes, pickles, onion)	tr-60
	Grain	2 Burger King BK Broilers	36-758
Full Satis. 5	**Protein**	(with extra sauces) (chicken)	
	Fruit	(tomatoes)	
Snack	**Water &**	12 oz.	
Dinner	**Water**	8 oz.	
	Vegetable	2 cups tossed salad/5 tb. lowfat dressing	11-300
	Grain	3 medium slices Pizza Hut Pepperoni Thick & Chewy Pizza slices	18-560
Full Satis. 5+	**Protein**	(pizza meat and cheese)	
	Fruit	large slice watermelon	0-100
		2 - 2 1/2" fudge brownies	14-300
		1 cup vanilla ice cream	14-280
Snack	**Water &**	12 oz.	
		6 cups buttered popcorn	11-210

DAY'S TOTAL ►

Calories:	3601
Fat Grams:	115
Percent Fat:	29*

124   *This day shows the worst you can be and still be okay with little or no fat gain
depending on the fat-burning capacity of your body. This is NOT a fat-loss day!*

© Dana Thornock 1

C = "Cholesterol" Day

LEAN&FREE 2000 PLUS™ — FAT-STORING MENU — C DAY

			FG/CAL
Breakfast	**Water**	2 cups coffee (cream/sugar)	6-116
	Grain	(biscuit)	
Full Satis. 3	**Protein**	1 Egg & Sausage Fast Food Breakfast Biscuit	35-529
	Fruit		
Snack	**Water &**	32 oz. diet cola/1 Snickers bar	14-290
Lunch	**Water**	16 oz. diet cola	0-0
	Vegetable	5 oz. coleslaw	27-289
		small fry	18-383
	Grain		
Full Satis. 4	**Protein**	2 fried fish fillets	20-350
	Fruit		
Snack	**Water &**	3.4 oz. plain M&M's	20-480
Dinner	**Water**	32 oz. diet cola	0-0
	Vegetable	50 potato chips	35-525
	Grain	1 white bun	2-140
Full Satis. 4	**Protein**	1 chicken hot dog	9-116
	Fruit		
Snack	**Water &**	1 cup dry-roasted peanuts	73-855

DAY'S TOTAL ►

Calories:	4073
Fat Grams:	259*
Percent Fat:	57*
Caffeine mg:	575*

Dana Thornock 1994

This is a very unhealthy day. It is high in fat, cholesterol, and caffeine; and it is low in nutrition.

125

LEAN&FREE 2000 PLUS™

EXTREME FAT-STORING MENU*

D DAY

			FG/CAL
Breakfast	Water	32 oz. diet cola	0-0
	Grain		
Full Satis. 1	Protein		
	Fruit		
Snack	Water &	appetite suppressant	
Lunch	Water Vegetable	small fry	18-383
	Grain		
Full Satis. 2	Protein		
	Fruit		
Snack	Water &	32 oz. diet cola	0-0
Dinner	Water Vegetable	32 oz. diet cola	0-0
	Grain	3/4 cup cookie dough	25-550
Full Satis. 4	Protein	fried fish sandwich	26-442
	Fruit		
Snack	Water &		

DAY'S TOTAL ▶

Calories:	1375*
Fat Grams:	69
Percent Fat:	45*
Caffeine mg:	614*

This day offers even more fat-storing stress than the "C" day because the body percieves even more caloric and nutritional starvation.

© Dana Thornock 199

LEAN&FREE 2000 PLUS™

FATAL FAMINE MENU* **F** DAY

			FG/CAL
Breakfast	**Water**	3 cups coffee, black	0-0
	Grain		
Full Satis. **1**	**Protein**		
	Fruit		
Snack	**Water &**	6 cups coffee	0-0
Lunch	**Water** **Vegetable**	3 cups coffee	0-0
	Grain		
No Signals (Numb).	**Protein**		
	Fruit	32 oz. diet cherry cola	0-0
Snack	**Water &**	sugar free gum	0-0
Dinner	**Water** **Vegetable**	6 cups coffee	0-0
	Grain		
No Signals (DEAD)	**Protein**		
	Fruit		
Snack	**Water &**	2 NoDoz tablets / 32 oz. diet cola /	0-0
		1/8 cup mint flavored mouth wash	0-0

DAY'S TOTAL ▶

Calories:	0*
Fat Grams:	0*
Percent Fat:	0*
Caffeine mg:	3644*

© Dana Thornock 1994

*A "D" day is bad, but an "F" day is even worse! And yes, there are people that live this way. This menu is not uncommon among chronic dieters.

It's important to understand that you don't have to score perfectly every day to succeed with this common-sense lifestyle. Scoring between 630 and 700 points a week still indicates that you are creating an efficient, fat-burning body. (But if you're a woman whose body fat is a healthy 20 percent and you want it to be 16 percent, you *may* have to be perfect to get there.) Scoring 560 to 629 points indicates that you are maintaining nicely and not regressing. Your goal is to improve your score as you proceed and never to "beat yourself up" or despair over disappointing days. After all, despair can only threaten your body. Your work is to develop a forgiving attitude toward yourself and your body and to enjoy how forgiving your new LEAN & FREE body is on your "C" days.

One of the great benefits of this program is what I call "splurge freedom." Gwen's story illustrates this point.

Gwen had suffered from chronic diarrhea and vomiting since her stomach bypass surgery five years before. She lost eighty pounds, then proceeded to regain that weight and more, although she was eating very small amounts of food.

Her first year following LEAN & FREE principles, Gwen's health problems completely disappeared and her survival system relaxed, allowing her to lose sixty-five pounds (much faster fat loss than is usual for a dieter). She was burning fat and feeling great. Her husband also lost forty-five pounds simply by sharing in the healthy, balanced meals she was preparing on this program. He didn't exercise at all.

Then the Christmas holidays came around. Gwen stopped exercising. She stopped snacking on complex carbohydrates and began snacking on sweets. Her meals increased from 20 percent fat to 50 percent fat. The only bad habit she didn't revert to was meal-skipping. Inevitably, her diarrhea and vomiting recurred.

Another year went by, and Gwen, who was feeling terrible, decided it was time to return to the sound, healthy principles she had learned on the program. When she did, she made a wonderful discovery. In spite of her bad habits, because she hadn't skipped meals or dieted, she had only regained fifteen pounds of the sixty-five she had lost. She didn't have to start all over. "If I had lost that sixty-five pounds by dieting, I would have gained it all back plus more," Gwen said. "I can't believe it. I am thrilled."

Her story is a perfect example of the "splurge freedom" you can enjoy on this program. It's not necessary to skip that birthday party or to show up at a dinner with your private bag of carrots to munch. In fact, if you do, you are not following this program. Do people a great service—show them you eat like a normal person.

Reverting to your old habits will slow your progress toward a lean, healthy body, but an occasional splurge will not destroy your progress. However, the more "A" days you have, the more quickly you'll reach your goal. So make a conscious effort to regularly eat an abundance of good food. And *never skip meals*. Although you may gain a small amount of body fat when your efforts fall into the "B-" range, this won't signal your body's survival system to resist fat-loss as meal deprivation will. And once you have perfected your LEAN & FREE habits, your fat will begin to decrease regularly and predictably.

On the back of your Daily Success Planner is a "Journal Entry" section for recording your thoughts and feelings of the day. Did you notice a change in your body? In your disposition? Were you happier, more energetic, less irritable, calmer? Did you feel better about yourself, more confident and optimistic? Did you lose inches on your stomach, hips, thighs? Was your blood pressure lower? Has your cholesterol level been reduced?

Some of these changes are very subtle but extremely important. Others are more dramatic and visible. Of course, every day will be different. If you feel that you had a "down" day, describe specifically how you felt. Then review what you ate, whether you avoided fat-storing stressors, what you did for exercise, and whether you received an adequate amount of sleep. This review will give you specific clues about the causes of "down" days and how to avoid them in the future.

The Daily Success Planner is your constant companion. When well maintained, it indicates clearly how well you're progressing and what changes you need to make in your habits and attitudes. But it is only a part of your overall plan. To score well in the "nourishment" section, you have to know what to eat.

Planning balanced meals is the next step in the plan. In the LEAN & FREE COOKBOOK SAMPLER section, you'll find delicious, economical menu plans that will guarantee you are receiving the essential nutrients and the balanced foods necessary to keep you lean and healthy. These menus feature delicious, "normal" food that can be easily and quickly prepared. They also feature excellent suggestions for occasions when you're dining out. In addition, you'll find a listing of fat grams and calories for each of the recommended dishes on the menu itself and in the recipe section.

Once you've sampled these foods, you can decide what best suits your personal tastes. Just remember, you're trying to learn to eat until you are fully satisfied, on a balanced and delicious menu. To do this, you must listen and respond to your body.

Now that you have a meal plan, you need a movement plan. Aerobic exercise has done almost as much to change my physical and emotional life as the changes in my eating habits have. I could never have managed the stress in my life and could certainly not have attained any reasonable degree of happiness and serenity without my program of aerobic dancing at least three days a week.

In chapter 5, I listed some recommended forms of low-impact aerobic exercise and described how they duplicate the seven specific movements that conditioned the bodies of our ancestors. Now it's time to select a form of exercise that is convenient for you to do three times per week (or more). This exercise must be moderate, low-impact, and aerobic, and ideally it must utilize your lower and upper body. It should be an exercise you can comfortably perform for forty-five minutes to an hour at least three times per week. If you can exercise for only five minutes when you start the program, that's fine. Your strength will increase as your condition improves.

If you suffer from severe obesity, you may want to initially split your exercise sessions into two daily sessions of five, ten, fifteen, twenty, or thirty minutes each. You may exercise once in the morning and once at night. For the very obese body, this is safer and less stressful.

In good weather, a wonderful exercise is brisk walking (including arm movements). It's a lot more fun if you can walk with a friend who moves at approximately the same pace you do. If you prefer to stay indoors, you can walk or march in place, do low-impact aerobic dancing, or use a stationary bicycle, stair-stepper, cross-country ski simulation machine, or treadmill. Any exercise will help create a fat-burning metabolism and will energize you, if that exercise is continuous, rhythmic, and involves your entire body (and you are eating nourishing foods to full satisfaction). Remember, if you can't talk while you're exercising, you're working too hard.

For many people, there are special advantages to aerobic dance classes. They're available in most areas, and they provide group support and a stronger motivation than many people attain exercising alone. That's why I've taught free and nonprofit community aerobics classes for more than ten years.

If you're just beginning an exercise program, check first with your doctor. (If you decide not to exercise, check with your doctor also. You may find you're too unhealthy not to!) Once you've received your doctor's approval, determine the most convenient time to exercise and make a schedule based on that time. If you can work out first thing in the morning, your chances of maintaining your exercise program are much greater. Later in the day, fatigue and distractions take their toll. The sooner exercise becomes a part of your regular routine (three to six days per week), the sooner you'll begin to notice positive changes in your body and health.

Write down what exercise you're planning to do, for what duration, and when on your Daily Success Planner. Remember to be moderate. Listen to your body. Don't allow yourself to become short of breath. As you become more fit, you'll be able to extend your exercise time to forty-five minutes or an hour.

Keeping a record of your thoughts and feelings is also essential. Schedule a

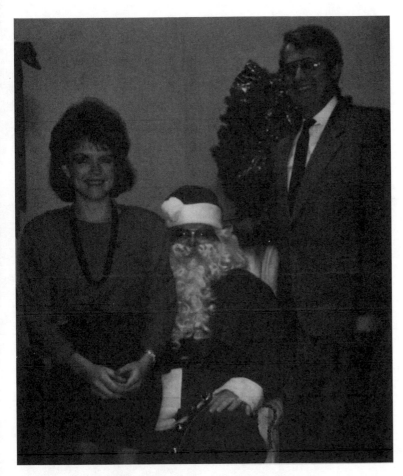

Planning ahead is imperative, especially when you attend parties. Eat lots of nourishing food before you go—then eat just a little junk—if you must. And remember to never eat dessert or sweets on an empty stomach!

If you're highly resistant to fat loss, delete the desserts and your rate of fat loss may triple. It did for me!

131

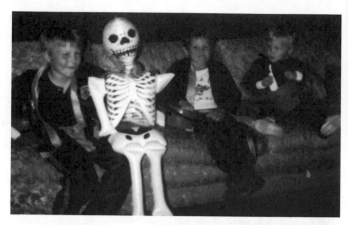

Yes, my kids even go trick-or-treating. Can you tell that the one in the middle has been a dieter? He's got that gaunt, starved-skinny look!

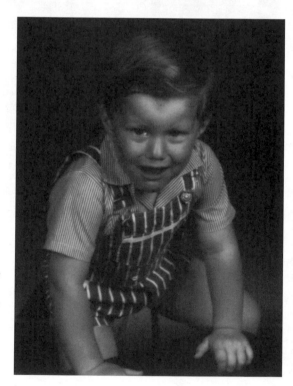

After eating all that candy, however, they are sometimes a little out of sorts.

time when you can take a few minutes to evaluate how you feel and what signals your body is sending. Then record those feelings in the "Journal Entry" section of your Left-Brain Planner.

Remember, for possibly the first time in your life, you're not being evaluated by how much you weigh. The measurements of progress in this program may at first be more subtle and are of utmost importance for your health, permanent leanness, and continued happiness. But you can learn to recognize them by recording the information outlined in your Planner.

Having a plan that details exactly what you're going to do each day is essential to your success. Once you've established your daily plan, write it down on one of your Planners. In your COOKBOOK SAMPLER, that begins on page 240, you will find my delicious GRAB 'N' GO and BUDGET meal plans that contain a wealth of time-saving information. They are perfectly balanced and already written out for you. Take advantage of them!

First, determine what meals you'll eat that day (either from the meal plans and menus provided or from your own sources). Then write them down. Next, check to see if you have the foods required to prepare the meals. If not, schedule a shopping trip.

Second, determine what kind of exercise you'll do that day (or even if it is an exercise day). Then set aside a convenient time for your exercise. Remember, this is a commitment, not an option.

Third, set aside time to evaluate your progress on the program and to write it in your Planner. Consider how you feel, your level of energy, your stress level, the appearance of your skin and hair, your blood pressure, and your cholesterol levels. Have your body fat tested every six months. Obviously, not every one of these factors can be checked every day, but it's worth an occasional checkup. You'll see wonderful improvements, and these improvements will motivate and inspire you to continue, and the longer you follow the LEAN & FREE principles, the more dramatic the improvements will be.

At the end of the day, complete your Left-Brain Planner and score yourself. If it was less than a "B" day, evaluate your activities to see where you can improve. The more complete and specific your recordings are, the better you'll be able to assess your progress. You'll love the exciting changes in your health, appearance, and disposition that will soon become apparent. And remember to be patient; you know now that quick fixes never work, except in reverse. Allow your body the time it needs to manifest permanent change, and it will reward you with a transformed life. (And remember to complete your 20-second Right-Brain Planner found on page 244, on days when time is short.)

In chapter 8, our final chapter, I'll show you specifically how to put your new plan into action, and we'll also review the critically important information you've learned in this book.

8. ACTION

GET EXCITED—GO FOR IT—DO ITNOW!

*D*uring the first six chapters of this book, you were given the foundation of knowledge that will support your efforts and strengthen your motivation as you implement the principles of the LEAN & FREE LIFESTYLE. In chapter 7, you were given a plan for that implementation, a structure for putting your knowledge to work so you can achieve your goals of becoming healthy and fit. With this final chapter, it's time for action! I call it the "do it now" chapter.

The late newscaster Eric Severeid is a good example of the "do it now" approach to life. Early in his broadcasting career he resigned from a lucrative position to write an epic-length book—a book that would eventually launch his career in network news.

But when he set out to write the book, he was overcome by the thought of the work ahead of him. He wondered: "Where should I start? This book requires so much writing, it will take forever. I'll never get it done." Faced with this monumental task, he felt discouraged and unsure; he found it difficult even to begin. Then he had a simple realization.

He found that the secret to starting and completing the book was in not trying to do it all at once. "I discovered that by focusing on one paragraph at a time and not being concerned with looking ahead at the entire task, the writing of the book took care of itself. And as a result of this little breakthrough in perspective, I was able to start and to stay committed to writing the book until it was completed five hundred thousand words later."

You're probably not thinking about writing a book. But any large project can be just as intimidating if you focus on the overall magnitude of it and not on the first immediate steps. I had an experience similar to that of Eric Severeid when I began creating this program, and, like him, I was able to accomplish my goal by first setting smaller goals and then consistently working to achieve them.

I had already completed much research and experience that I needed to design an effective fat-loss program. But when I was asked to teach that program, my responsibilities multiplied. I was training teachers, writing my first book, and trying to fulfill my obligations as a wife and the mother of four small children. I knew I had to share this wonderful new information about health and fat loss; in fact, I was bursting at the seams to do so—but how should I go about it, and how could I balance it with my other tasks?

I did it by taking one little step at a time. I did it by breaking my larger tasks and responsibilities into smaller manageable tasks. I did it by setting immediate deadlines and goals rather than aiming at the long-term goal. And I did it by scheduling my tasks.

Each day I dedicated a specific time to my project. Each day I also scheduled specific time with my family. I set aside a certain night for teaching. I also set aside a night each week to go out with my husband. And I set aside important times every day and all day Saturday to spend with the children.

When I did this, suddenly all the tasks that were so intimidating before became manageable and attainable. However, at times I would feel overwhelmed because I wasn't prioritizing very well. Then I would slow down and stop running faster than I could walk and take things one day at a time. Whenever I felt overwhelmed, I remembered a lesson a friend of mine told me about planning and time.

"If you decided to plant a garden," he said, " you wouldn't plan to complete it in one day. Suppose you selected a plot of ground that was thirty by twenty-five feet and was full of weeds. At first, you might be overwhelmed. That's 750 square feet of weeds to eliminate before you can even start a garden. How would you ever find time to get that done?

"You could decide that you had fifteen minutes a day to spend at this task. Then you might find that in fifteen minutes you could clear a five-by-five foot plot, or twenty-five square feet. Thirty days later, you'd have a twenty-five-by-thirty-foot garden plot ready to plow and plant. And a few months later you'd have an abundance of vegetables.

"Clearing your garden plot," he said, "wouldn't be drudgery. It would be exciting. Why? Because you'd be able to see your progress. Each time you cleared a five-by-five plot, you'd become more excited because you could measure your progress against the work that remained without becoming intimidated. And the more you progressed, the more clearly you'd be able to imagine the fresh vegetables your garden would eventually produce."

I have learned that all learning and growing experiences follow the same pattern. When you learned to speak or read, you didn't do it overnight. You learned a little more each day, a word here, a phrase there, until you had mastered the language.

It's the same way with the LEAN & FREE LIFESTYLE. You may feel overwhelmed by the task of implementing what you have just learned. It may seem even more overwhelming than writing a 700-page novel or clearing a 750-square-foot garden plot. But as you become more familiar with the principles and as you complete your daily planning sheets, your new wellness lifestyle will develop comfortably and naturally. This is partly due to the fact that you'll be working with your body, in harmony, meeting its real needs and living as we were intended to live to maintain health and fitness. It is simple, basic, common sense.

You didn't get fat overnight, and you won't become lean overnight either.

However, if you take it one step at a time, if you monitor each day's activities and carefully observe what you're accomplishing, you'll soon see positive results. And each positive change will excite and motivate you to accomplish the next steps.

Throughout this book we've focused on six steps to leanness. They are: (1) knowledge; (2) commitment; (3) nurturing; (4) nourishing; (5) movement or exercise; and (6) service.

Let's look briefly at the actions required to get you started on each step.

Step 1 is knowledge. You've already begun the program and taken step 1 by reading this book. In fact, the knowledge you've gained has motivated you to continue reading to this point. That knowledge has given you the power to change. To sustain that power, you need to read and re-read this book as well as articles and books that I have listed in the References section. Also, look for articles on new research. Schedule these activities. Set aside time each day to re-read parts of this book or other related materials. And make sure you record anything you've learned or come to newly understand in the journal section on the back of your Daily Success Planner. Remember that your metabolism can gradually adjust downward when you decrease calories and upward when you gradually eat more balanced, nourishing food and exercise moderately.

Step 2 is commitment. Your commitment to the program grows as you experience success. Once you begin noticing physical and emotional changes, staying with the program becomes much easier. Your Physical and Emotional Health Chart and your Body Measurement Charts are on the following pages. You will record your physical and emotional changes on these charts.

Every week you should recheck and record your physical and emotional health changes and your measurements until you have achieved your LEAN & FREE goals. Measure yourself in front of a mirror or with a friend. Make sure you measure in the same location each week to ensure accurate results.

Once you've completed your progress chart for this week, write a brief statement of how you feel on the "current feelings" sheet on page 139. Then paste in recent photos of yourself on the "current pictures" sheet on pages 140.

Next, write a brief statement on the "ideal feelings" form on page 141. It should describe how you would like to feel when you have become lean and healthy. Then, on the "ideal pictures" sheet on page 142, attach pictures of yourself when you were leaner, or attach pictures of other lean, healthy people who represent your ideal.

Physical and Emotional Health Chart

TIME LINE	WEEK 1	WEEK 2	WEEK 3	WEEK 4	WEEK 5	WEEK 6	WEEK 7	WEEK 8	WEEK 9	WEEK 10	WEEK 11	WEEK 12	WEEK 13	WEEK 14	WEEK 15	WEEK 16	16 WEEK GOAL	ULTIMATE GOAL
DATE																		
Resting Heart Rate																		
Energy Level																		
Depression																		
Self-Esteem																		
Zest for Life																		
Desire to Serve																		
Ability to Sleep																		
Complexion																		
Hair																		
Eyes																		
Nails																		
Muscle Tone																		
(Blood Pressure)																		
(Cholesterol)																		
(Blood Sugar Lvl)																		

Permission granted to enlarge and copy this chart.

137

Body Measurement Chart

TIME LINE ▶	WEEK 0	WEEK 1	WEEK 2	WEEK 3	WEEK 4	WEEK 5	WEEK 6	WEEK 7	WEEK 8	WEEK 9	WEEK 10	WEEK 11	WEEK 12	WEEK 13	WEEK 14	WEEK 15	WEEK 16	16 Week Approx. Goal	Ultimate Approx. Goal
DATE ▶																			
Neck																			
Under Chin (Ear to Ear)																			
(Rt. Arm Flexed)																			
Rt. Arm Relaxed																			
Forearm																			
Right Wrist																			
Upper Chest (Under Arms)																			
Chest/Bust																			
Rib Cage																			
Waist																			
Abdomen																			
Hips																			
Right Thigh																			
Right Knee																			
Right Calf																			
Right Ankle																			
(Estimated Body % Fat)																			
(Weight)																			
Total Weekly Inch Loss																			
Running Total Inch Loss																			

Permission granted to enlarge and copy this chart. Remember to measure in exactly the same locations each week for accuracy sake. When adding inches lost, remember to double inch loss pertaining to arms and legs because you have two of each. (Example: 1/8 inch lost in right calf = 1/4 inch loss for both calves.) Do not add or subtract the flexed arm measurement to your overall total. Circle measurements you show

138

Use this page to explain in detail how you are feeling physically and emotionally right now, before beginning the LEAN & FREE 2000 PLUS ULTIMATE WELLNESS/WEIGHT CONTROL LIFESTYLE.

On this page, place several pictures of yourself currently. Record the way you feel on audio or video tape for future reference—a great idea! If you don't, you'll wish you had.

Write in detail how you would ideally like to feel both physically and emotionally.

Place several pictures of yourself on this page that exemplify the way you would ideally and realistically like to look and feel. If you do not have pictures of yourself that exemplify this ideal state, cut pictures from magazines of people with height and bone structure similar to your own. You could even cut your face out of a photograph and glue it on top of the shoulders of a lean, healthy body to make a very exciting, personal visual.

This may sound simplistic to you, yet imagining yourself as LEAN & FREE can create tremendous emotion that can truly speed your journey toward a healthy and lean body.

By completing these forms, you establish benchmarks by which you can compare and rate your progress later. As you become leaner and more energetic, this positive comparison will dramatically increase your commitment to the principles you're learning. Every energy increase will motivate you. Each smaller clothing size will spur you on. Remember, you need to check these measurements every week. And also remember, if you have a fat-storing body to begin with, your measurements may *increase* at first. You're rehydrating (restoring optimal water balance) and increasing your muscle mass before you can begin burning excess fat. Don't be alarmed—this rehydration is what will transform you from a dried, wrinkled prune into a lush, smooth plum!

Your commitment is built on a daily basis by completing the simple four-step vision exercise you learned in chapter 2. Schedule a time for this exercise every day.

Step 3 is nurturing. The action you can take for this step is to practice "body talk." Make certain you talk (or think) positively toward your body every day. Tell your body you love, understand, and appreciate it. Look at your body in the mirror and remind it that you have committed yourself to a program that is making it healthy, lean, and happy. And start becoming your own best friend.

Step 4 is nourishing. Take action *now!* Start by beginning to eliminate foods from your kitchen that are excessively high in fat, sugar, and the other fat-storing stressors. Clear out your refrigerator and your pantries. Then look at the menus and shopping lists in your LEAN & FREE COOKBOOK SAMPLER section and plan a trip to the grocery store so you can purchase normal, delicious, and nourishing foods. Then prepare some of these recipes. They not only provide the high-quality calories and nutrition you and your family need every day, but they're also tasty and easy to fix. As you become more and more knowledgeable, you'll have fun designing your own healthy menus and recipes. See the recipe healthification section in the cookbook.

Step 5 is movement or exercise, and to begin action at this step, you need to establish a regular exercise program. Without exercise, your chance of becoming optimally healthy and lean diminishes greatly. If you're already in fairly good condition, take a brisk half-hour-to-an-hour walk. If not, walk, dance, march, or use the rhythmic aerobic exercise machine of your choice. Work out as long as you comfortably can, even if it's only five minutes. Remember, if you can't talk comfortably while exercising, you're working too hard. Keep a close eye on your pulse rate (60 to 90 percent of the maximum heart rate you determined in chapter 5). Strenuous exercise burns mainly sugar, not fat.

Step 6, the final step, is service. And the simplest action you can take immediately is to do something for someone else. Service to others is good for everyone. It makes others feel better, and it dramatically boosts your self-esteem.

143

If you're like most people, it will probably take a few months before you're weight stable — that is, you will have converted your body from a fat-storing state to a neutral state in which you are eating large amounts of good food without gaining weight. Don't be discouraged by this phase. During this time you'll notice seven positive changes in how you look and feel. It is these changes that will help keep you motivated to stay with the program.

1. You may begin to notice an increase in energy. You may tire less easily and be able to accomplish more.

2. You may notice an improvement in how you look Your skin may be smoother, your hair thicker.

3. Your disposition may improve. You may be able to handle the stress of daily life with more equilibrium and be less nervous and irritable.

4. If your cholesterol levels have been high, you may notice a significant reduction in them.

5. Your muscle tone may significantly improve. You may notice soft, flabby areas of your body becoming firm and strong.

6. Even though your weight may at first increase or remain constant, you may notice a significant firming and tightening of your body.

7. Many pear-shaped people may begin to lose inches from their hips and thighs. This generally happens before they lose inches from their waist and areas above it—just the opposite of the results they get from low-calorie diets. And apple-shaped people may lose inches in the torso first while adding shape and tone to skinny arms and legs.

Remember, the secret to successfully becoming LEAN & FREE is eating an abundance of healthy, balanced food and exercising moderately. Over the next several weeks, you will be building a new unique and wonderful relationship with your body. You're becoming a friend and partner with your body and you'll actually be *listening to each other*, perhaps for the first time in your life! You may progress from a fat-storing survival metabolism to a weight-stable metabolism and finally to an energy-releasing, fat-burning metabolism.

The longer you can continue to eat an abundance of nourishing foods, the more you'll be relaxing your body's fat-storing starvation defense. Eating such foods will become easier and easier because soon you'll develop actual cravings for them. Your desire for fats and sweets may greatly decline, and even when you do eat them, they may not trigger fat-storing, starvation responses as they once did.

Monitor your progress by filling out a Right or Left-Brain Success Planner every day. Review them each morning to develop awareness of your progress. And ignore the scales. Your goal is to be lean and healthy and to increase your energy. You're transforming the shape of your body from fat and saggy to curvy and firm. If weight must be lost in the process, it will take care of itself. *Feed yourself lean and healthy—and your family too.*

If you're responsible for the nourishment of others besides yourself, you can be assured that the changes in your cuisine will be beneficial to all your family members, whether they're overly fat, overly thin, or just right, from age two to age ninety-two. When consistently followed, the LEAN & FREE principles can benefit and satisfy everyone. Entire families can see each member improve both physically and emotionally as all their nutritional needs are met. Fat five-year-olds firm up; tubby twelve-year-olds gain energy; and self-conscious eighteen-year-olds find themselves with new, lean bodies, increased confidence, and a more active social world. All of this is accomplished while mom and dad and grandma and grandpa begin looking and feeling younger than they've looked or felt in many years. Cholesterol levels may drop; depressed folks start to smile; diabetics may decrease their need for insulin; chronic fatigue is replaced by vitality; and arthritis sufferers may experience dramatic relief—all because their new focus is on optimal physical and emotional health, not dieting. *Leanness is the natural side-effect of excellent health*!

However, since you're asking your family to make profound changes in what they eat, you must employ a little tact. Here are ten ways to convert your family to the LEAN & FREE LIFESTYLE so that the conversion is easy, amiable, and alot of fun!

1. Don't talk a lot about the program. It's wonderful to be excited about it, but nothing repels people more than a barrage of information about how great it is.

2. Begin by slightly "healthifying" recipes. Example: If your family is used to eating white bread, buy cracked-wheat bread that is half white and half wheat. Mix your macaroni noodles—half white and half whole wheat. Or just use white pasta and top it with nutritious, lowfat sauces.

LEAN & FREE FAMILY CHANGES

1. Don't talk a lot about the program.
2. Begin by slightly "healthifying" recipes.
3. Ask your family members what they would like to eat and encourage them to participate in selecting menus.
4. Pay attention to the colors in a meal.
5. If your family is used to "whole" dairy products, gradually change to 2% fat products, then 1%.
6. If your family really loves pepperoni pizza, include it now and then.
7. Let them know you love them the way they are, whether they decide to participate in these lifestyle changes or not.
8. Give quiet praise if they embrace new, healthier habits.
9. Approach it lightly. Try to introduce a spirit of fun with the changes.
10. Most important, always respect your family's feelings. Lead quietly through example, not aggressively through force.

3. Ask your family members what they would like to eat and encourage them to participate in selecting menus. And prepare their favorite foods often, gradually healthifying them little by little.

4. Pay attention to the colors in a meal. Aim for a variety of colors; you'll increase the visual appeal and most likely the nutritional value. Example: Have a plate of purple cabbage and green grapes with your spaghetti dinner rather than the muted tones of applesauce or cauliflower.

5. If your family is used to "whole" dairy products, gradually convert to 2-percent fat products, then 1 percent.

6. If your family really loves pepperoni pizza, include it now and then. Don't make an event of it; just put the relish tray or tossed salad on the table first, when they're hungriest. Then put a large fruit plate on the table with the pizza.

7. Let your family know you love them just the way they are, whether they decide to participate in these lifestyle changes or not.

8. Give quiet praise when family members adjust to the new cuisine. If you over-dramatize it, you may embarrass them, or they may feel that the purpose of positive change is simply to gratify you.

9. Approach changes lightly. Try to introduce a spirit of fun with the changes. Scolding or insistence may create stress, which can encourage more fat gain through resistance and rebellion. This may lead family members to consciously make unhealthy food choices.

10. Most important, always respect your family's feelings. Lead quietly through example, not aggressively through force. Always remember to love and accept them regardless of their food and exercise choices. Special note: If a certain member of your family constantly tries to discourage your progress by saying, "Everyone knows if you want to weigh less you have to eat less," just smile and encourage the person to read this book or listen to the audio tapes. Tell the person that you're doing the right thing for your mind and body this time and that you won't talk the person's ear off about it. Ask the person to please support you in what you've chosen to do.

An example of unproductive behavior in working with family members is a friend of mine I shall call Lucy. Though a nutritionist, Lucy has always starved herself thin. She has a perfectly flat stomach at age fifty-five. But her thirty-one-year-old daughter is overly fat, which is distressing for Lucy. She says: "I tell her to hold her stomach in and pull out her blouse. I tell her to stand straight and smile. Then she gets depressed, eats even more unhealthy foods, and gets fatter and fatter."

I asked Lucy how big her daughter was. She answered, "Oh, I'd say Cecilia's at least twenty to thirty pounds more than she should be." (I was expecting her to be sixty or seventy pounds too high, the way Lucy had carried on.) She continued: "She has no social life and no self-esteem. I don't think my daughter likes herself very much, and it's because she's overweight. I'm always telling her to lose weight, but she doesn't seem to have any willpower. She won't listen to me anymore. Maybe you could talk to her."

I wondered how I should respond to Lucy. In reality, she herself is a skinny, starved calorie-counter whose entire self-worth is based on her size and her weight, and even on the weight of her adult child. Her problem is that her daughter, Cecilia, doesn't fit her own starved image. I knew Cecilia actually has very little weight to lose; instead she just needs to reduce her percentage of body fat.

Cecilia highly resents the fact that her mother's approval (or lack of approval) is based on her appearance. She would like to be lean, but neither she nor her mother has the knowledge to accomplish it. And her mother's persistent badgering is causing stress that contributes to Cecilia's fat-storing tendencies.

147

If I told them what Cecilia needed to do, I doubt if either would believe me. So I did the next best thing; I gave them a copy of my book. I hope they'll read the book, act on its principles, and achieve permanent fat loss. I hope, too, that it will create a bonding experience and restore their relationship.

Cases like that of Lucy and Cecilia are not uncommon. One often sees starved, skinny moms trailed by a little band of chubby children. The mothers have repeatedly warned these children, "Don't eat too much or you'll get fat." So the children constantly crave fats and sweets, are lethargic, and would rather watch TV than participate in active sports or even moderate exercise. Their youthful survival systems are causing them to store what they eat as fat.

Because of the attitudes and ignorance of parents like these, the family meal has become one of the casualties of the "diet age." Such families seldom sit down to enjoy meals together; mom resists cooking delicious foods because she's afraid she'll overeat and gain weight. Instead, she feeds the children peanut-butter sandwiches (which aren't that bad—but not every day!). Yet families who don't eat together and share their day's experiences have a much harder time staying together. The benefits of balanced meals go far beyond enjoyment; they are critical to physical and mental health as well as family unity and nurturing.

In this chapter, I've given you specific actions to take every day in each of the six components of this program: *knowledge, commitment, nurturing, nourishment, motion,* and *service.* Now it's time for you to take action. You have the knowledge and the plan, so *get excited and go for it.* There's nothing that can stop you, now that you know how your body functions and what you need to do to effectively free it.

Now, let's review what you've learned in this book.

In the introduction I told you my personal story. You learned how I took my knowledge, my studies, and the experience I've had with many others who needed to lose fat to develop the LEAN & FREE LIFESTYLE.

In chapter 1 you were given the knowledge you need to become lean and healthy and to help build commitment and motivation. You learned that storing fat is your body's natural response to life- and health-threatening stress. You learned the twelve fat-storing stressors and how to eliminate them from your life. You learned that by restricting the amount of food you eat, as you do when you diet, you may signal your survival system that a famine is coming, encouraging your body to store fat. And you were introduced to changes you need to make in your life if you hope to become lean, healthy, and happy.

In chapter 2 you learned how to create a vision of yourself as a healthy, lean, and free person—a vision that can motivate you to start and stay with this program.

You learned why hating your body can actually prevent fat loss. And you learned a system called "body talk" that can help you develop a loving and nurturing attitude toward your body, an attitude that will actively promote health and leanness.

In chapter 4 you were introduced to food plans designed to nourish your body by providing you with abundant, balanced, high-quality calories each day. These plans include an ideal amount of protein, approximately 10 to 20 percent dietary fat, an abundance of complex carbohydrates, and an ample intake of water.

You also learned why eating to comfortably-full satisfaction is critical to preventing your body's fat-storing survival response. You learned why balance is the key to nutrition, and you learned the "five fingers of balance" that are the basis of nutritious meals—water, vegetables, grains, proteins, and fruit.

In chapter 5 you learned the benefits of exercise and why it plays a critical role in changing your body from a fat-storer to a fat-burner. You learned that a low-impact, aerobic exercise program is most efficient at fat burning; why walking is a focus for many people; why you shouldn't exercise so strenuously that you can't talk or breathe easily; why excessively strenuous exercise burns mainly sugar, not fat; how to determine your target pulse rate; and alternative exercises you can do if walking doesn't suit you. You also learned how to duplicate the seven specific motions that our ancestors used in their daily survival activities. I believe that duplicating these motions helps to signal our body's survival system to burn excess fat because they simulate the movements used in the hunting and gathering of food.

One of the major benefits of this program may be a dramatic increase in energy. In chapter 6 you learned that service to others provides a natural outlet for your newfound energy. You learned that service freely given not only helps others but also boosts your own self-esteem. And the more positive you feel about yourself, the more successful you will be with this program.

In chapter 7 you were supplied with a plan to implement all you had learned. You were introduced to the Daily Success Planner, which is your anchor for success following the LEAN & FREE LIFESTYLE. It keeps you aware of the changes occurring, including many important, subtle signs of success not experienced with low-calorie diets.

You learned how to complete your Right and Left-Brain Success Planners and why the information they provide can directly motivate and teach you how to become lean and healthy. In your LEAN & FREE COOKBOOK SAMPLER, you'll discover delicious menus and recipes. The majority of these wonderful foods require five or ten minutes to prepare and can fit into very tight budgets. And you have an invigorating effective exercise plan that meets the guidelines of this program.

Finally, in this chapter you were given a specific plan of action that focuses on each of the six elements of this program—knowledge, commitment, nurturing, nourishment, motion, and service.

The reward for following the principles you've learned in the LEAN & FREE LIFESTYLE is freedom—freedom from diets, unpalatable foods, excess body fat, depression , uncontrolable fatigue, and multiple health problems.

The LEAN & FREE LIFESTYLE can free you from the all-consuming slavery associated with being overly fat. You'll never again have to worry about feeling deprived. You may be less irritable; your susceptibility to many forms of disease and illness may be reduced; you may feel more confident and empowered; and you may relate to people better and have the energy to serve yourself, your family, and your community; you'll look more vibrant, and you'll dramatically increase your chances of living a long, healthy, purposeful life.

Everything you'll be doing on this program is based on solid, scientifically-valid studies that have taken many years to research. Nothing recommended in this book should put you medically at risk. My students and I are living proof that these principles work. You can see from my story in the introduction that I personally experienced many of the problems you're experiencing now. And, you'll find numerous inspirational stories in the chapter entitled "LEAN & FREE Success Stories—Acquiring a Personal Vision of Success" that you can use as models for your own accomplishment.

My hope is that by learning from my experiences and research, you can avoid the frustrations and mistakes that delayed my own progress. I offer you a blueprint for health and happiness that is honest, detailed, and extremely effective. I've put the research and common sense together for you. Incorporate what you've learned into your own life. I know it will serve you well, as it has me, my family, and thousands of other people like you.

In the "LEAN & FREE COOKBOOK SAMPLER," you'll find delicious, fast recipes, shopping lists, fat gram and calorie charts, extra Right and Left-Brain Success Planner sheets, and other information that will help you make the LEAN & FREE 2000 ULTIMATE WELLNESS/WEIGHT CONTROL LIFESTYLE your new standard for living. This is the first day of your new LEAN & FREE life. Make it a joyous, grand adventure!

QUESTION: *I'm used to living on two diet shakes and a frozen dinner. I don't know where to start. I'm overwhelmed. What should I do?*
ANSWER: *Read pages 239 through 244 very carefully. Follow the PERFECTLY SIMPLE Right-Brain Planner on page 244. It's as easy as that. And start by eating breakfast. If you can pour milk on cold cereal and open a can, you can do this program! And remember to mix and match the "quick and easy" meals on the menus. Eat what you like and choose the meals that fit your time and budget needs.*

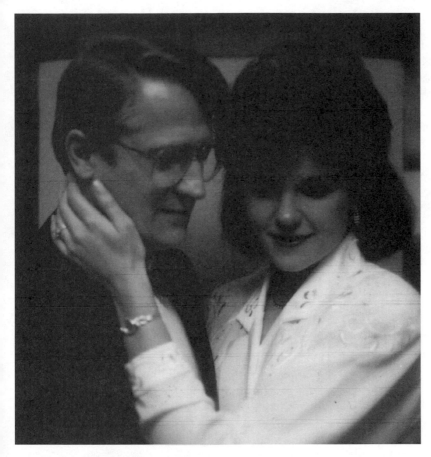

Enjoying the freedom to eat means enjoying
your life. I love my life. You can love yours, too!

QUESTION: *Who is Danmar Health Corporation?*

ANSWER: *Danmar stands for Dana and Marty. My husband Marty and I are the sole investors. It is a family corporation with me being president and the majority owner. We believe so strongly in the principles of LEAN & FREE that we have dedicated our own personal assets in bringing this program to you.*

151

IF YOU HAVE A LAPSE,
WILL YOU GAIN EVERYTHING BACK?

During the last four and a half years, my life has been tremendously stressful. There was little opportunity to focus on myself or my personal needs. I exercised only three days a week. And there were times, due to illness or the injuries from our accident, that I didn't exercise at all. I averaged a "B–" as an eater, although I managed never to slip to a "C," "D", or "F." I ate three reasonably well-balanced meals everyday and I never skipped meals or ate dessert on an empty stomach. But an average day might have included a menu something like this:

Breakfast:	"A" or "B" Choice cold or hot cereal with honey, banana and 1% milk.
Snack:	Cold cereal and 1% milk (notice the lack of veggies)
Lunch:	Wendy's chicken sandwich with extra veggies and no sauce, a large Frostie, and water
Dinner:	2 slices pepperoni and cheese pizza 4 slices all-veggie and cheese pizza Peaches canned in lite syrup 1 large ice milk shake with fat free hot fudge and malt Water
Snack:	Lots of popcorn with a little butter Water

On a day like this, I averaged 3,500 to 4,000 calories and about 80 to 120 fat grams. If you round nine calories in one gram of fat up to ten (for simplicity's sake), then 10 to 20 percent of 4,000 calories is 40 to 80 fat grams (for an A day); and 30 percent (for a "B" day) is 120 fat grams. So I averaged between 20 and 30 percent fat calories. And I was eating far too much sugar. Did I gain? Yes, I did. But I was amazed at just how little I gained. In four years, I went from a loose size 4 to a snug size 6 and I stayed there. Now, not all people will gain so little when they let their habits slip. Some will decidedly gain more—but they will NOT put on 50 pounds! If their habits are still reasonable and they don't skip meals, they can expect a minimal change in weight and shape.

Minimal or not, when that period of stress was over, I felt the need to take this program to the maximum. Three months ago, I decided to kick into "A+" habits again and to shed the excess. The first two weeks of that effort were tough—really tough. I eliminated all desserts except "A" Choice ones. I completed my Success Planners regularly. But the effort was well worth the result. Now I'm feeling considerably more freedom than I did with those "B" habits and I'm wondering why on earth I didn't do this a year ago. It's so much fun! I've lost over 30 inches in three months and that's with only twelve pounds lost ("morning" weight that is...with no "make-up"). I lost inches every week regardless of whether my weight went up or down. (Refer to my chart on the following page.) This astounded even me. From the second week of my new program through today, I've lost only 7 1/2 pounds—yet I look like I've lost 20. Now, most people estimate my weight at between 105 and 130 pounds!

This most recent effort supports what I've always known—that it requires just as much determination to drop from a size 6 to a size 4 as it does to drop from a size 18 to a size 16. I know, because I've done both. Some people will never have to make that comparison because they're very lean at a size 12—your ideal size and weight depends entirely on your bone structure and what looks and feels right for you.

I wish I could describe to you how exciting it is to be an "A" student everyday and to be able to count on that inevitable inch loss every Tuesday morning. This amazing process happens every time I really kick in and give the program my best...and it stays dormant, and ready to be reclaimed, every time I give less than my best. For me, "B+" habits simply don't give me the optimum benefits. Perhaps the most important key to my success is maintaining my Right-Brain Planners and especially my Left-Brain Planners. It's being able to see, taste, and touch that success in detail, before I actually achieve it.

You can do this too! I know you can because I've done it and so have thousands of others just like you. Always remember that you are the one in control. And if you listen to your body and give it 200%, you can't fail. In some ways, this program is like driving a car. When you first took driving lessons, you may have been overwhelmed by all you had to master. You couldn't imagine how you'd ever do it. Yet after a few lessons and a lot of personal effort, it started to get easier. And after a few months, it was hard to even remember that it ever took any effort at all. Driving had become totally second nature—a spontaneous habit, like breathing. This isn't the case with low-calorie dieting. Dieting gets harder and harder as you escalate your fight against the natural caloric and nutritional needs of your body. But LEAN & FREE is like driving—it gets easier and more natural the more you do it. That's because your body is supporting you 100 percent. The only fight taking place is against old, destructive habits. Yet after only two weeks of 200 percent effort, you'll begin to sail into freedom. You'll feel the welcome surge of new energy, the thrill of leanness, and an overall infusion of joy into your life. It's so amazingly fun and easy. So get excited now! Take it one day at a time, and do it!

Body Measurement Chart

TIME LINE ➤ DATE ➤	WEEK 0 6/29	WEEK 1 7/6	WEEK 2 7/13	WEEK 3 7/20	WEEK 4 6/27	WEEK 5 8/3	WEEK 6 8/10	WEEK 7 8/17	WEEK 8 8/24	WEEK 9 8/31	WEEK 10 9/7	WEEK 11 9/14	WEEK 12 9/21	WEEK 13 9/28	WEEK 14 10/5	WEEK 15 10/12	WEEK 16 10/18	16 Week Approx. Goal 10/18	Ultimate Approx. Goal 11/29
Neck	13 1/2	13	13	12 7/8	12 3/4	12 3/4	12 3/4	12 1/2	12 1/2	12 1/4	12 1/4	12 1/4	12 1/8	12 1/8	12 1/8	12 1/8		12	12
Under Chin (Ear to Ear)	8 1/2	8 1/8	8 1/8	8	8	8 7/8	8 7/8	7 7/8	7 7/8	7 3/4	7 1/2	7 1/4	7 1/4	7 1/4	7 1/4	7 1/4		7	7
(Rt. Arm Flexed)	(12 1/4)	(11 7/8)	(11 7/8)	(12)	(12)	(12)	(12)	(12)	(11 3/4)	(11 3/4)	(11 1/2)	(11 3/8)	(11 1/2)	(11 5/8)	(11 5/8)	(11 3/4)		11 1/2	10 1/2
Rt. Arm Relaxed x 2	11 1/2	11 1/4	11 1/4	11	11	11	11	11	10 3/4	10 3/4	10 3/4	10 3/4	10 3/4	10 5/8	10 1/2	10 1/2		10	9
Forearm x 2	10 1/4	10 1/8	10	10	10	10	10	9 7/8	9 7/8	9 3/4	9 3/4	9 3/4	9 3/4	9 3/4	9 3/4	9 3/4		9 1/2	9
Right Wrist x 2	6 3/8	6 3/8	6 3/8	6 3/8	6 1/8	6 1/8	6 1/8	6 1/8	6 1/8	6 1/8	6 1/8	6 1/8	6 1/8	6 1/8	6 1/8	6 1/8		6 1/8	6
Upper Chest (Under Arms)	36 5/8	36 1/2	36 3/8	36 3/8	36	35 7/8	35 3/4	35 3/4	35 3/4	35 5/8	35 5/8	35 1/2	35 1/2	35 1/2	35 1/2	35 1/2		35 1/2	35
Chest/Bust	38 1/2	38 1/4	38 1/4	38 1/4	38	38	38	37 5/8	37 1/2	37 1/2	37 1/2	37 1/2	37 1/2	37 1/2	37 1/2	37 1/2		37 1/2	37
Rib Cage	33	32 3/4	32 3/4	32 3/4	32 5/8	32 5/8	32 1/2	32 1/4	32 1/4	32	32	31	30 1/2	30 1/2	30 1/2	30 1/2		30 1/2	30
Waist	27	25 1/2	25 1/2	25	24 3/4	24 1/2	24 1/4	23 3/4	23 1/2	23	23	23	23	23	23	23		23	22
Abdomen	35 1/4	35	35	35	33 3/4	33 3/4	33	32 1/2	32 1/4	32	32	31 1/2	31 1/2	31 1/2	31	30 1/2		30 1/2	29
Hips	40	39 1/2	39 1/4	39 1/4	38 3/4	38 1/2	38 1/2	38 1/4	37 7/8	37 7/8	37 7/8	37 3/4	37 1/2	37 1/2	37 1/2	37 1/8		36 1/2	35
Right Thigh x 2	23 3/4	23 1/2	23 1/2	23	23	22 7/8	22 3/4	21 7/8	21 7/8	21 7/8	21 1/2	21 1/2	21 1/2	21 1/2	21 3/8	21 1/4		21	19
Right Knee x 2	16	15 7/8	15 3/4	15 3/4	15 1/2	15 1/4	15 1/8	15 1/8	15 1/8	15 1/8	15	14 3/4	14 3/4	14 3/4	14 3/4	14 3/4		14 1/2	12 3/4
Right Calf x 2	15 3/4	15 1/2	15 3/8	15 3/8	15 3/8	15 3/8	15 3/8	15 3/8	15 3/8	15 3/8	15 1/8	15	15	15	15	14 7/8		14 3/4	13
Right Ankle x 2	9 3/8	9	9	8 7/8	8 7/8	8 7/8	8 7/8	8 3/4	8 3/4	8 5/8	8 5/8	8 5/8	8 5/8	8 5/8	8 5/8	8 5/8		8 1/2	8
(Estimated Body % Fat)	19	18.5%	18.5%	18%	18%	18%	17.5%	17.5%	17%	17%	16.5%	16%	16%	15.5%	15.5%	15%		15%	14%
(Weight)	160	155 1/2	155 1/2	155	156	155	156	154	154	152	150	147	148	146	148	148		no goal	no goal
Total Weekly Inch Loss		6 1/4	1 1/8	2 1/4	3 5/8	1 1/2	1 3/4	4 1/4	1 1/4	2	1 3/4	2 3/4	7/8	2 1/4	1	1 3/4			
Running Total Inch Loss		7 5/7	9 7/8	13 1/2	15	16 3/4	21	22 1/4	24 1/4	26	28 3/4	29 5/8	29 7/8	30 7/8	32 1/4				

BODY MEASUREMENT CHART
INSTRUCTIONS

1. WHEN? Measure once a week, preferably on the same morning before breakfast. I measure every Tuesday morning. This motivates me to be an "A" student over the weekend. And it gives me Monday to really gear into my best habits.

2. WHERE? Measure in front of a full-length mirror. Make certain to measure at the same location each week. This includes: neck—about in the center; under your chin—from ear lobe to ear lobe; right flexed arm at the fullest part of the flexed bicep; right relaxed arm at the same location; right forearm at the fullest location; right wrist at the smallest location; upper chest—under the arms, just above the bust or chest; chest or bust at the fullest location; ribs just under the chest or bust; waist—usually at or just above the umbilicus or belly button; abdomen at the fullest location; hips at the fullest location; right thigh at the fullest location; right knee around the knee cap; right calf at the fullest location; and right ankle at the smallest location.

3. ADDING INCH LOSS? When adding inch loss, make certain to multiply arm and leg measurement losses by two. And neither add to nor subtract from your total your flexed arm measurement. Aim for at least a one-inch difference between your flexed and relaxed arm measurement.

If you have other measurements that you'd like to see increase, neither add to nor subtract these from your total inch loss as well. For instance, it's not uncommon for starved-skinny, apple-shaped individuals (with full torsoes and spindley arms and legs to see a marked decrease in their waist and abdomens while their chests or busts, arms, legs (especially calves), and skinny necks fill out, becoming much more shapely and supple. In the case of an individual such as this, it would be wise for them to keep two seperate running totals including one category for areas they desire to lose in and another category for areas they want to see increase.

4. WEEKLY INCH LOSS TOTAL AND RUNNING INCH LOSS TOTAL? Make certain to keep a weekly inch loss total and a running inch loss total. Example: Let's say you lost 1/4 inch in your right relaxed arm, 1/2 inch in your waist, and 1/4 inch in your right thigh this week. Multiply the arm and leg measurement losses by two. Then add the waist measurement losses for a total of 1 1/2 inches lost this week. If you also lost 1 1/2 inches the week before, your two week running total inch loss is 3 inches! And believe me, it adds up quickly. It's so much more motivating than the bathroom scales. This is such a fun, new process of change. Cherish your journey to a healthier, leaner life. And enjoy the freedom!

5. BODY WEIGHT? Write down your weight every sixteen weeks for the sake of comparison. Other than that, it's up to you whether or not you weigh each week. It's always my goal to weigh as much as possible at my ideal size and appearance. This means that my body hydration, bone mass, and curvy muscle tissue are optimal along with my skin suppleness and energy level. As people study LEAN & FREE, the new trend is to amaze people with how much they weigh at their new ideal size. When someone refers to them as dense, they simply say, "Thank you very much!"

6. BODY FAT PERCENTAGE? Hydrostatic weighing can measure both subcutaneous and intramuscular fat, unlike calipers which ignore intramuscular fat all together. Hydrostatic weighing is discussed in the QUESTION/ANSWER section of this book. Your local hospital or fitness center may offer hydrostatic weighing at a very reasonable price. Call them and inquire about this effective procedure.

QUESTION: *I understand that dieters and meal-skippers often eat more calories as they become LEAN & FREE. Do "stuffers" eat fewer calories?* **ANSWER:** *Most definitely. I've been both a "starver" and a "stuffer". After starving, I ate more calories as my metabolism increased. However, when my calories were 4,000 and my fat intake was 30 percent, my calories came down with my fat percentage, even though the amounts of food I was eating remained about the same.*

ANSWERS
TO FREQUENTLY ASKED QUESTIONS

• KNOWLEDGE (BODY FAT & FAT-STORING STRESSORS)
• COMMITMENT • NURTURING • NOURISHMENT • MOTION
• SERVICE • MISCELLANEOUS

KNOWLEDGE: BODY FAT

1. Q: What is the best way to test my body fat level?

A: Hydrostatic or underwater weighing is generally considered to be the most accurate way to measure body fat percentage. Fat floats while bone and muscle sink. A person's buoyancy is, therefore, an excellent indication of body fat level. Contact your local hospital or fitness center to see what body fat measurement procedures they have available. (A pulmonary lung function test assures a much more accurate hydrostatic measurement.)

2. Q: What percentage of body fat should I have?

A: For most men, between 10 percent and 20 percent body fat. For most women the ideal is between 15 percent and 25 percent. These are generous ranges and allow for the fact that larger-framed men and women and small breasted women tend to have lower percentages of body fat. Conversely, small-framed men and women and women with larger breasts tend to carry a slightly higher percentage of body fat.

3. Q: I'm a twenty-five-year-old woman. Will I lose my periods if my body fat percentage gets too low?

A: Body fat percentages lower than fifteen percent are often associated with loss of menstruation. However, this seems to be linked to extreme low-calorie dieting and excessive, exhaustive exercise rather than the body fat percent itself. Staying between 15 and 25 percent body fat is a good "secondary" goal, but your "main" goal should be to focus on optimal health and energy. Then the ideal body fat percentage for you can naturally follow.

KNOWLEDGE: FAT-STORING STRESSORS

4. Q: I crave sweets and high-fat foods all the time. How do I get rid of these cravings?

A: Most people notice that their cravings subside in less than one month after consistently eating balanced meals (water, vegetables, grains, proteins, and fruits) to full satisfaction. Your body craves fats and sweets when it is not fully satisfied by enough calories and nutrients. Fats and sweets are more easily stored in your fat cells, and fat is your body's protection against starvation (dieting). So eat more and balance your meals.

5. Q: What foods contain the most caffeine?

A: The following table lists the amount of caffeine in many common foods.

Caffeine Content of Beverages, Foods, and Drugs[1]

Product	Range of Milligrams
Coffee (5 oz. cup)	
Brewed, drip method	110-150
Brewed, percolator	64-124
Instant	40-180
Decaffeinated (brewed or instant)	1-5
Tea (5 oz. cup)	
Brewed, major U.S. brands	20-90
Brewed, imported brands	25-110
Instant	25-50
Iced (12 oz. glass)	67-76
Soft Drinks (12 oz. can)	
Regular cola	30-58
Caffeine-free cola	0-trace
Jolt Cola	72
Mountain Dew, Mellow Yellow	52
Big Red	38
Cocoa Beverage (5 oz. cup)	(avg = 4) 2-20
Chocolate Milk (8 oz. glass)	2-7
Milk Chocolate Candy (1 oz.)	(avg = 6) 1-15
Dark Chocolate	
Semisweet (1 oz.)	(avg = 20) 5-35
Baker's Chocolate (1 oz.)	26
Chocolate Flavored Syrup (1 oz.)	4
Cold Remedies (standard dose)	
Dristan	0
Coryban-D, Triaminicin	30
Diuretics (standard dose)	
Aqua-ban, Permathene H_2Off	200
Pre-mens Forte	100
Pain Relievers (standard dose)	
Excedrin	130
Midol, Anacin	65
Aspirin (plain, any brand)	0
Stimulants	
Caffedrin, NoDoz, Vivarin	200
Weight Control Aids (daily dose)	
Prolamine	280
Dexatrim, Dietac	200

NOTE: Because products change, contact the manufacturer for updates of changes in caffeine milligram content.

6. Q: Is it stressful on my body to drink tea?

A: Most teas have significantly less caffeine in them than is found in coffee. However, some evidence suggests that tea drinkers have a higher rate of esophageal and gastric cancer[3] because of the "tannic acid" found in many teas. Tannic acid is used to tan the hides of animals and toughen blistered skin. Tea consumption has also been linked to worsened symptoms of PMS.[2]

A good test for tannic acid in tea is the "fuzzy tongue" test. If your tongue feels fuzzy, the tea you are drinking contains tannic acid, a definite stressor.

7. Q: How do I cut out my coffee?

A: Let me answer this question with the following story:

Carol, a former resident of Florida, and her daughter, Lori, attended one of my classes. I thought I heard Carol incorrectly when she approached me after the first class and informed me that she drank an average of 25 cups of coffee per day. She asked me what she should do. I counseled her to certainly not end her coffee consumption all at once, but to decrease the amount gradually; perhaps slash the amount by 5 or 6 cups per week and then after one month she would be down to two or fewer cups per day.

The next week, I received the following report from Lori (approximately age thirty-five) about her mother (approximately age sixty) (this is not word for word): "My mom is a very determined lady. When she sets her mind to doing something, she does it all the way, and she does it right. She wanted to drop three dress sizes and feel better. She cut out her twenty-five cups of coffee right after the first class last week. We went walking the next day, and she looked awful, like she was going to die or throw up. I stopped her in the middle of our walk and said, 'Mom, I'm going to say a prayer for you right now.' After that she looked and felt better. She has felt really good ever since."

By the end of two months, Carol had dropped more than two sizes, and her complexion had literally changed from gray to peach. She looked and felt like a new, much happier lady.

COMMITMENT

8. Q: I weigh more than 300 pounds, and I have a very resistant, fat-storing body. I have dieted for twenty years! How can I ever wait two or three whole years to turn it around?

A: The positive changes start the day you begin on this program, not in two years. While a fully efficient fat-burning body will not appear by next week, you can begin enjoying life right now. Imagine that there are two magic pills available.

One would make you thin tomorrow, but in two years you would gain 100 pounds and never lose it again; the other would slowly and subtly begin changing your metabolism tomorrow, and in two years you would be lean for life, even when you eat high fat and sugar foods. Which pill would you choose? The LEAN & FREE LIFESTYLE won't wither you artificially skinny in a couple of months. It is designed to create a permanently fat-burning body and a healthy, happy individual.

9. **Q: What do I say when a friend says to me, "Well, I've lost thirty pounds over the past three months on my diet. How much have you gained on your program?"**
    A: Just congratulate the person and tell him or her the story of the Tortoise and the Hare. Since the person is losing water, lean muscle tissue, and probably bone mass, you may be leaner and healthier already.

NURTURING
10. Q: What if I eat for emotional reasons?
    A: It's okay to eat, even when you're not hungry–just grab *good* choices. The chart on the following page illustrates emotional reasons for eating coupled with old diet solutions versus LEAN & FREE LIFESTYLE solutions.

NOURISHMENT
11. Q: I hate to cook and clean up. Can I do this program?
    A: Most certainly. Just follow the fast food, convenience food, and "quick and easy" meal suggestions. Also use paper plates, cups, and bowls. You may also plan to have just one cooking day each week. Double or triple recipes and freeze portions of them for the next week. I do this all the time.

12. Q: Is it helpful to take vitamin and mineral supplements?
    A: If you are already eating well and exercising regularly, it is not generally essential for you to take a supplement. But, if you decide to do so, your body will most likely absorb and use much more of the supplements than if you ate poorly and did not exercise. Consult your doctor. In chapter 5, the vitamin and mineral charts show the symptoms of vitamin and mineral deficiencies and excesses. Do not overuse supplements! A moderate amount of supplementation may help restore nutritional satisfaction more rapidly, thus encouraging your survival system to relax and trigger excess fat loss. Large amounts of supplementation can be very stressful to your body and promote serious side effects.

Emotional Reasons for Eating

Old Diet Solutions	LEAN& FREE 2000 PLUS Solutions
BOREDOM	
Don't eat—work	Work and grab a LEAN & FREE sandwich or two!
LONEINESS	
Don't eat—read	Read and eat good healthy snacks!
SADNESS	
Don't eat—listen to inspiring tapes or music	Listen to inspiring tapes or music while enjoying a big bowl of whole-grain cereal, fruit, and 1% milk.
STRESS	
Don't eat after 6 p.m.—exercise	Exercise; then eat a nourishing dinner.
NERVOUSNESS	
Don't eat—socialize	Eat good food before you socialize or party. Then eat a "moderate" amount of party goodies.

---

13. Q: I have very uncomfortable gas and bloating. Can you help me?

A: You are most likely adding whole grains, beans, raw vegetables, and fresh fruits into your eating program in too large a quantity too quickly. You may also be eating too much of one food, such as wheat. Try part whole-grain breads and cereals and wheat-free breakfast cereals. Concentrate more on using cornbread, brown rice, and barley soups. Steam your vegetables and use more canned fruit rather than fresh fruit initially. It may take your body many months to fully adjust to more complex, nutritious foods. A natural food enzyme found in many pharmacies known as "Beano" drops can also be of great help to some people. Also, be certain to avoid foods to which you are allergic, because they stress your body and can encourage excess body fat gain.

14. Q: Will eating often and snacking help me lose more fat?

A: Eating frequent meals and snacking on good food seems to do six things:[1-6]

1. Eating frequent meals seems to encourage your body to store less fat.

2. Frequent meal consumption encourages fat-burning and the retention of lean muscle. (Remember, muscle "curves." Fat "hangs.") Muscle is the machinery where that saggy fat is burned, so eat often. Keep the muscle and burn the fat.

3. Total blood cholesterol levels, low-density lipoproteins (the bad cholesterol), and triglyceride levels may be significantly reduced when meals are eaten frequently.

4. Eating often helps prevent low blood sugar, which may lead to fatigue, poor concentration, memory loss, and blood-sugar disorders.

5. Frequent meal consumption encourages lower serum insulin levels. Insulin is a hormone released by the pancreas to help metabolize the food you eat. It is lovingly known as the "fat hormone" because it "knocks" on the fat cell wall to let the calories you have eaten be stored in your fat cells.

6. Eating often may also help to control or alleviate gas and bloating.

When you skip a meal or go long periods between meals, your blood-sugar level drops markedly. Then, when you do eat, your insulin level rises significantly and may drive much of what you have eaten directly into your fat cells, thus giving you added fat storage to help carry you through long periods between meals or missed meals. So eat often and burn more fat. You'll enjoy the energy!

15. Q: I always grab an apple, grapes, or banana between my meals. Is that okay?

A: Fruit is the least complex of the complex carbohydrates. It takes less effort for the body to digest than vegetables, legumes, and grains, and it's high in natural sugar. When introduced into an empty stomach, it may cause a direct rise in your insulin level to balance your higher blood-sugar level. Insulin is the "fat hormone," so it may drive more of the glucose manufactured from fruit directly into your fat cells. The best advice is to eat fruit with a meal or for dessert, not on an empty stomach. But keep in mind, an apple or banana is a *much* healthier snack than a candy bar.

16. Q: What about eating fruit until noon and never combining a solid and a liquid food?

A: This is a suggested practice dismissed by most professionals as quackery. The food combinations of water, vegetable, grain, protein, and fruit will not "ferment" in your stomach as some people claim. After you've followed this program for a couple of months, you may decide to try eating only fruit until noon. If you do, you'll most likely feel dissatisfied, light-headed, weak, and dizzy as you approach noon. Fruit also triggers highs and lows in your blood-sugar level that may lead to more fat-storage of the foods you eat later in the day.

17. Q: Can juice or milk replace my water drinking?

A: No. A minimum of six eight-ounce glasses of water is essential for optimal health. You'll notice that fruit and vegetable juices are included only occasionally in the LEAN & FREE menus. This is because the majority of fiber is removed when you juice a whole food, and the natural sugars absorb more quickly into your system. Fiber can help inhibit excess fat storage. If you buy a juicer, use it only once in a while, unless you have a system that cannot tolerate whole foods.

18. Q: To succeed on this program, do I have to eat raw broccoli until I'm green or raw carrots until I'm orange?

A: Certainly not, and you actually could turn orange from an overdose of carotene. Give yourself many months to adjust to eating vegetables and grains by initially eating more steamed vegetables and part-whole (cracked-grain) breads and cereals.

19. Q: What foods are the highest in fiber?

A: The table on the following page lists the top 100 most fibrous foods.

20. Q: There is a new diet drink out that's selling like gangbusters. It's supposed to speed up your metabolism and burn fat. When I drink it, I feel an increase in energy almost immediately. What do you think about this product?

A: First of all, read the ingredients. If a word ends in "ose" (like sucrose, dextrose, etc.), it is a form of sugar. It offers quick energy and, in excess, fat-storing stress. Also look for caffeine. Many times caffeine will occur naturally in one of the ingredients listed. Therefore, it will not be listed as a separate ingredient. In addition, the fiber often added to these drinks is not the "whole food" that was the source of the fiber, yet the whole food is much greater than the sum of its separate parts. Most of these supplemental drinks supply you with negative stresses that will most likely encourage a reduced-energy, fat-storing body in the long run. Fat cannot be burned by dietary supplements any more than it can be squashed, rubbed, shaken, pressed, rolled, or melted away. Fat can only be burned in the muscles of a fat-burning body.

Top 100 Fiber Foods

Item	Serving	Fiber Grams
GRAINS		
bulgur, raw	1 ounce	5.2
barley, raw	1 ounce	4.9
oat bran, raw	1 ounce	4.5
cornmeal, whole-grain	1 ounce	4.3
wheat flour, whole-grain	1 ounce	3.6
wheat germ	1 ounce	3.0
oats, rolled dry	1 ounce	2.9
millet, hulled, raw	1 ounce	2.4
LEGUMES		
baked beans,		
vegetarian, canned	1/2 cup	9.8
kidney, cooked	1/2 cup	9.0
pinto, cooked	1/2 cup	8.9
black-eyed peas, cooked	1/2 cup	8.3
miso (a fermented soybean product)	1/2 cup	7.5
chick peas (garbanzos)	1/2 cup	7.0
limas, cooked	1/2 cup	6.8
navy, cooked	1/2 cup	6.8
lentils, cooked	1/2 cup	5.2
white, cooked	1/2 cup	5.0
green peas, cooked	1/2 cup	2.4
NUTS & SEEDS		
almonds, oil-roasted	1/4 cup	4.4
pistachio nuts	1/4 cup	3.5
mixed nuts, oil-roasted	1/4 cup	3.2
peanuts	1/4 cup	3.2
pecans	1/4 cup	2.3
RICE, PASTA, TORTILLAS		
pasta, multigrain		
with quinoa, dry	2 ounces	8.0
with triticale, dry	2 ounces	6.5
with oat bran, dry	2 ounces	6.0
whole-wheat, dry	2 ounces	6.0
wild rice, cooked	1/2 cup	5.3
brown rice, long-grain, cooked	1/2 cup	1.7
tortilla, corn	2 shells	3.1
SNACKS		
crackers, stoned-wheat	1 ounce	3.9
crisps, thin oat	1/2 ounce	3.2
crisps, thin rye	1/2 ounce	3.0
hearty wheat	4 crackers	3.0
whole-wheat saltines	5 crackers	1.0
cookies, oat plus fruit	2 crackers	3.0
oat bran	2 cookies	2.8
fig bars	2 cookies	1.3
graham crackers, oat bran	1.2 ounces	3.0
popcorn, gourmet	1/2 ounce	2.0
VEGETABLES		
artichokes	1 medium	6.7
brussels sprouts, boiled	5 sprouts	4.5
mixed vegetables, frozen, cooked	1/2 cup	3.5
sweet potato, baked	1 potato	3.4
corn, cooked	1 ear	2.8
parsley, chopped	1 cup	2.8
parsnips, cooked	1/2 cup	2.7
broccoli, raw, chopped	1 cup	2.5
potato, with skin	1 medium	2.5
carrots, raw	1 carrot	2.3
turnip greens, broiled	1/2 cup	2.2
spinach, broiled	1/2 cup	2.1
asparagus, cut	1 cup	2.0
cauliflower, cooked	5 florets	2.0
zucchini, cooked	1/2 cup	1.8
cabbage, raw, shredded	1 cup	1.7
green beans, string, cooked	1/2 cup	1.6
tomato, raw	1 medium	1.5

Sources: "Soluble and Total Dietary Fiber in Selected Foods" and "Provisional Table on the Dietary Fiber Content of Selected Foods," USDA Human Nutrition Information Service; Fiber Facts, Chicago, Illinois, The American Dietetic Association, 1986 (reprinted in "Dietary Fiber and Health," *Journal of the American Medical Association,* July 1989); "Dietary fiber content of selected foods," *American Journal of Clinical Nutrition,* 1988; Plant Fiber in Foods, James W. Anderson, 1986, HCF Nutrition Research Foundation, Inc.; *Prevention Magazine,* vol. 41, 11.

21. Q: What types of oil are best to buy?

A: The words "cold pressed" on the label of an oil do not always ensure that the oil has not been damaged by mechanical extraction methods that expose the oil to temperatures ranging from 140 to 160 degrees. Your best bet is to look for the words "expeller pressed" or "crude" on the label to ensure the most natural, unrefined type of oil you can buy. Check the regular oil section in your grocery store, the health-food section, or your local health-food store to purchase expeller pressed oil.

The best expeller pressed oils to buy are:

1.	Olive oil	4.	Sunflower oil
2.	Peanut oil	5.	Corn oil
3.	Safflower oil	6.	Soybean oil

Canola oil goes through a different expelling process. It is high in monounsaturated fats and linoleic acid but does not perform well when heated to high temperatures. For long-term storage, I buy partially hydrogenated corn oils such as Mazola. These oils have a longer shelf life.

22. Q: What about artificial fats?

A: **Olestra:** A noncaloric artificial fat made from sucrose and fatty acids; formerly called "sucrose polyester."

Simplesse: The trade name for a protein-based, low-calorie artificial fat, approved by the FDA for use in food.

Olsetra and Simplesse are scientifically manufactured substitutes for nature's fats. The idea behind these fats is to create low-calorie (as in the case of Simplesse which equals 1 1/3 calories per gram) or no-calorie (Olsetra passes through the digestive tract unabsorbed) fat replacements. Olestra can serve as a partial replacement for cooking fats. Simplesse cannot, as it gels when heated.

Some currently reported side effects during the brief use of artificial fats have been diarrhea and interference with vitamin E absorption.

The entire premise of the Lean & Free 2000 Plus Lifestyle program is that when the body receives an abundance of good, natural, well-balanced calories, it will not then have a need to store excess fat. We have just discussed some of the essential roles of good fat for health and fat loss. I do not recommend artificial, man-made fats. There are numerous fat free products on the market that contain no artificial fats.

23. Q: You use real butter and regular cheese because it's more natural. What about real mayonnaise?

A: I mix fat free mayonnnaise and fat free salad dressing together for a more balanced flavor. Butter and cheese are "real" foods to start with, while mayonnaise is manufactured and not all ingredients are natural. I prefer a no fat "man-made" food to a high fat "man-made" food. It's a matter of taste and mathematics. I'd rather save my fat grams in high fat mayonnaise for a little more cheese and butter. Other people have different preferences.

I recently heard a report on the radio that indicated a stronger link between the use of margarine and heart disease than between the use of butter and heart disease—not surprising!

24. Q: What exactly is cholesterol?

A: Cholesterol is a soft, waxy substance manufactured in the body and also found in animal products such as meat, eggs, and dairy products. Cholesterol and triglycerides are not the same thing. Triglycerides are food fats in the blood.

High blood cholesterol is implicated as one of the main predictors of a person's likelihood of a heart attack or stroke.

Reducing cholesterol by one-third may decrease a person's risk of heart disease by one-half.

The cholesterol in foods may not affect blood cholesterol levels nearly as much as the fat in foods, especially the saturated fats.

25. Q: Is there anything good about cholesterol?

A: Yes:
1. It helps the body manufacture adrenal hormones and sex hormones.
2. It indirectly aids in fat digestion.
3. The brain is 80 percent cholesterol.
4. It helps insulate nerves.
5. It lubricates artery walls.

26. Q: What is HDL and LDL?

A: HDL stands for "high-density lipoproteins" or the "good"cholesterol. It is a protein-like substance in the blood that helps carry food fats or triglycerides out of the body. LDL stands for "low-density lipoproteins" or "bad" cholesterol. LDLs facilitate the storage of triglycerides along artery walls, which can lead to atherosclerosis or hardening of the arteries and eventual heart attack or stroke.

27. Q: How do I increase HDL, reduce LDL, and/or reduce total blood cholesterol?

A: Do the following:

1. Reduce total fat intake, especially saturated fat.
2. Increase high-fiber, complex-carbohydrate food intake.
3. Increase fish intake that is high in essential fatty acids.
4. Exercise aerobically three to six days per week for thirty to sixty minutes.
5. Avoid smoking.
6. Think positive thoughts and reduce stress in your life.
7. Unless directed by your doctor, do not totally avoid foods containing cholesterol. Just use them in moderation.

28. Q: I hate fish. What should I do?

A: If you have an overall moderate cholesterol level (approximately 100 plus your age—a little more if you are under fifty), your HDL is at the high end of the correct range, and your LDL is at the low end of the correct range, then you may get along fine without adding fish to your diet. However, if this is not the case, ask your doctor what he recommends. He may recommend fish-oil capsules along with exercise, increased fiber, and decreased saturated and overall dietary fat intake.

29. Q: How much protein do I need?

A: Study the following chart.

The recommended dietary allowance (RDA - 1989) for protein:

	WGT	HGT	AGE	GRAMS
Infants				
	13 24	0 - 0.5	13	Your protein RDA will vary
	20 28	0.5 -1	14	depending on height and weight.
Children				To figure your protein RDA:
	29 35	1 - 3	16	1. Find your body weight.
	44 44	4 - 6	24	2. Convert pounds to kilograms
	62 52	7 - 10	28	(Pounds divided by 2.2= kg)

The recommended dietary allowance (RDA - 1989) for protein: (cont'd)

WGT *	HGT*	AGE	GRAMS	
Males				
99	62	11 - 14	45	3. Multiply by .08g/kg to get
145	69	15 - 18	59	your RDA in grams/day.
160	70	19 - 24	58	*For example:*
174	70	25 - 50	63	1. Weight = 150 lbs
170	68	51+	63	2. 150 / 2.2 = 68 k
				3. 68 x 0.8 = **54 grams**
Females				
101	62	11 - 14	46	The National Research Council
120	64	15 - 18	44	requirements are met if a 150-lb.
128	65	19 - 24	46	person consumes not less than 54
138	64	25 - 50	50	grams of protein per day and not
143	63	51+	50	more than 108 grams or double
			90	the minimum amount.
Pregnant				
Lactating				
First six months			65	* Weights given in pounds.
Second six months			62	* Height given in inches.

There are four calories in one gram (g) of protein. Therefore, a twenty-five to fifty-year-old woman would need fifty grams times four equaling 200 calories of protein per day. Fifty grams of protein would be very easily obtained by eating:

2 cups nonfat milk =	16	g protein
1 cup oatmeal cereal =	6	g protein
4 oz. broiled salmon =	28	g protein
TOTAL =	50	g protein

The National Research Council recommends that the RDA for protein be used as the minimum intake standard and that the maximum intake of protein be *not more than double the RDA*. Therefore, a twenty-five to fifty-year-old woman would meet requirements of her protein intake ranged between 50 and 100 grams per day, or 200 to 400 calories from protein.

The LEAN & FREE 2000 LIFESTYLE recommends that you keep your animal protein intake around 10 percent with your total protein intake not exceeding 15 percent of your total calories. Notice how perfectly this fits into these national requirements. A woman beginning this program may be consuming 2,000 calories for full satisfaction. Ten percent of 2,000 is 200 calories or 50 grams of protein. I consume between 3,000 and 4,000 calories per day. Ten percent of 3,000 is 300 calories or 75 grams of protein. Ten percent of 4,000 calories is 400 protein calories or 100 grams of protein.

By following the LEAN & FREE LIFESTYLE, you will not need to worry about counting protein grams. Just follow the quick, delicious meal plans and the Five Fingers of Balance, and you'll be assured an ideal amount of protein.

30. Q: I would like to store food for a rainy day. What should I store ?

A: Review the chart on the following page.

For storage purposes, make certain to buy foods you normally eat. It is important to like these foods and have a digestive system that is already adjusted to them.

31. Q: What kind of wheat should I buy?

A: My favorite is the new, softer white wheat. It makes up into bread products that are lighter in color, flavor, and texture. Most people assume that these bread products are half whole-wheat and half white flour because of the lightness.

White wheat is as high in nutrients and fiber as hard red wheat, which makes into heavier, darker bread with a stronger flavor.

White wheat can be found in kitchen centers, mill and mixer, health food, and food storage stores. Many grocers will also order large sacks of it for you.

32. Q: Do I need a wheat grinder?

A: A wheat grinder is a *must* if you want the luxury of delicious five-minute *Three Bear Porridge, Cracked Wheat* hot cereal, and wonderful muffins, pancakes, and breads. I have a large wheat grinder with several different texture settings. Prior to purchasing this, I used a small electric coffee grinder that cost about $15. Purchase a grinder that suits your budget and your grinding needs. It may pay for itself in a month or two as you enjoy fresh ground hot cereals over the more expensive cold cereals.

MOTION
33. Q: Will I really live two years longer if I exercise regularly?

A: Not necessarily. You may get hit by a Mack truck tomorrow. But let us assume that you are forty years old today. If you begin exercising today, and you exercise six days a week for the next forty years, and you die at age eighty instead of seventy-eight, you will have spent nearly one and a half of those two extra years

169

LEAN & FREE 2000 PLUS Food Storage Items for One Adult for One Year

WATER	360 gallons (30 gal./month)
VEGETABLES	50 Lbs.— Variety of canned 70 Lbs.— Variety of dried beans peas, lentils (low fat refried beans)
GRAINS	300 Lbs.— White or red wheat (will need grinder) 150 Lbs.— Other grains-(brown and white rice, oats, hard yellow popcorn, barley, millet, etc.) 50 Lbs.— Variety of whole grain and white pastas
PROTEINS	100 Lbs.— Nonfat dried milk 20 Lbs.— Variety of low fat canned meats (tuna in water, canned chicken, turkey, lean beef, etc.) 10 Lbs.— Powdered eggs 10 Lbs.— Peanut butter
FRUITS	50 Lbs.— Canned fruit (in own juice)
FATS	20 Lbs.— Vegetable oil 6 Lbs.— Butter (frozen)
SWEETENERS	15 Lbs.— Sugar 15 Lbs.— Honey 20 Lbs.— Variety of canned, frozen fruit juice concentrates (no sugar or artificial sweeteners added)
SALT	5 Lbs.— Iodized salt

of life exercising. The real point is not that exercise extends your life but that it greatly enhances the *quality* of that life. If you exercise regularly, you reduce your chances of spending the last two, five, or ten years in a rest home or hospital. Your present and later years will be more productive and joyful. And, you'll feel much more fulfilled than those leading sedentary lifestyles.

34. Q: What if I want to exercise more than the A+ schedule provides?

A: If you opt for a more rigorous schedule, it is my suggestion that you make it the exception and not the rule. After all, life is meant to be enhanced by exercise; it is not meant to be exercise. One hour six days a week will more than meet your health and fitness needs. After that, exercise becomes sport. And if you are in "training," make certain to significantly increase your calorie and nutrient intake to assure optimal growth and repair of lean muscle tissue, and be very sensitive to your increased risk of exercise-induced injury.

35. Q: My stomach muscles are shot after three normal births and a cesarean section. What can I do to tighten and flatten my stomach?

A: Do your regular aerobic exercise to create a fat-burning metabolism along with your 2000 PLUS balanced eating. Then, do two or three minutes of half sit-ups with your knees bent and your hands behind your head. Lift from the lower back, keeping your chin up, your forehead back, and your stomach flat. Breathe out as you rise up (during the effort).

Another excellent way to flatten your abdominal muscles is to wear a snug pair of jeans around the house that are just snug in the lower abdominal area, not the waist. They will remind you to hold your stomach in all the time and will actually *help* you flatten your stomach. Abdominal muscles are very "moldable." They get pushed out during a pregnancy and after years of poor eating and poor posture. Snug jeans help to push them back in and flatten the muscle—not burn fat. In one to three days, you may notice a marked difference.

Finally, remember to consciously keep your lower abdominal section "tucked in." Not only will this help you to look fifteen pounds leaner, it will help to strengthen your lower back. And don't forget to practice deep (not shallow) breathing throughout the day. Oxygen is essential for optimal health and fat loss.

36. Q: I understand that no exercise can threaten my health and increase my body fat. But I am so obese (more than three hundred pounds) that movement is extremely difficult, and a walk to the front door leaves me short of breath. What should I do?

A: First, check with your doctor. If he or she gives you the go-ahead, turn on your favorite TV show. Stand in front of it and move toe-heel, toe-heel with your feet without lifting them off the ground. Bend your right knee, left knee, right knee, left knee. Gently push your arms up and down, right and left. Start with five minutes in the morning and five minutes at night. Add about a half minute per day until you are doing two twenty-minute sessions, then two thirty-minute sessions. Eventually, as your body fat decreases, work up to forty-five to sixty-minute sessions, three to six days a week. Remember, you didn't get fat overnight and you won't get lean and healthy overnight either. If standing is impossible, sit in a straight chair, lift right heel (toe stays down), left heel, right heel, left heel as you perform varying arm movements.

SERVICE

37. Q: How do you find time to do service projects when you're fixing two or three meals a day for your family?

A: It's my feeling that one of the greatest services you can perform is to provide healthy, delicious meals for your family and thoughtfully involve them in menu planning, cooking, and cleaning up. It's great training. The families I know that eat *together* at least once or twice a day seem to develop a much stronger bond than those who do not.

When I used to diet, I didn't want to cook because I was afraid I'd eat what I cooked. I didn't have the energy to cook either.

The LEAN & FREE LIFESTYLE has made cooking a pleasure again, and I also have the energy to enjoy preparing meals.

There is a much better feeling in our home now that we usually eat together; because when you *eat together,* you *talk together,* and you have the energy to be nice to one another.

Serve your family first. Then they'll all have the physical and emotional energy to expand their service as well. Many hands can perform more service than just your two hands alone.

MISCELLANEOUS

38. Q: I'm shaped like an apple with skinny arms and legs and a full torso. My sister is shaped like a pear with a thin upper body and fat hips and thighs. When I used to diet, my arms and legs would get skinnier, and my torso was the last area to trim down. My sister would get tiny in her waist but always had full thighs. Will this continue to happen with this program?

A: Eating to be "naturally lean" is entirely different than starving to be artificially skinny. If you are apple shaped, you may start to notice firmness and muscle definition developing in your arms and legs while your torso gradually firms, tightens, and reduces in size.

If you are pear shaped, you may notice inch loss and firming in your arms and legs with a slight increase in your "starved skinny" torso at first (because food takes some room). Then you'll gradually become proportioned and continue losing inches all over.

At more than two hundred pounds, I wore a size 14 dress and a tight size 18 pant. As I began losing my body fat correctly, I became a size 10 all over for the first time in my life. Then I continued to drop to a size 4 pant and a size 6 dress—just the reverse of my former "pear" shape.

Whatever your shape, you *can* optimize your body's health and appearance potential by nourishing, not starving your body. Just follow the LEAN & FREE LIFESTYLE principles; and remember, never compare yourself to someone else. The end goal of this program is service and happiness. Happiness doesn't come from having a model perfect figure. It comes from being the best person you can be.

39. Q: What if a person needs to gain weight? What does he or she do?

A: The principles are basically the same: simply follow the LEAN & FREE LIFESTYLE health principles. Such people should increase their fat intake to 30 percent of total calories (mostly from "good" fats in nuts, seeds, fish, etc.) and build lean muscle tissue though exercise. In addition to their regular exercise, they can bulk up on off days with moderately heavy weight lifting. They should build up slowly. Most important, they should simply focus on good health and increased energy.

40. Q: My husband and I travel a lot. I always return with my clothing so tight I can hardly zip my pants. I go days without a bowel movement. What can I do?

A: First of all, my guess is that you're cutting calories, skipping meals, or eating lightly in order to slim down before you travel. As a result you have already developed a fat-storing metabolism. Thus, the foods you eat on vacation can quickly and easily be stored as fat. My first suggestion to avoid this discomfort in the future is to never diet or skip meals. Then, when you eat "C "choices on your vacation, your body may store only one or two pounds of body fat instead of ten to twenty.

Second, while on vacation eat as normally as possible. Never eat desserts on an empty stomach, and try to get in at least thirty minutes of brisk walking every day. (Walk or march in place in your hotel room while watching TV.) Make sure to pack your aerobic shoes and a supportive exercise outfit. Find a grocery store close to your hotel and purchase whole-grain breads, lowfat whole-grain crackers, cold cereals, vegetables, fruits, and 1% or skim milk to put on ice in your hotel room.

You may also want to pack a gentle laxative prescribed by your doctor. Before I discovered the principles of the LEAN & FREE LIFESTYLE, I would go two or three days without a bowel movement. Now this is never the case unless I'm traveling and forget to take necessary precautions.

Most important, eat at least three balanced, high-fiber meals every day when you travel and wear loose, comfortable clothing. Eat to enjoy your vacation.

41. Q: How do I figure out how many fat grams and calories are in my own homemade recipes?

A: Look up each recipe ingredient in your fat gram/calorie charts in the back of this book. Then total the fat grams and calories. Divide each of those numbers by the number of servings the recipe makes.

Example:

Pork Chow Mein

Calories	Fat grams	
120	14	1 Tb. vegetable oil
150	4	1 cup extra-lean pork, cubed
58		1 cup chopped onion
20	t	1 cup celery, slant cut
18	t	3/4 cup bamboo shoots
70	t	1 small can mushrooms
16	t	1 cup bean sprouts
45	t	1 1/3 cups chicken soup stock
20	0	1/2 tsp. sugar
14	t	2 Tb. soy sauce
60	0	2 Tb. cornstarch
0	0	3 Tb. cold water
1824	40	4 cups chow mein noodles

Total = 2415   62 (Approx.) (1 cup = 1 serving)

Look at the recipe and see how many cups you have added. In this recipe we have added almost eight cups of vegetables, meat, and soup stock. This will help you determine how many servings and the serving size. Now take the total number of calories and divide by the number of servings. Do the same to determine the number of fat grams per serving.

2,415 ÷ 8 = approx. 302 calories/serving

62 ÷ 8 = approx. 8 fat grams/serving

Therefore:
   Calories per serving = 302
   Fat grams per serving = 8
   Number of servings = 8
   Size of serving = 1 cup vegetable mixture plus 1/2 cup noodles

To determine the fat percentage for this recipe:
   8 fat grams x 9 calories = 72 fat calories
   72 fat calories ÷ 302 total calories = 24% of total calories from fat
(Count two "traces" as one fat gram when figuring recipes. In this recipe, 61.5 is rounded to 62 fat grams.)

You may include an oriental vegetable soup and a fruit plate with this dish. Both are under 10 percent fat. The overall meal will easily have 20 percent or fewer of its calories coming from fat.

42. Q: What are the best ways for me to save money and still eat right?

A: Cook more from scratch and buy fewer convenience items such as cold cereal and canned soup. Buy wheat, beans, rice, corn, oats, and barley in bulk and use your food storage items. Buy canned goods on special by the case. Also purchase fresh fruits and vegetables in season and buy them by the half or whole case if you can eat that many before spoilage occurs.

LEAN & FREE can be the cheapest wellness lifestyle in the world. Not only will you be saving bundles of money by avoiding junk food items such as soda pop, candy, and chips, but you may also save tremendously on medical bills. You may enjoy amazing increases in your physical and emotional stamina, thus enabling you to earn more money. Your decreases in excess body fat and illness may precipitate marvelous increases in many other areas of your life, such as increased happiness, self-esteem, energy, wellness, and financial security!

43. Q: How do I know when my body has switched from a *neutral* state to a *fat-burning* state?

A: Your body is in neutral when you are relatively size stable, even if you go on vacation for a week. If you can also read signals from your body such as hunger, comfortable-satisfaction, low-energy, and high-energy, you can kick into fat-burning acceleration tomorrow by becoming an A+ student. Remember that an A+ student listens closely to his or her body's individual needs and increases exercise duration, fiber, and calories very gradually. And be sure to take your measurements *every* week!

LEAN & FREE SUCCESS STORIES

The following case studies summarize the experiences of real people who have followed the principles of the LEAN & FREE LIFESTYLE and have made significant changes in their lives. In most cases, their names have been changed to protect their privacy. The quotations indicate direct, unaltered comments and feelings from the individuals.

Subject: JANE
Age: 34
Height: 5-feet 1-inch
Weight Lost: 24 Pounds (206 to 182 so far)
Size Change: 14 to 10
Special Benefit: *Painful cramps have subsided.*

Jane's History: Jane had been battling a body-fat problem for many years and eventually found herself about forty-three pounds overly fat. She had uterine cramps every day; she felt tired, depressed, and discouraged. She was diagnosed with endometriosis and was told by her doctor that the solution was a hysterectomy.

Jane's Challenge: Jane did not want to have the operation, so she vowed instead to make an extreme effort to lose weight.

Jane's Solution: "I went on a liquid diet under a doctor's supervision. After one week, I hadn't lost a pound, so I cut my liquid supplement from three drinks a day to two drinks a day. At the end of the second week, I still hadn't experienced any weight loss, so I cut my drinks to one a day. At twenty-one days I proudly, but very weakly, stepped on my doctor's scales. I hadn't cheated once in those three weeks, but the scales showed I had gained three pounds. I broke down in tears. All the doctor could say was, 'It must be your thyroid.' But he checked it and found it normal."

After the liquid diet failed, Jane tried every alternative she could think of to lose weight. She joined an aerobics class, but the cramps became so painful she couldn't continue. Then, just when she was about to give up and have the hysterectomy, she was introduced to the principles you've just learned in the LEAN & FREE 2000 PLUS program.

The LEAN & FREE Solution: "I immediately noticed an increase in energy." Jane says. "The difference was so drastic, I canceled an appointment with my doctor to discuss the hysterectomy." Jane was apparently suffering from symptoms of poor nutrition, not endometriosis as was thought to be the possible cause of her painful cramps. She said, "Since I had seen immediate results, I had no trouble remaining committed to the program. So far I have lost twenty-four pounds and dropped from a size 14 to a size 10 dress, and I feel wonderful.

"I'm looking forward to being a size 5 again. I have saved a pair of size-5 pants for over eight years waiting for a miracle. Now I've found it."

Subject: MARGE
Age: 54
Height: 5 feet 9 inches
Weight Lost: 35 pounds
Size Change: 16 to 5
Special Benefit: *Depression has subsided.*

Marge's History: Marge suffered depression from her long years of struggling with her weight. She says, "One day I was in a grocery store, and I became aware of the many middle-aged women that were passing me. They were wearing polyester pants and pullover tops trying to cover large abdomens and lots of fat. I had gone up to 160 pounds, and I did not want to wind up like those women."

Marge's Challenge: She didn't believe in dieting and was searching for another method that would enable her to effectively and permanently lose weight.

Marge's Solution: "For a year I watched what I was eating. I ate small portions and no desserts, but by the end of the year I had lost only ten pounds. I looked at myself when I got home and said, 'What can I do?' I didn't want to continue to buy larger-sized clothing (I had just bought a size-16 blue suit). Finally in desperation, I mentioned my situation to a friend, and she recommended this program."

The LEAN & FREE Solution: "Since I had never fully believed in dieting, I was fascinated by the emphasis on eating. I really wanted to know how I could eat and still lose weight. I enrolled in an eleven-week class, which began what was to become one of the most thrilling times of my life. When Dana Thornock came to class and told me she was my height, weighed 150 pounds, but was a size four, I was absolutely amazed. I started the program with total inches of 231.5 (adding up measurements from neck to ankles). In six months my total inches were 228.5. After a year they were just 211, and my weight had stabilized at 125 pounds.

"Now I love to eat and exercise. In fact, I gave away all my large clothes because I knew I wouldn't "grow" back into them. My ultimate reward came when I went shopping at a wonderful store where I had my own private clerk help me select a huge pile of clothes I really liked. For two hours I tried them on without looking at the sizes. Wow, was I excited when I got home and read the size-5 labels.

"Every week someone comes up to me and says how nice I look. I feel so wonderful physically, and my mental health has improved a lot. I am really glad to be alive. By the way, I've had that size-16 blue suit taken in professionally twice now, and it's still too big. Guess I'll have to give it away."

Subject: LOIS
Age: 45
Height: 5 feet 7 inches
Weight Lost: 20 pounds (257 to 237 so far)
Size Change: One full slack size (in first three months)
Special Benefits: *Rash is gone and self-esteem has greatly improved.*

Lois's History: At forty-three years old, Lois weighed 257 pounds and was extremely unhappy. She ate three to four Snickers candy bars daily and was also taking caffeine pills for energy. Almost everything she ate contained artificial sweeteners. Her arms were covered with a rash that itched intensely.

Lois's Challenge: She felt she couldn't continue on this path. She was exhausted and unhealthy and felt desperate for help.

Lois's Solution: "I tried every diet I could find, but nothing worked."

The LEAN & FREE Solution: "The more I learned about the program, the more and more excited I became. I felt at last I had found a program that really dealt with my dilemma and my feelings. I learned to eat right. I learned to exercise. I learned to love and nurture my body. In three months I have already dropped a size in my slacks and lost twenty pounds (I thought about not weighing myself, but I was so curious I couldn't stand it).

"I feel good about myself, and I know that what I am doing is the right thing for me. I have also improved my self-esteem by telling others about this program and watching them succeed. My three sisters, my sister-in-law, my boss and his wife, and several friends are currently on the program. I am not bashful about spreading the excitement I feel. I have many other people who are cautiously watching to see if it really works, and that is just fine with me.

"Now the rash is gone. I do not even crave a Snickers bar; I do not eat anything with NutraSweet in it, and no caffeine. I feel great. I feel free. This program was the turning point in my life."

Subject: JANELLE
Age: 40
Height: 5 feet 7 inches
Weight Lost: 165 pounds (325 to 160 and still dropping)
Size Change: 50 to 10
Special Benefit: *Cholesterol – 301 to 178*

Janelle's History: Janelle has been plagued by a weight problem her entire life. In high school they called her "Janelephant." Later, after four pregnancies in five years, she weighed 325 pounds and had a cholesterol level of 301. She has an inherited tendency to be obese. Both of her parents weighed well over 300 pounds and died in their early fifties of associated complications.

Janelle's Challenge: She needed to understand and believe that she could overcome her genetic history, that she did not have to be fat, and that she could successfully become lean and healthy without ever dieting again. She also needed to find a healthy, economical lifestyle that she could believe in that would help her make the desired transformation.

Janelle's Solution: "From age fourteen on, I tried everything—starvation diets, diet pills, diet shots. Nothing worked. Finally, out of desperation, I had my stomach stapled but only lost forty pounds. I was discouraged and ready to accept that I was going to lead a miserable life." So Janelle stopped dieting four years before beginning this program and became neutral, or weight stable, at 325 pounds.

The LEAN & FREE Solution: "Eating like a normal person and exercising have made all the difference for me. After just eighteen months on this program, I weigh 165 pounds; I have gone from a size 50 to a size 10. My cholesterol dropped to 170 after eight months, and it's still there. And all this after I had given birth to four children in five years.

"Sometimes it's still hard for me to believe I'm this lean. I can't remember being this small. I feel great, and I am able to do things I've never been able to do before. For the first time, I really like myself.

"It is really wonderful to eat like a normal person and to look like a normal person. I can handle so many stresses in my life and be calm. I am really happy. And now my whole family is on the program. We all feel great. What a blessing to know that I can prevent the pain of extreme obesity in their lives."

(Examine Janelle's lifetime diet roller coaster on the next page.)

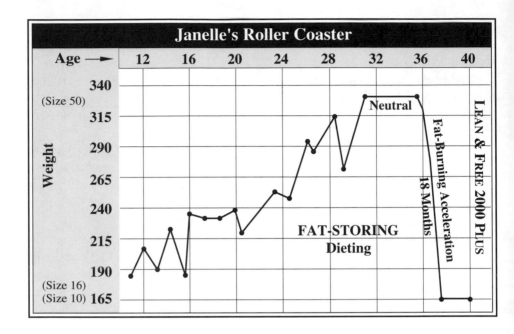

Janelle's Roller Coaster

Subject: LUANN
Age: 61
Height: 5 feet 5 inches
Weight Lost: 22 pounds
Size Change: 16 to 12
Body Fat: 32% to 29% (so far)
Special Benefit: *Life has changed!*

LuAnn's History: LuAnn had her own method for eating "balanced meals" before she discovered the LEAN & FREE 2000 PLUS LIFESTYLE: "I used to love hot dogs. Sometimes I'd cook three hot dogs and eat them without the buns. And, of course, I'd have my veggies—a handful of potato chips for a grand total of 62 fat grams in just one meal. I weighed 183 1/2 pounds, my body fat was 32.8 percent and I was a large size 16. I couldn't stand to see my reflection in a mirror."

LuAnn's Challenge: She needed to find a balanced eating program that provided the nutrition she needed for optimal health and energy.

The LEAN & FREE Solution: LuAnn writes: "Dana, I'd like to thank you for a wonderful program that has really changed my life. Five and a half months ago, I weighed 183 1/2 pounds, my body fat was 32.8 percent and I was a large size 16.

After three and a half months on the program, I weighed 168 pounds and had reduced my body fat to 30.6 percent. Now I weigh 163 pounds, I'm a proud size 12, and I'm still working toward my goal of 20 to 25 percent body fat and whatever size that will be. I'm totally dedicated to the program. It's exciting to go around the house and see my reflection in the mirror or a window and go, 'Yes! Yes'! It sounds crazy, but it's fun. I just crack up inside when I think about the way I used to eat. No wonder I was fat."

Subject: CAROL ANN
Age: 46
Height: 5 feet 5 inches
Weight Lost: 88 pounds (228 to 140)
Size Change: 24 to 10
Special Benefits: *Abdominal cramps and diarrhea have subsided.*

Carol Ann' s History: Throughout grade school and junior high, Carol Ann was the smallest and leanest person in her class. She excelled in advanced ballet and tap, even performing in the Nutcracker ballet. Then in the ninth grade she stopped dancing, and her body changed. In one year she went from 110 to 150 pounds. After that her weight fluctuated as she went on and off diets. Then when she was pregnant with her first child, she became very conscious of her health and the health of her baby and ate balanced foods, something she did not normally do.

She says, "Consequently, I gained only eighteen pounds during my pregnancy and lost thirty-six pounds after I had the baby. At that point I should have realized that eating more good food, not less, was the key to controlling my weight. But as I was nursing my baby, I began eating less and less good food. I was drawn to eating more French fries and sweets, and I gained the thirty pounds back.

"With my second and third pregnancies, the same thing happened. I ate good food, didn't gain too much weight, and lost weight after the births. But I ate lousy between pregnancies and gained a lot of weight. Finally, I got tired of feeling guilty about the way I ate. I decided to just give up and try to be fat and happy. The only problem was that I was fat but I wasn't happy."

Carol Ann's Challenge: Find a consistent, long-term solution to her weight problem.

Carol Ann's Solution: "I decided to do something drastic. I had gastric by-pass surgery. After the surgery I could eat only a small portion of food the size of an egg. I panicked. I was afraid I would starve to death, and I was totally consumed by thoughts of food. I would try to eat more, but my heart would pound extremely rapidly, and I would lie on my bed in severe agony from abdominal cramps alternating with diarrhea. At that point I promised myself I would never do bad things to my body again. I knew to be healthy I had to eat good foods as I had during my pregnancies."

The LEAN & FREE Solution: "Once I discovered Dana's program, it confirmed everything I learned during my pregnancies. I started eating good food, and I quit beating myself up emotionally when I wanted to eat goodies. Eating desserts after full satisfaction is one of the best things about this program. It has really helped me meet my psychological needs.

"My stomach has gradually increased in capacity. I can eat many more good foods now, and I walk three to five days a week for an hour and love it. Following the eating and exercise guidelines in this program has dramatically increased my energy level. This program is truly the way to go. At a size 10, I not only have freedom from my excess body fat, but I also feel free to eat the foods I love to eat. And I love healthifying new recipes. Don't ever damage your body like I did. Just follow this program."

Subject: LEE ROY
Age: 51
Height: 6 feet 2 inches
Weight Lost: 30 pounds (199 to 169)
Waist Change: 38 to 31
Special Benefit: *People say he looks younger than his actual age.*

Lee Roy's History: Lee Roy had always been lean and active. But when he turned forty, he noticed a change. His activity level decreased, and he began putting on abdominal fat.

Lee Roy's Challenge: Firming his stomach and regaining his energy level.

Lee Roy's Solution: "I ignored it because I figured it must be unavoidable as you get older."

The LEAN & FREE Solution: He tells us: "My wife had been a yo-yo dieter. For years she had eaten practically nothing. Then she discovered this program and began feeling wonderful. Now she looks beautiful, and she is so much less emotional."

"Two months after she started feeding me this delicious food, I had lost thirty pounds and five inches off my waist. I wasn't even exercising except for a basketball game once a week. The rapid weight loss worried me, so I went to the doctor to see if I was sick. He asked me how I felt. I said, 'Great! I've never had more energy.' My blood pressure and cholesterol were perfect. He asked me if I'd been dieting. I said, 'No, in fact I'm probably eating twice what I used to eat!' He sent me home with a clean bill of health."

"I don't look skinny in the face and neck, and thanks to my thirty-one inch waist, many people think I'm quite a bit younger than 51. I sure do love feeling so great and eating this way. Thanks to this program, I don't think I've ever felt better in my life."

Subject: GIB
Age: 60
Height: 6 feet
Weight Lost: 40 pounds (250 to 210 so far)
Waist Change: 48 to 40
Special Benefit: *Blood Pressure – 160 over 105 to 128 over 84!*

Gib's History: Through most of his life, Gib gave no thought to what he ate. He loved sweets and never exercised.

Gib's Challenge: He was chronically tired (from the extra weight), and he could never rest well.

Gib's Solution: Fortunately, Gib had never considered dieting or any other ineffective solution.

The LEAN & FREE Solution: "I've been following this program for only five months, and I'm thrilled with how I've changed. Now I walk for sixty to seventy minutes three to four days a week, up and down the hills in my neighborhood, and I absolutely love it.

"My wife does a wonderful job with her delicious new recipes. I always eat until I'm full, then eat her wonderful desserts afterward. We are both aware of fat grams and know how to read labels. My wife is doing very well too. Her skin and hair look very healthy and nice. She is losing weight more slowly than I, probably because she is a former dieter.

"However, I must confess that my wife deserves all the credit for my success. She did all the reading, studying, and cooking surrounding this program. All I had to do was follow along. I'm retired, and it's just wonderful to feel so good. I have a very large frame, and I'm six feet tall. I think my ideal weight will be around 190 pounds, but I don't care how much I weigh as long as I look and feel so good.

"I might mention that I sure enjoy the freedom of not having to be perfect. I went on vacation, ate lots of junk food, and didn't exercise. I gained only about three pounds. As soon as I got home and tuned up my habits, I lost those three pounds in a week.

"My thirty-year-old son, who is widowed with three children, is also doing this program. He has dropped fifteen pounds and several inches, has much more energy, and is feeling much less stress."

Subject: CHARLENE
Age: 37
Height: 5 feet 9 inches
Weight Lost: 126 pounds (266 to 140)
Size Change:
Body Fat: 77% to 14%
Cholesterol: Down 105 points
Special Benefit: *No more problems with bulimia.*

Charlene's History: In high school Charlene weighed 180 pounds and dieted constantly. Once she lost 25 pounds in one week by abstaining from food and drinking only water and diet pop. Then she was scared, embarrassed, and totally amazed when she gained back the 25 pounds in about ten days. She says: "When I was dieting I felt crabby and awful all the time. I was always mad at myself and other people around me."

Charlene weighed 160 pounds when she got married, had eight children in twelve years, and gained extra weight with each child by dieting between each pregnancy.

Charlene's Challenge: Determining what to eat. "After a while, I couldn't even lose weight on an 800-calorie diet when I never cheated," she says.

Charlene's Solution: "I finally got so angry with my fat body that I'd make a chocolate cake and eat the whole thing, one piece at a time. Then I'd make cookies and eat the whole batch myself. Then I'd make myself throw up. Even though I kept throwing up for several years, I kept gaining weight. I started having severe heartburn regularly, and I got a bad hernia."

The LEAN & FREE Solution: "I've dropped from 266 pounds to 140. I love to eat, and I never crave sweets even though I eat them for dessert (after full satisfaction, of course). I've learned to nurture and love my body, and loving it has helped me feel wonderful. I don't feel angry with myself or other people. I'm so much nicer and calmer, and I really like myself.

"I save a bundle on doctor bills. I've dropped 105 points on my cholesterol (in addition to losing 126 pounds) in eighteen months, and I've been there for four years now. My husband has lost 100 pounds and looks and feels really great. He loves to eat a lot too.

184

"Oh, did I mention I'm expecting my ninth child in about three weeks? This time I've gained only 33 pounds instead of 60. I can't tell you how thrilled I am that something really works for me and my whole family."

Subject: GERALDINE
Age: 47
Height: 5 feet 5 inches
Weight Lost: 30 pounds
Size Change: 14 to 6
Special Benefit: *Loves vacationing now!*

Geraldine's History: Geraldine was always fairly trim until she reached age forty. Then she gradually began to put on weight. About five years ago she and her husband decided to go on a Caribbean cruise, and she got serious about losing weight. "I went to a quick weight-loss program, ate their small packaged foods, and was really hungry. My metabolism slowed down. I lost eighteen pounds the first month, eight pounds, the second month, and four pounds the third. This didn't make sense because I was doing the exact same thing each month. By the way, I spent almost $1,400 to lose thirty pounds. When I went on the ten-day cruise, I ate very little of the wonderful food available, and gained eighteen of the thirty pounds back."

Geraldine's Challenge: Geraldine needed to overcome and resolve her anger while also finding a permanent solution to her weight problem. "I was so angry, angry at myself for being so helpless, angry at the diet people for all the money I wasted, and angry at life for being so unfair and not allowing me to eat. Then I proceeded to put on seventeen more pounds over the next few months."

The LEAN & FREE Solution: "A year later I discovered Dana's program. I dropped thirty pounds in nine months instead of three. My face and neck aren't skinny at all, and I just love to eat. I think it's interesting that I weigh five pounds more now at a size 6 than I did when I was a size 10 after my diet. I have so much more energy, and I love to eat.

"Not only have I been a solid size 6 for three years, but a few months ago my husband and I went on another cruise. This time I ate about five times more food than the last time, and I wore my size-6 pants both on and off the cruise ship. When I got home I had gained only two pounds, and I lost them within a week. It's wonderful to party and vacation and eat whatever you want and stay a size 6.

"I exercise only three days a week now for an hour. I did six days while I was losing. I just love not having to be a perfect eater to stay lean. My friends can't believe all the good foods and desserts I eat."

185

Subject: JULIA
Age: 36
Height: 5 feet 8 inches
Weight Lost: 92 pounds (230 to 138)
Size Change: 28 to 10
Special Benefit: *No longer needs blood-pressure medication.*

Julia's History: Through grade school, junior high, and high school, Julia was heavier than the other children and the subject of cruel name calling. She survived because she had supportive parents who worked hard to build her self-esteem. During her senior year in high school, she lost 30 pounds and then gained it right back, eating lots of candy. She was the epitome of a yo-yo dieter. Once she lost 50 pounds over two years only to regain every pound and more. "With my first baby I gained to 160 pounds. Later, after I had gained even more weight, I lost 80 pounds, only to put it back on and more."

Julia's Challenge: Kicking the yo-yo diet habit and freeing herself of that excess fat. "After five babies and numerous diets, my body had taken so much abuse that my weight just kept going up and up."

The LEAN & FREE Solution: "About two years ago, a girl friend of mine told me about Dana's program. I was so excited I got the whole family in on it. I knew I had finally found the right, common-sense way of life. As I followed the plan, my cravings for sweets completely left. Now I love whole-grain breads and cereals. I used to be a complete chocoholic. Now people don't believe me when I tell them I haven't had any sweets for many months — not because I can't; I can, but I really don't want them at all.

"I now have bundles of excess energy. I race walk for fifty minutes at five o'clock every morning. Then I use my stair climber for fifteen minutes. Emotionally this program is so satisfying and peaceful. I never eat something different than my kids. I'm completely off my blood-pressure medication. My blood pressure was 148 over 100; now it's 98 over 70. My kids love this program too. They even eat kidney and garbanzo beans like they were popcorn.

"I'm saving a ton of money on food because I buy my grains and beans in bulk quantities. Diets don't teach you to eat; they just want you to buy their high-priced foods. I eat real food now, and I will for the rest of my life. I'd feel so empty every time I'd finish a diet, not just physically but emotionally, that I used to suffer from severe depression. Now I'm completely satisfied. I know food was meant to be eaten and I was meant to eat it. I feel contentment. I have hope, energy, and excitement for life. I no longer feel panic stricken or obsessed with food because I know I can have all I want. Since I dropped from a size 28 to a size 10, I'm actually pretty cute, and I have a wonderful new life."

Subject: JOSEPH
Age: 47
Height: 5 feet 11 inches
Weight Lost: 77 pounds (272 to 195)
Waist Size Change: 52 to 38
Special Benefit: *Diabetes is under control.*

Joseph's History: Years of misguided eating habits and a lack of consistent exercise had left Joseph overly-fat, out of condition, and extremely concerned about a worsening case of diabetes.

Joseph's Challenge: Find a program that would help him improve his physical condition and control his diabetes.

The LEAN & FREE Solution: "When I started Dana's program I began exercising three days a week. I kept it very low impact and simply walked through the aerobic dance movements at first.

"Now I've been doing this for nine months, and I've already lost my stomach, seventy-seven pounds, and my taste for sweets. My doctor is thrilled with my progress. He's got me down to one-fourth the amount of insulin I used to depend on. I can move much better, and I feel more successful about my whole life. Thanks to this program, I really feel great."

Subject: CORINE
Age: 39
Height: 5 feet 5 inches
Weight Lost: *25 pounds (207 to 182 so far)*
Special Benefit: *Children are also losing body fat.*

Corine's History: During high school, Corine's weight rose from 140 to 180 pounds. Her mother, who was 100 pounds overweight, wouldn't let her diet because Corine's fat was insurance that she wouldn't get involved with boys. "We always had cookies, cakes, and sweet rolls around. The more I ate, the better my mom and I got along." During college, Corine's weight dropped to 140. Along with the weight loss, she got attention from boys, got married, and had a daughter.

"After the birth of my daughter, my yo-yo life really started. I weighed 160 pounds before and after her birth. Then I went to Weight Watchers and got down to 120 pounds. During this time my mother accused me of being a sex symbol for my husband. When I went to her house, she wouldn't cook food I could eat, so I wouldn't eat. We did not get along.

"After the birth of my second child, I weighed 165. I couldn't get back with the Weight Watchers program. I tried shots and diet pills, but I didn't lose weight until I (unexplainably) dropped to 140 after my divorce.

"When I married the second time, I weighed 136, and my husband thought I was fat. I went to the Weight Loss Clinic and lost 20 pounds in six weeks. I'm 5-feet-5, and I had to keep my weight under 120 to be the size I wanted, about a 9. I was small on top with a normal bottom. My face and neck looked hollow. People asked me if I'd been sick. The thinner I got, the fatter I thought I was. I went on liquid diets. I got my weight down to 107. I wouldn't (couldn't) exercise. I wouldn't eat for days, and when I did, I would make myself throw up. I would go to bed hungry. I would not eat after 5:00 p.m. I kept my weight down for a couple of years doing this. If I did eat, I would cook two meals, one for me and one for my family.

"During this time I had bladder infections and strep throat. Sex was impossible. Slowly my weight crept back to 130. After a change from a physically active job to a desk job, my weight went up to 170. During this time I went back to Weight Watchers, tried Diet Center, NutriSystem, everything. After being married seven years, my second husband and I decided to have children. This time (my third child) I delivered at 196 pounds.

"I went back to my Diet Center Program and added exercise. I didn't have to worry about being interrupted because I was so mean that my kids were afraid to bother me during my hour of torture. I was miserable, and I let everyone know it. I got my weight down to 150 and joined Celestial Bodies. I got my weight down to 135, and my husband thought I looked great.

"Then we decided to have our second child (my fourth). I stopped worrying about what I ate and gained fifty pounds by the time I got pregnant. I was 217 pounds when I delivered."

Corine's Challenge: Finding a program that worked. Each former diet had encouraged her body to create an even more efficient fat-storing metabolism.

The LEAN & FREE Solution: "When I heard about your program, I weighed 207. Now after five months of eating well, I weigh 182, and my life is totally changed because I finally understand how my body works, what I should eat, and why. With this program it was easy to make a commitment and stay with it. I am never hungry, my energy increases daily, I am less tired, and now my kids love to be around me. I eat what I want and when I want. I exercise for an hour a day and really enjoy it. For the first time in my life, I feel I have a good relationship with food. I enjoy eating, and I eat plenty. And just as important, I am able to serve those around me instead of being consumed by my own problems. My son has lost six pounds, and my oldest daughter has come down from a size 18 to a size 13. She rides her bike for exercise, and I am encouraging her to eat properly.

"Your program has been the answer to my prayers, and praying is something I do not normally do."

Subject: MARSHA
Age: 51
Height: 5 feet 6 inches
Weight Lost: 50 pounds (size 24 to size 14)
Special Benefit: *No more cravings! Single: almost never cooks.*

Marsha's History: As a youngster, Marsha and her sister always ate the same foods, but she was "chunky" while her sister stayed thin. In high school, Marsha was about twenty pounds overly fat, and after high school she continually fluctuated between 130 and 160 pounds.

Marsha's Challenge: How to maintain a stable weight.

Marsha's Solution: Marsha felt she had tried everything. She tried the ice cream diet, the grapefruit and egg diet, the "only water and diet drinks" diet, and more. Then she tried what she called "a real winner" :

"I would fast for ten days, then eat for two or three days, then fast for ten days again."

One day in a movie theater, Marsha thought the picture went dark gray. Then later, when driving home, everything went dark gray again. She stopped the car and had her friend drive her home. When she consulted a doctor, he told her that extreme dieting will affect the most vulnerable part of the body. In her case, it was her eyes. After that experience, Marsha didn't resort to extreme fad diets anymore. However, she did lose 75 pounds on Weight Watchers, only to regain it later. And she experimented with a self-designed 1,200 calorie diet in which she also lost and regained weight. Wisely, she quit dieting altogether about ten years ago.

The LEAN & FREE Solution: "I guess not dieting for a long time converted my body from fat-storing to weight stable, because when I started following Dana's program eight months ago, fat loss wasn't slow for me at all. I've already dropped 50 pounds, and I'm down to 20 percent body fat. My size (14) is smaller than I've ever been at this weight, and my cholesterol has dropped from 220 to 140. I used to be a size 24.

"People constantly tell me how pretty I look. I have a wonderful complexion, and my face and neck aren't dry like they used to be when I dieted. And the best thing about this program is that I don't crave sweets because my body isn't looking for quick energy.

"I'm single and I don't like to take time to cook for myself, so I eat lots of very simple things like wheat-free spaghetti (I'm allergic to wheat), brown rice, canned chicken or tuna, sandwiches made with corn tortillas rolled up, lots of mixed vegetables (frozen), baked potatoes, halibut, cold cereal, and foot-long sandwiches on wheat-free bread. I also love my walking and aerobics five or six days a week. When I used to exercise, I felt very weak. Now I exercise, eat a lot, and feel a great increase in endurance. This is really fun. Even my legs and feet don't ache anymore."

Subject: ARDITH
Age: 57
Height: 5 feet 7 1/2 inches
Weight Lost: 38 pounds (183 to 145)
                18 to 10
Body Fat: 35% to 20%
Special Benefit: *The entire family eats the same delicious, healthy food.*

Ardith's History: Before Ardith had her children, she weighed about 118 pounds. She had always had a hearty appetite and came from a family where the women were excellent cooks and everyone enjoyed eating. While her family members tended to be tall and lean, her husband's family was short and stocky. It was her husband who became concerned about the quantities she ate, so she began to cut back. When she had children, she gained weight with each baby, until finally she had a weight problem. Then as a grandmother her weight problem persisted.

Ardith's Challenge: How to reclaim her naturally lean self and satisfy her family as well.

Ardith's Solution: Two years ago, Ardith started eating packaged diet products and lost thirty-seven pounds and twenty-six inches. But these products were expensive, they reduced her energy level, and they weren't something the whole family could use. She felt guilty about the expense of her food, particularly since it wasn't benefiting the family. She tried other diets but kept gaining weight. Finally, because of her weight and lack of optimal calories and nutrition, her knees and feet became so sore she couldn't continue her walking program. She went to a foot specialist and was treated with injections, but nothing worked. She was simply too heavy for her frame. She was hungry all the time and very shaky. And she was afraid to cook any of the foods she liked because she feared that if she ate them they would make her fat.

The LEAN & FREE Solution: "Once I was introduced to this program, my husband said, 'Honey, this is just what we've been looking for.' And it has been. I started eating lots of good food, and now I have the energy to do what I need to do in my life. In the first three weeks I lost eight inches, never to be found again. I have introduced the program to my daughters, and my oldest daughter, who is now expecting her third baby, had lost eight pounds. Now I can feed my family good, healthy food. I can cook and I can eat too. I tell everyone who tells me I look great about this program. I feel like I was let out of prison."

Subject: CLARISE
Age: 36
Height: 5 feet 3 inches
Weight Lost: 25 pounds (so far)
Size Change: 24 to 18
Special Benefits: *Headaches, fatigue, depression, and diabetic symptoms have subsided.*

Clarise's History: Not too long ago, Clarise suffered from mental, physical, and emotional problems. She had many symptoms of diabetes, which seriously frightened her. She had unexplained headaches and fatigue and was plagued with monthly bouts of PMS. She was depressed, she didn't like herself, and she was angry. She found herself yelling at her children, whom she loved dearly.

Clarise's Challenge: She was overweight, unhappy, and extremely unhealthy. She needed to make a profound change in her life.

The LEAN & FREE Solution: "THE LEAN & FREE program has changed my life. All symptoms of diabetes have disappeared totally. I have much more energy, and I cannot remember when I last had a headache. These improvements in my life are great, but they are only part of the benefits. The best thing is that I like myself now. I no longer call myself fat. I have learned to love and nurture my body. I never tell myself that I am a failure. If I falter I don't give up. I have gained quite a bit of patience, and my whole family is much happier because of it. Additionally, I've lost twenty-five pounds and reduced my pants size from 24 to 18. I know I'm just going to keep losing on this wonderful program."

Subject: KARLA
Age: 33
Height: 5 feet 2 inches
Size Change: 16 to 5
Special Benefits: *Bulimic tendencies and depression have subsided.*

Karla's History: Karla has battled a weight problem all her life. In the third grade she was one pound from being the heaviest child in her class. Her embarrassment at this was exacerbated when her teacher once yelled out each student's weight. At twelve, her mother enrolled her in a spa, where, unfortunately, she learned to diet. At that time, she weighed 130 pounds and was five feet tall. By age eighteen, Karla, now 5-feet-2 and an experienced dieter, weighed 172 pounds. While in college, she got involved in another spa and was put on a 500-calorie diet while working out four to six hours a day. She got her weight down to between 98 and 103 pounds but was tired and constantly sick with strep throat and canker sores. Later she gained to 110 pounds, and her mother took her to a doctor. He put her on diet pills and vitamin shots. The doctor prescribed a stronger dose of diet pills each week, and her weight dropped to 98 pounds, but the medication disrupted her sleep pattern; she went three weeks without sleeping more than one hour per night. Finally, Karla quit the spa and ballooned again to 170 pounds. She continued to diet through her marriage and two babies. Finally, after her third baby, the weight wouldn't budge, even though she was exercising two hours a day and starving herself.

Karla's Challenge: Find an alternative to diets that would provide permanent fat loss while also improving her health.

Karla's Solutions: Karla watched a television show on bulimia and started to drink Ipecac. After two months of throwing up, she was weak, ill, and very depressed. This dark secret was a horrible nightmare.

The LEAN & FREE Solution: "Dana's program was just like the lights going on. The neatest thing about the program was that it took the guilt away. For the first time in my life I knew that being fat was not my fault. I was so excited, I read Dana's materials in one night. I told my husband everything and began. When I sat down to eat, he said, 'Is this what you're going to eat for the next two weeks?' I answered, 'No, this is just one meal.' Now he loves to take me out to eat with friends just to show off how much his size-5 wife can eat.

"Now I'm six months pregnant with my fourth baby, I wear a size 7 in maternity clothes, and this time the weight is only in my tummy. I have no problems with my back, and I can't tell you the last time I was sick. I have dropped from a size 16 pant to a size 5 when I'm not pregnant. My husband, who is a diabetic, now takes half the insulin he used to take thanks to our new eating habits. Now we can eat the same things together, and we're almost never sick. It is so neat to feel free to eat."

Subject: PATTY
Age: 55
Height: 5 feet 7 inches
Weight Lost: 48 pounds (168 to 120)
Size Change: 18 to 8
Body Fat: 31% to 23%
Special Benefit: *Weakness and virtual paralysis have subsided.*

Patty's History: When Patty was sixteen she couldn't buy a formal because, she says, "the lady said they didn't make it in my size." By age thirty-five Patty was in terrible condition. She had tried every diet. Once she lost thirty pounds in six weeks only to gain back forty in the next five weeks. She went to a doctor, spent $1,000 on tests, and found no solution. He just sent her home. She was extremely weak, could hardly walk, and was virtually paralyzed.

Patty's Challenge: Patty needed guidance and correct information about her body. When she couldn't find outside help, she turned to her own solutions.

Patty's Solution: She completely eliminated sugar, white flour, and red meat from her diet. She began eating more vegetables and grains. Seven months later, with the use of a cane, she was able to help at a girl's camp. A year later, her husband was able to buy her a size 10 coat, down from size 18. Her program was working, but she wavered from time to time because she didn't fully understand what was happening to her body.

The LEAN & FREE Solution: "Dana's program is similar to what I had been doing except that it really tightened up my habits. I increased my exercise from fifteen minutes to thirty minutes, cut out diet drinks, ate even more vegetables, and drank more water. I followed the success plans very faithfully, and I dropped from a size 10 to a size 8 in nine weeks. It blew my mind because I'd been a solid 10 for fifteen years. The freedom this program gives me makes me ecstatic. Even on vacation I gain only one or two pounds. Now that I know how to cook good foods, everyone loves my cooking. My three-year-old grandson always wants more. A wellness test I took recently said I was three years younger physically than my real age of fifty-five."

Subject: LISA
Age: 26
Height: 5 feet 4 inches
Weight Lost: 10 pounds (140 to 130)
Size Change: 14 to 4-5
Special Benefit: *Problems with anorexia and bulimia have subsided.*

Lisa's History: Lisa grew up the oldest of five children, a skinny kid in a skinny family. Weight wasn't a concern until she reached age fifteeen and got a job in a candy store. Then she expanded from a size 4 (108 pounds) to a size 14 (138 pounds). Since she was on several dance teams and couldn't bear the thought of dancing in front of her peers looking so fat, she began to diet. She dieted until she weighed eighty-seven pounds and wore a size 0. Through college she counted every calorie. She lived on diet colas, raw vegetables, and candy. She began to force herself to throw up any time she ate more than 600 calories per day. This anorexic/bulimic behavior continued for several years. Her life revolved around her weight, her size, calories, and food. She would go to the library for eight-hour study marathons, thinking that her studies would keep her mind off food. She resented eating and was angry at anyone who tried to force her to eat. She exercised every spare moment and even studied while exercising on a mini-tramp. Finally, her toes became so depleted from over-exercising that they split. She had to have bone chips grafted from her ankle to repair the damage. After Lisa married, she was told by doctors that she would never be able to have children. Her extreme dieting and exercise habits interfered with normal menstruation; she hadn't had a menstrual period in four years. She began to take a variety of fertility tests but also continued to diet and exercise. In spite of her regimen, she began to gain weight again. Finally her weight crept up to 140 pounds, and she was once again a size 14.

Lisa's Challenge: Lisa's lifelong approach to weight management through dieting, exercise, anorexia, and bulimia was destroying her health and happiness. And she was extremely frustrated and upset by the possibility that she might not be able to have children.

The LEAN & FREE Solution: "When I discovered Dana's program, I knew it was the answer to being truly happy, healthy, and permanently lean. I jumped right in and never looked back. Three months later I could not see a difference in my size so my enthusiasm for the program wavered just a little. Then I got the wonderful news: I was pregnant! To me it was the greatest thing I could ask for. At that point I began to eat to nourish the little one instead of worrying about how soon I could lose inches. As long as I ate well and exercised regularly, I felt great.

Eight months later, I had a beautiful baby boy in only an hour and a half of labor. I lost about a size a month after Jamison was born, and I was feeling great. My weird and destructive eating and exercise habits were gone. I lost to about a size 8; then I got stuck. I was starting to get frustrated just when I learned I was pregnant again. My husband joked that this program should be called 'Eat and get pregnant.' Eight months later I had a beautiful baby girl.

"I cannot describe well enough the incredible changes that have occurred in my life because of Dana's program. I often look back and wonder if that sickly 90-pound fanatic was really me. My life is so full and meaningful. Very rarely do I spend time thinking about food, weight, calories, or size. I love to tell people I wear a size 4-5, weigh 130 pounds, and eat more than 3,000 calories a day, then watch their eyes pop out." (Remember, at that same weight, Lisa was once a size 12.)

Subject: LAURA
Age: 36
Height: 5 feet 6 inches
Weight Lost: 32 pounds (189 to 157 so far)
Size Change: 22 to 14 (in four months)
Special Benefits: *No more flu-like feelings; more patient as a mother.*

Laura's History: Until she began having children, Laura had no problem with her weight. By the time she was pregnant with her third child, her weight had risen from 128 to 155 pounds. When she found out she was pregnant with her fourth child, she weighed 178 pounds. She had not seriously pursued diets during these years, although she had tried a few programs that were ineffective. Embarrassed by her size, Laura began to withdraw from life. She didn't want to see anyone, and she didn't want anyone to see her. She and her husband did go to Hawaii, their first trip together in thirteen years. She was a size 22, weighed 189 pounds, and was too humiliated to fully enjoy herself. Her enjoyment was further hampered by intense headaches and frequent flu-like feelings. Laura vowed never to be that weight again, and she longed to feel healthy and well.

Laura's Challenge: Find a program that would help her regain her self-esteem and offer a common-sense approach to excess fat loss and health.

The Lean & Free Solution: "This program seemed to fit right into what I thought I should be doing. I dropped thirty-two pounds and twenty inches. I feel like I have not only learned to eat but also to be drug free. I haven't had any Elavil (medication for headaches) since March. The headaches, which are now seldom, are not often intense. I take only an occasional Advil three times a month. The flu feelings are gone, and I have more energy than I've had in ten years. Everyone I know comments on my weight loss. When they ask how I did it, I tell them I'm eating and exercising and enjoy it. I do aerobic dance or Nordic Track for one hour each day. My family loves the new meals, and I feel I am a kinder, more patient mother now because I feel better. My weight's on its way down and I'm on my way up. I'm not at all reclusive now. I'm so excited! I love it. This is the way you're supposed to eat and live."

SPECIAL CASES
(Significant Health Changes)

Subject: JOHN
Age: 6
Special Benefit: *Constipation has subsided.*

John's Story (in the words of his mother, Mary): "One year ago my six-year-old son, John, was diagnosed with encopresis, a severe form of constipation. He suffered from severe stomach cramps, bleeding in his stools, and, worst of all, partial loss of control of his bowel movements.

"John's condition led to great frustration and anxiety on the part of not only John but also our whole family. Doctors and specialists put him on mineral oil and encouraged him to eat a high-fiber and low-sugar diet. But how? I struggled for a year on my own and became very frustrated. Then I found this program and put him and myself on it. To my complete delight, one week later he was totally free from any sign of the disease. No follow-up was necessary with specialists, and he was able to start first grade as a normal child.

"I can't express to you the joy we feel or the great happiness my son feels. The sparkle is back in his eyes, and he's healthy and very happy."

Subject: KYLE
Age: 64
Special Benefits: *Blood Pressure and cholesterol are excellent.*

Kyle's Story: "I had dieted for fifty years, losing and regaining up to 600 pounds before discovering the principles of this program. I'm thrilled to tell you that as a result of living these principles, I've lost the last seventy pounds of my 600 excess pounds and have kept it off for four years.

"Best of all, at age sixty-four, my blood pressure is 108 over 64, my pulse rate is 59, and my cholesterol level is 157. Don't wait sixty years like I did before you apply this wonderful information to your life!"

Subject: CARY
Age: 26
Special Benefits: *No more bloating, depression, or hay fever.*

Cary's Story: "I had suffered from extreme bloating every day from 1:00 p.m. on, during the past three years. I've been on this program only eleven weeks; my bloating is gone and my depression is lifted. I am also not suffering from bad hay fever, which amazes me.

"I have triple the energy, I've lost inches, and for the first time in five years, I like myself again. I'm excited about my life and my future. Thank you!"

Subject: JANET
Age: 67
Special Benefits: *Cholesterol—293 to 210 so far (in two months).*

Janet's Story: "I've always taken care of myself, and my husband doesn't. But when we got our cholesterol checked, his was normal and mine was 293. Talk about unfair.

"Well, the doctor told me to increase my fiber and my exercise and decrease my fat. I did all that and more, but six months later my cholesterol had gone up six points.

"Then, I heard about Dana's program. It's been only two months since then, and my cholesterol is already down to 210. This program is simple, common sense. It rings true. It works. Life isn't fair, as you can see in the case of my husband and me. But this program helps even it out. By the way, I've never been overweight."

Subject: TONI
Age: 29
Special Benefit: *Enjoyed a wonderful pregnancy!*

Toni's Story: "I started this program when I was four months pregnant. I ate lots of great food and lost inches—while I was pregnant. Lots of people commented on how much thinner I looked in my hips, face, and arms when I was seven to nine months pregnant.

"I've just had the baby. I was back in "pre-pregnancy clothes" within a week.

197

By two weeks I was even wearing clothes I couldn't wear last winter because they were too tight. At my two-week checkup, I was fifteen pounds lighter than when I got pregnant. These changes in my body are entirely from changes in my eating. I have not changed my exercise routine."

Subjects: CURT and GREG
Ages: 17 and 15 (respectively)
Weight Lost: Curt, 25 pounds; Greg, 20 pounds
Special Situation: *Olympic swimming contenders!*

Curt and Greg's Story: "I'm seventeen years old and I'm working toward qualifying for the Olympics in swimming. Two years ago my fifteen-year-old brother, Greg, and I were struggling with too much extra body fat that was slowing us down a lot when we swam. My grandma began following Dana's program and was so excited about her health changes—no more depression, weight and size loss— that she talked about the program all the time.

"Greg and I started eating about twice as much food and less meat and fat, and in two weeks we had both lost two inches in the waist and significantly decreased our swimming times. I've lost twenty-five pounds and Greg has lost twenty, and neither of us was fat to start with.

"I eat whatever I want. I like whole-wheat breads, muffins, and cereals and lots of pasta and beans. I love pizza and Mexican food. I also love desserts, but I don't eat sweets when I'm hungry. They make me sick. I'm sure I eat more than 5,000 calories a day, including 100 to 150 fat grams. My endurance is greatly improved along with my speed. My whole family loves not having to worry about calories anymore. My mom's a great cook, and my friends love to eat at our house. They think it's great we all eat together and that we all eat the same things. And they can't believe how much our family eats and stays so thin."

Subject: MELLY
Age: 54
Height: 5 feet 2 inches
Weight Lost: 8 pounds (118 to 110)
Size Change: 8 to 4-6
Special Benefits: *Energy and sense of well-being have greatly increased.*

Melly's History: Ever since she was a teenager, Melly stayed thin by cutting back on what she ate (dieting) and exercising (when she had time). She virtually starved herself to lose weight and keep it off—usually eating fewer than 800 calories a day.

Melly's Challenge: She never achieved a sense of well-being or vitality no matter how much or how little she weighed.

The LEAN & FREE Solution: "I eat loads of food, good healthy food, and I feel so much better and look better too. I actually wear a smaller size (4 or 6, depending on the clothes) than I did when I was dieting. I know what Dana says is true because all the good things that are promised in this program have happened to me. The first thing I noticed was that I felt so good. I gained four pounds at first (as Dana said I might), but I knew I wasn't going to give up because I felt so good. After four months I lost those four pounds and more. I really enjoy walking and aerobic exercise. I like to alternate them. I tell everyone about this wonderful program. If we would raise our children eating like this, wouldn't we be doing a wonderful thing for them? I'm slimmer and trimmer than I've been since I was a teenager, and I've never eaten so much before—ever."

Subject: RENEE
Age: 64
Height: 4 feet 11 inches
Size Change: 16 to 12
Special Benefit: *Enjoys being an energetic grandma!*

Renee's History: Renee has never been a dieter. She loves being a grandmother and had never really concerned herself about body fat until she noticed one day that she was becoming a very "round" grandmother.

Renee's Challenge: Since she wasn't a dieter, Renee wanted to know how she could still eat all she wanted and lose weight. "I hate being hungry," she says. "It makes me really cross."

The LEAN & FREE Solution: "Ever since I discovered this program, I've been shrinking. I eat five or six times a day and a lot more cereals and breads and soups and stews and fruit. I've found I really like to eat. I'm also doing aerobics and walking. It's a lot of fun, and I've become a pretty spunky grandma. I'm not going to let myself get old. I don't need to. I've got a good body and now, thanks to the knowledge I've gained in this program, I know how to take care of it and not let it get fat or too skinny and wrinkly. I look and feel just about right."

Subject: BETTY
Age: 42
Height: 5 feet 6 inches
Weight Lost: 10 pounds (156-146)
Size Change: 18 to 8
Body Fat: 32% to 19%
Special Benefit: *Stomach has flattened.*

Betty's History: Betty had never been much of a dieter or meal skipper, but after six pregnancies in ten years, she had lost the muscle tone in her stomach. "My back hurt, and I looked five months pregnant all the time. People asked me when my baby was due."

Betty's Challenge: "I was embarrassed by how I looked and by people thinking I was pregnant. And when I told them I wasn't pregnant, they were embarrassed too. I needed to find a way to strengthen my stomach and to improve my overall conditioning."

The LEAN & FREE Solution: "Now I do sixty minutes of aerobics or forty minutes of Nordic Track faithfully six days a week. I probably eat twice as much as before. I have desserts three or four times a week, and I can't believe I've lost so much because I'm not a perfect eater — about a "B" on my success sheets. My stomach looks much flatter, and I've lost five sizes (18 to 8) and only ten pounds. I absolutely love being lean and free."

Subject: KENT
Age: 52
Height: 6 feet
Weight Lost: 71 pounds (236-165)
Waist Change: 47 to 34
Body Fat: 34% to 9%
Special Benefit: *Cholesterol—166 down to 120; HDL: 33 to 48; LDL: 107 to 70*

Kent's History: Although Kent had a long history of being overly fat, he resisted diets because he instinctively knew they were not the answer to permanent fat control. Finally, though, he reached complete exasperation with his weight. "I had no energy, my clothes were tight, I couldn't go skiing and enjoy it, and besides, I didn't like the way I looked and felt. Something was definitely going to have to change."

Kent's Challenge: He knew that exercise affected fat and weight, but he wasn't sure how or why. Several years earlier he had exercised on a mini-trampoline for forty-five minutes per day. "I didn't lose weight, but I felt really good, and I didn't gain any either. For some reason I quit using the mini-trampoline and, over a period of years, my weight increased." Kent needed to increase his awareness of the benefits of exercise and the relationship between exercise and fat so he could establish an effective and committed exercise program.

The LEAN & FREE Solution: "I discovered this program, bought a Nordic Track, and changed my eating patterns, and today I am running 10K (6.2 mile) races and feel great. I've even won some ribbons for best in my age group. As my aerobic exercise continued to build, my body became an even better fat-burner. My weight dropped to 170 pounds, then stabilized between 165 and 168 pounds. I feel the key is persistence and doing the right things. I have consistently eaten the right foods and have not restricted the amount I have eaten. My wife and I make our own bread and many special recipes.

"During one period of time, I worked preparing rich foods for a restaurant. The foods were high in fat and not conducive to weight management. I ate a lot of deep-fried and other high-fat foods because that was all that was available. This program taught me that once your body becomes a fat-burning machine, it can handle periods of time when you aren't eating good food. My experience at the restaurant proved it. My body fat did not change much at all. When I was able to return to correct eating, however, I definitely felt much better. Today my body fat is 9 percent. I've never felt better."

Subject: CLAIR
Age: 37
Height: 5 feet 4 inches
Size Lost: 12 to 5
Special Situation and Benefits: *Clair gained nineteen pounds and one size at first, while her high blood pressure, high cholesterol, chronic fatigue, and severe depression were alliviated.*

Clair's History: Clair was a "perfect" dieter for twenty years. She lived on two protein drinks and a small salad for four years. Eventually she was diagnosed with chronic fatigue syndrome and severe depression. She was on medication for high blood pressure and high cholesterol levels.

Clair's Challenge: "I thought I was going to die. I needed to find a solution to my health problems."

The LEAN & FREE Solution: "I immediately began eating *six times* more food than I had eaten in twenty years. (A much more gradual increase is highly recommended.) My chronic fatigue and depression were virtually nonexistent after only three months. After six months my doctor took me off of my high cholesterol and high blood pressure medications. I felt wonderful. I gained nineteen pounds, but I increased only one dress size. I looked in the mirror one day and realized how much better my body looked as a size 12. I'd lost most of that jiggly, cellulite look, and I looked at least seven or eight years younger. Even the lines under my eyes were almost gone." (Clair had gained approximately fifteen pounds of water as her body became fully hydrated, about two to three pounds of muscle, possibly a slight amount from increased bone mass, and about one to two pounds of fat). "I decided that being a size 12 would be fine. Then fourteen months into the program I dropped from a size 12 to a size 5 and lost twenty-three pounds in less than two months. I wear the same size clothes as my daughter who is on her college drill team. I'm healthy, have great energy, and have a very nice figure." (Note: Clair looks like a beautiful young woman in her middle 20's.)

Examine Clair's roller-coaster chart on the following page.

Clair experienced the "lose - maintain - gain" diet cycle as her metabolism continually adjusted to twenty years of dieting. Then she went through the LEAN & FREE 2000 PLUS metabolic process as her metabolism gradually geared back up and she became optimally healthy. (See comparison chart on page 204.) Clair's body chemistry changed from fat-storing, to neutral, and then to fat-burning. She then dropped twenty-three pounds and four dress sizes in two months. For the first time in many years, Clair became naturally lean, not starved skinny.

Subject: MARSHA
Age: 55
Height: 4 feet 11 inches
Weight Lost: 38 pounds
Size Lost: 20 to 12 (so far)
Special Benefit: *Diabetes is under control.*

Marsha's History: When Marsha was expecting her last baby twenty-six years ago, she developed headaches and would become shaky between meals or if she didn't eat on time. Medical tests indicated nothing unusual even though she occasionally had convulsions. She was given tranquilizers and psychiatric care, but both were ineffective. She found that if she ate more, she felt better and the

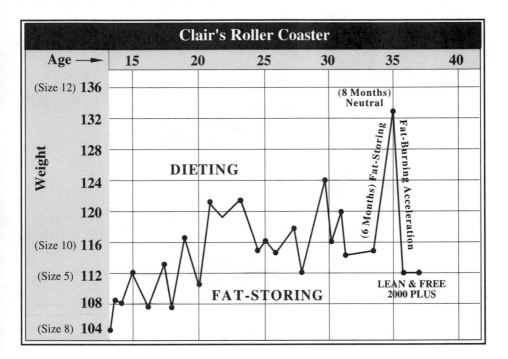

Clair's Roller Coaster

convulsions ceased. But when she ate more, weight became a problem. So she would diet, and the convulsions would recur. Finally she was diagnosed with hypoglycemia and was told to eat protein six times a day. This seemed to be a solution until, after a while, she began to gain even more weight.

Marsha's Challenge: Finding a solution to her health problems that did not promote excess fat gain.

Marsha's Solution: She tried liquid diets, no-carbohydrate diets, Weight Watchers, the American Heart Association diet, NutriSystem, the grapefruit diet, and so on. She says they nearly did her in. Then Marsha discovered she had developed diabetes, and she was put on a diabetic diet. She felt shaky and had "the sweats" all the time.

The LEAN & FREE Solution:"I lost thirty-eight pounds and felt like a happy, healthy person. I forced myself to exercise. All I did at first was five minutes on a stationary bike. Now I do forty minutes four or five days a week. My diabetes is now under control, and I'm down to a size 12 and want a size 8. I don't always eat correctly, and I still need to lose more, but I'm on the right track. I feel wonderful."

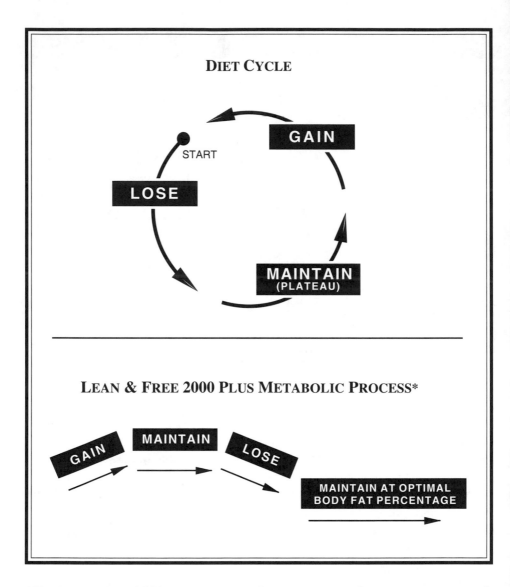

DIET CYCLE

LEAN & FREE 2000 PLUS METABOLIC PROCESS*

THE LEAN & FREE 2000 PLUS METABOLIC PROCESS occurs when a person is severely calorically or nutritionally starved. I gained seven pounds the first four months that I began to gradually increase my calories. I increased one inch in my waist and decreased one inch in my hips—just the opposite of dieting. Then I began to lose, and in one year's time, I decreased from a size 18 pant to a size 4 pant, and I've been size stable for more than eleven years, even when I don't eat perfectly! I can't tell you what an amazing relief it is to splurge now and then and not increase in pant size! And I don't look lined and shriveled in my face and neck.

Subject: LA RANE
Age: 41
Height: 5 feet 2 inches
Size Lost: Three dress sizes
Special Benefits: *Off of all medications and sleeps very well.*

La Rane's History: La Rane felt she had tried just about every diet available. She found them to be difficult and frustrating because none of them provided lasting success. In addition, she was taking several medications for a variety of ailments, including allergies. She felt terrible.

La Rane's Problem: Find a program that would enable her to control her fat while also feeling healthy and well.

The LEAN & FREE Solution: "I started this program, and within ten days I was off all medication, had good energy, slept well, had a good appetite, and felt wonderful. By taking a two-and-a-half mile walk every day and staying on the program, success, health, and well-being are mine. Thanks for a new way of life. I can't tell you how nice it is to finally feel good."

Subject: LILIAN
Age: 48
Height: 5 feet 6 inches
Weight Lost: 26 pounds (184 to 158)
Sizes Lost: 16 to 10
Special Benefit: *Cholesterol—299 to 222*

Lilian's History: Lilian was never what she describes as a "good dieter." She tried Dexatrim for a week, chewable tablets and diet drinks, and many other gimmicks and fads. No matter what she did, she gained fat. She hated to be hungry and would go from dieting to eating large orders of French fries and big juicy double cheeseburgers. She was eating two foot-long hot dogs and at least one or two candy bars almost every day.

Lilian's Challenge: She wanted a "program for life," not a diet. She had seen too many people get even bigger from dieting.

The LEAN & FREE Solution: "After the first three months following this program, my cholesterol dropped from 299 to 272, my body fat went from 32.8

percent down to 30.2 percent, and my size dropped from 16 to 14. In the next three months, my cholesterol dropped to 220, my body fat was 28.6 percent, my weight reduced to 158, and I became a terrific size 10. I feel so good. I haven't had a high-fat hot dog for ten months now, and I never will again. I went from eating 90 to 100 fat grams a day to around 45. I'm eating more now than I ever have before. Thank you again."

PIZZA AND ICE CREAM
WHY LEAN & FREE 2000 PLUS IS SO EASY TO LIVE

*G*iving up the foods you really like to eat has long been considered a prerequiste for losing excess body fat. But not on the LEAN & FREE 2000 PLUS LIFESTYLE.

This point is illustrated by a conversation between Kay, who has become lean and energetic by following the 2000 PLUS principles, and Robyn, who would like to be lean and free but fears she'll have to sacrifice too much.

ROBYN: "You look wonderful, Kay. I ought to follow your program too, but I just don't have time to cook special foods. And I hate "all natural" foods. I'm just not into that fat-free, no-sugar stuff. My favorite meal is pizza and ice cream. I guess I'm just destined to be fat because I don't have any willpower."

KAY: "It doesn't take willpower to be lean and free. All it takes is about five minutes of planning each day. Have you studied this program much?"

ROBYN: "Well, I haven't really had time to get into it yet."

KAY: "You'll be surprised and excited when you do. You don't give up the foods you love. You don't eat all fat-free, sugar-free foods. You won't believe the freedom. I eat out all the time, and I buy convenience foods, too! I follow the LEAN & FREE 2000 PLUS menus every day. Most of the meals take fifteen minutes or less to fix. Oh, I even go to parties quite often."

ROBYN: "Really? I didn't think you could do that and look like you do."

KAY: "You can. And I feel so much better too—I have a lot more energy than I ever had before. But I never deprive myself. Let's, for example, take your favorite meal—pizza and ice cream. I have two kinds of days when I eat pizza and ice cream—"A" days when I'm really into being perfect, and "B" days when I'm just maintaining or coasting along."

"On an A day, I buy whole-wheat hamburger buns, split them in half, and put canned pizza sauce, fresh mixed stir-fry vegetables (prepared in advance), and skim mozzarella cheese on top. Then I bake these pizza wheels at 400 degrees, and in just eight minutes they're ready. My family loves them. Then for ice cream, I blend frozen peaches with frozen peach-juice concentrate and skim or 1% milk. It makes the most delicious ice cream you've ever tasted. I eat at least four mini-pizzas along with a cup and a half of the "ice cream." When you add a glass of water, you have a completely balanced A+ meal of water, vegetable, grain, protein, and fruit all prepared in less than fifteen minutes.

ROBYN: "Sounds delicious, but what if I don't even have 15 minutes?"

KAY: "In that case, I order a plain cheese pizza and a pepperoni pizza (on the kids' request). I also order an all-vegetable-and-fruit pizza with tomatoes, onions, green peppers, mushrooms, pineapple, and just a few olives (I look on my fat-gram list for lower-fat pizzas). Before the pizza comes, I put a plate of mixed raw vegetables and lowfat dip on the table along with a pitcher of water. The whole family attacks the vegetables while the pizza is in transit. When the pizza arrives, I usually have two vegetable slices, one cheese slice, and one pepperoni slice along with some delicious fresh or canned fruit."

"Then for dessert I pull out the "premium lite ice milk." It has only eight fat grams per cup, and it tastes great—not like that icy, fat-free kind. I sometimes add a lowfat fudge topping. And there you have it—a great B meal with your favorite foods: pizza and ice cream."

ROBYN: "But what about the white flour in the pizza crust? What about the sugar in the ice cream? And the whole thing sounds like lots of fat and calories."

KAY: "That's what I love about this program—you don't have to be perfect. I don't lose fat on a B day like some people do (such as my husband), but I don't store excess fat either. I can even enjoy myself at a party where all the wrong food is served, because an occasional splurge doesn't set me back. It just means I coast a little. Anyway, when you've been lean and free as long as I have, you automatically select the best food available at parties and other events that serve rich food. And before I go to a party, I eat good foods at home until I'm satisfied. That way I never gorge on goodies, and those I do eat are not easily stored as fat because my blood sugar level isn't low. Also, the fats and sugars combine with the other, more complex foods I've eaten, which encourages much less fat storage. And I've eaten a lot to develop a "fat-burning" body, not starved to develop a "fat-storing" body.

ROBYN: "It's obvious I need to learn a lot more about this program. Right now I can't imagine how I can eat pizza and ice cream and still be successful. Will you help me Kay?

KAY: "Of course. I have so much extra energy. I'd just love to share what I've learned with you."

If you have a friend who has the mistaken notion that being lean and free is too hard or demanding, share with them some of the points that Kay made, or let them read this section in your book. It may open the door to a whole new life for them.

OVERCOMING YOUR FEAR OF EATING
THE MYTH OF FOOD ADDICTION

*T*here are people who, overwhelmed by the stress in their lives, resort to the abuse of substances such as alcohol, drugs, or food. But I feel that the vast majority of people who are being led to believe that they are "food addicts" are simply people who are victims of misinformation and ignorance about the essential needs and functions of the human body. Calling most people food addicts makes no more sense than calling them air or oxygen addicts; because, like oxygen, food is essential to life. You must eat and breathe to live.

To illustrate my point, there is a story I like to tell about a person I call "Joe." Joe is placed in a room where there is very little oxygen. Soon Joe becomes weak, light-headed, and lethargic. He continually gasps for air as though he is trying to consume all the oxygen in the room in one breath. (Joe seems downright "gluttonous" when it comes to air.)

Behind a one-way glass window sits an "air-addiction" expert named Kim who talks to Joe through an intercom. He suggests that since Joe is so desperate for air, he must have some type of unfulfilled need that he is trying to fulfill by hoarding oxygen. "Perhaps, Joe," Kim says, "you were an unloved child. Maybe you don't like yourself and you're trying to punish yourself by abusing air. Your chronic fatigue may actually be a manifestation of this self-hate and lack of confidence in yourself. Do you think that any of these psychological problems may be creating your oxygen addiction?"

Joe thinks for a minute as he slumps to the floor. "Well maybe you're right (pant, pant). I didn't ever feel I was popular in school (pant, pant). Maybe that did some permanent psychological damage that causes me to abuse oxygen (pant, pant)."

Kim then suggests some "behavior modification" techniques that may help cure Joe's psychological sickness. "First of all, Joe, I want you to breathe very slowly. Breathe in through your nose to the count of sixty and then exhale through your mouth. Do this for one hour. Then take a deep breath and wait twenty minutes before blowing it out. This will help send a message to your brain that you are getting enough oxygen. It will also teach you self-control. Do this twenty-minute breath-holding exercise at least three times per day."

Furthermore, he adds, "Being an 'air-addiction' expert, I have learned that addicts are more successful if they don't breathe at all after 6:00 P.M. This helps them to crave less air the next day.

"Finally, I want you to love yourself and speak kindly to yourself. Tell yourself that you don't need very much air and that you will be healthier without it. Tell yourself you have lots of energy and are always happy. Remind yourself that you are a real success and that you can do it. And reiterate to yourself that it is ridiculous, gluttonous, and wasteful to use up that much air."

"Thank you," Joe pants, "I know (pant) I can do it. I knew it must be psychological all the time (pant, pant). I'll try your 20-minute self-control, (pant) willpower exercise right now." Joe inhales deeply and holds his breath.

Kim walks down the hall. Then he remembers he has forgotten his briefcase and goes back to get it. He looks into Joe's room one more time, only to find him lying face down on the floor. "Darn," Kim exclaims. "Another failure. But I do succeed with one out of every 200 people I work with. That's pretty good you know."

Joe's survival system was screaming for air just as a dieter's survival system screams for food. Diet behavior modifications such as "put down your fork after each bite of food," "never eat after 6 p.m., " "leave the table slightly hungry and wait 20 minutes to let your brain register fullness," are all about as logical and effective as what you've just read. And, for most people, the term "food addiction" makes about as much sense as "air addiction". Without either, we simply die.

QUESTION: *I'm a diabetic. If I eat more calories from carbohydrates, won't this increase my blood-glucose level, causing me to need more insulin?*
ANSWER: *Write down exactly what you are eating right now on page 237 in this book. Then very gradually increase your calories and high-fiber complex carbo-hydrates over a period of months as you respond to your increase in hunger, muscle mass, and energy level. Work closely with your doctor to monitor your need for insulin and your increase in good food.*

Most diabetics notice a significant increase in their energy level as their excess body-fat and need for insulin markedly decrease. The American Diabetic Association recommends an increase in high-fiber foods (complex carbohy-drates), along with a moderate amount of fat and animal protein. They also recommend moderate exercise which can help to stabilize blood-sugar levels.

Make certain you are balancing your meals with all of the essential vitamins, minerals, and amino acids found in water, vegetables, grain, protein, and fruit. And completely avoid refined sugar and artificial sweeteners. Remember to eat fruit with your meals, not on an empty stomach. Enjoy concentrated fruit-juice sweetened desserts in moderation. You'll lose your sweet cravings and enjoy tremendously increased energy and sense of well-being, along with a lot less body fat.

OVERCOMING YOUR FEAR OF EATING
OVERCOMING ANOREXIA AND BULIMIA

*T*he age-old myth that the only way you can lose weight is by eating less is the myth that may now be directly responsible for thousands of cases of anorexia and bulimia throughout the world.

Too many people still think: "If I eat a little less I'll lose a little weight. If I eat nothing, I'll lose a lot of weight."

As you've learned in this program, these assumptions are completely false. By eating less, you can trigger your body's survival system to store fat to protect you from an impending famine. That's why most obese people eat much less than lean people and still continually get fatter.

I've seen anorexic women weighing as little as seventy pounds who were 30 percent body fat. They have skinny, withered, fat little bodies. Quite a contradiction, isn't it?

The survival systems of anorexia sufferers are literally screaming at them to eat. "Eat anything and everything," the survival system yells. "You're going to die!" Food becomes the focus of every thought; fat and sugar cravings become all consuming; life either revolves around the desire to eat or the total "avoidance" of the perceived enemy—food.

It's at this point that many people make the mistake of believing they can have the best of both worlds. They can eat what they want *and* stay thin, simply by purging themselves afterwards. Bulimics may eat enormous amounts of sweet and fatty foods, sometimes hundreds of dollars worth in a single day. Then they force themselves to throw up.

Jane states, "I became such an expert at throwing up that all I had to do was look at the toilet and it would trigger a purging response. I learned what foods to eat that I could easily throw up, and I got so I thought that no one would ever suspect. However, I did worry about the smell."

Jane was a perfectionist at home and at work. Everyone thought she was in complete control of her life. But she was entirely out of control. "I hated myself and my hidden secret," she says. "I felt so ashamed."

For those with eating disorders, it is a frightening task to relearn normal eating. "Eating was very difficult for me at first," Jane said. "I was really scared to eat and keep it down. Since I experienced no clear signals of hunger or fullness at first, I set up a time schedule and ate when the clock said eat—at 7:00 A.M., 12:30 P.M., and 6:00 P.M. for meals, and at 10:00 A.M., 3:30 P.M., and 9:30 p.m. for snacks.

After about a year and a half, Jane dropped from a size 16 to a size eight which she says, is smaller than she's ever been before. She looks and feels like a new person. She says, "I'm no longer haunted by my eating disorders because I know that eating a lot of healthy calories is making me lean and healthy. Now I eat more than 2,000 calories a day, and I know when I'm hungry or full."

Darla, who suffered from anorexia for more than seven years, said she was scared to death to eat. "When I started the LEAN & FREE LIFESTYLE, I could hardly force food down, and I couldn't stand to drink water," she says. "It took me a half hour to eat a celery stick, a half piece of whole-wheat toast, a tablespoon or two of canned chicken mixed with fat-free mayo, and an orange slice. And I just about had to force it down."

"Now I can eat like a real person again —a whole foot-long turkey and veggie sandwich and a big glass of water. I feel and look like a real person, too. I'm 5-feet-8 and used to weigh eighty-eight pounds. The largest part of my thigh measured fourteen inches around. People tell me now that I used to look like I'd just walked out of a prison camp."

Today Darla weighs a healthy 144 pounds and wears a size 5 dress and pants. She says: "My kids think they have a new, 'nice' pretty mom. My husband is so thrilled. He thinks I'm just beautiful. It's like I've been let out of prison."

The key for any former dieter or meal skipper following the LEAN AND FREE LIFESTYLE, is to increase food intake *very gradually* and never worry about calorie numbers—just energetic satisfaction!

If you're a stuffer, you'll lose that desire to be miserably full on improper balance because you'll be comfortably satisfied on perfect balance. And you'll have the freedom to eat any time, any where, and any place you choose. Just slow down, balance, and enjoy! Use of the Daily Success Planners is essential in your quest for optimal health, complete freedom from eating disorders, and permanent leanness. As you faithfully use your invaluable Success Planner sheets and follow the LEAN & FREE quick and easy menus, you may begin to recognize feelings of peace about food, about yourself, and about life in general that you may not have experienced in years.

Eat the way you probably did as a child—relaxed and happy. Like a child, stop when you feel comfortable, not before or after. Balance your meals. By following these guidelines, you can signal your body's survival system to relax, and you'll begin developing a wonderful, high-energy, fat-burning body that can be free from eating disorders and food preoccupations for life!

Overcoming Your Fear of Eating

The Devastation of Dieting

I have reiterated throughout this program that eating less can make you fatter. But studies show that the biggest threat of limited-calorie diets isn't fat gain — it's illness, disease, and even premature death.

One study of 850 women showed that the women within that group who suffered fatal strokes ate an average of 361 calories less per day than the other study participants. According to the traditional diet theory, the survivors should have weighed an average of thirty-five pounds more than the stroke victims, yet they actually weighed less.[9]

In another study of 8,000 Puerto Rican men ages forty-five to sixty-four, those who died of heart disease and other "natural" causes ate up to 277 calories *less* than the survivors.[10] And hypertension victims were found to consume an average of 302 calories a day *less* than the normal study participants.[11]

In an English study of three groups of men, those who ate the least had three times the incidence of coronary artery disease than those who ate the most.[13]

My favorite study, though, was conducted by the Human Subjects Institutional Review Board of the University of Illinois at Chicago. The study investigated two groups of sedentary, weight-stable women. These women were non-exercisers before and during the study and had not had major weight fluctuation for at least a year (they had not been dieting). One group was obese. The other group was not obese.

For six months all participants were fed from a metabolic kitchen to maximize the accuracy of the results. The obese women ate about 2,000 calories a day. The non-obese women consumed approximately 2,250 calories daily. Both ate approximately 37 percent fat through the first month. Then dietary fat content was decreased to 20 percent over the last five months.

The researchers continually adjusted caloric intake to keep the participants' weight stable. By the end of the study, both obese and non-obese women were eating 2,500 calories per day and had lost an average of 3 percent body weight and 11.3 percent body fat. They also had a significant increase in lean body mass, the muscle tissue that burns fat, with no exercise at all. Weight decreased earlier in the obese women (five to eight weeks) than in the non-obese women (thirteen to sixteen weeks), but at the end of the study both groups were at 97 percent of their initial weight.

The researchers could not account for the fact that such a large increase in calories did not result in weight gain, especially since there was no visible form of energy expenditure. To balance the increase in calories, they estimated that the obese women would have had to exercise for two and a half hours a day to prevent weight gain. They estimated that the non-obese women would have had to exercise two hours per day. Yet neither group exercised at all.

The study also concludes that the effect of eating plenty of good food may be more pronounced as the duration of the eating program is extended. After four months, there were less noticeable results, but after six months the weight and body fat began to drop off steadily. At this point, these previously neutral women's body chemistries were actually changing to create a fat-burning metabolism.[29]

Study after study proves that eating less results in weight gain, not permanent weight loss, thus fully supporting the principles you're learning in the LEAN &FREE 2000 PLUS LIFESTYLE.

These studies also suggest that:

1. Your body's ability to burn calories at rest may decrease during and after dieting. [1]

2. When you return to normal eating following a diet, the majority of the weight you regain is fat.[1]

3. Lean children and adults eat significantly more than obese children and adults. This seems unrelated to differences in activity levels.[1, 2]

4. According to a study of thousands, fat people may eat considerably fewer calories than lean people.[4]

5. Dieting may lead to a constant preoccupation with food, chronic fatigue, lethargy, apathy, and a significant decrease in activity.[5]

6. Constant feelings of dissatisfaction seem to accompany dieting.[5]

7. Subjects force-fed up to 8,000 calories a day experienced little weight gain; and when they resumed normal eating, they returned to normal weight without any need for dieting or calorie restriction.[6]

8. After a force-feeding episode, subjects are able to lose weight even when eating more calories than they had eaten before the episode.[6]

9. Gradual, substantial increases in caloric intake may not increase original weight[7] and may increase lean body mass.[29]

10. Animal studies indicate that after caloric restriction a subject may gain weight up to twenty times faster than before the diet, even though the subject is eating the same foods and the same number of calories as before.[8]

11. Subjects have been documented with weight gains of as much as 10 pounds in hours when they resume normal eating after a low-calorie diet.[5,8]

12. More than 90 percent of dieters return to their previous weight within two to three years of their diet. Estimates are that after five years only one in 200 people stays "skinny." The other 199 put the weight back on plus about 10 percent more! Having experienced the threat of starvation, the body is now looking for extra insurance.

13. Dieting, rather than excessive caloric intake, may be one of the major contributors to high blood pressure, stroke, heart disease, and other degenerative diseases.[9-13] An increase in the incidence of gallstones may also be linked to dieting.

14. All the following symptoms have been noted in people who regularly eat less than 1,600 to 2,000 calories a day (women, 1,600 calories; men, 2,000 calories): weakness, poor endurance, irritability, insomnia, digestive disturbances, diarrhea, frequent urination, swelling, chilling, lack of concentration, food preoccupation, and depression.[14] Since food, water, and oxygen are the main elements used in the building of cells and the sustaining of life, it follows that an abundance of nutritious, balanced food would greatly contribute to an increased life span.[5]

15. Sustained aerobic exercise is known to increase the post-exercise metabolic rate (calorie burning after exercise), but when a person diets, this benefit of exercise may be lost.[17] The average person burns 30 calories in thirty minutes in a state of rest. If moderate exercise has been performed earlier in the day, this rate may increase to 90 to 240 calories in thirty minutes of rest. However, restricted-calorie dieting may cancel the metabolically stimulating effects of exercise.

16. Dieting may increase muscle dysfunction and risk of injury because of muscle loss.[5,19,21]

17. Overfeeding with complex carbohydrates, but not with fat, may actually protect against excess fat gain because complex carbohydrates may stimulate your metabolic rate.[26] Intake of fat and complex carbohydrates must be measured against your total intake. For instance, if you eat 200 fat calories in a 1,000-calorie meal, you are eating only 20 percent fat. But, if you eat 200 fat calories during a 400-calorie meal, your fat intake is 50 percent. If you eat excess fat or sugar, eat more good food afterward.

18. Studies suggest that obese and non-obese individuals would be leaner, even without exercise, if they ate more nutritionally balanced calories.[29] Eating to full satisfaction on high-quality food will create a much leaner, healthier body than if you diet.

19. Lean body mass (muscle) may increase even without exercise when carbohydrate and protein intake is increased and dietary fat is decreased.[29]

20. The effects of eating to full satisfaction become more pronounced the longer the practice is maintained.[29] For past dieters, six months may barely show results, but twelve to twenty-four months may show pronounced results.

21. Two to four-year studies would be useful in confirming the long-term metabolic benefits of eating to full satisfaction in proper balance.

22. More good calories increase health, add energy, and decrease body fat.[14-29]

23. A healthy body is naturally lean, not starved and skinny. Remember, you have to eat to become permanently lean and free from ever worrying about excess body fat again. With that freedom from worry also comes the freedom from self-blame. Perhaps the greatest disservice of the $30-billion diet industry isn't the counterproductive effects of metabolic slow-down or the vast array of health problems dieters experience; instead, it may be the tremendous guilt that dieters are burdened with. Many of them adhere to their diets with amazing discipline, particularly considering the deprivation and misery those diets can cause. And when they gain their weight back, they blame themselves. The LEAN & FREE LIFESTYLE can release you from the futile and self-destructive path of guilt and self-hatred. Eat, have energy, love yourself and others, and be lean and free to love life.

Common 2000 Plus Calorie Concern

QUESTION: *Okay, so I won't diet. But why on earth would anyone even want to eat 2,000 calories? That's such a huge amount of food.*

ANSWER: Dieters and meal-skippers ask this all the time. Remember that this program is about listening to your body and responding to its hunger and energy needs, not manipulating calorie numbers. You should eat often until you are comfortably satisfied not stuffed or still hungry. And remember that one hundred calories from a lowfat food takes up a lot more space than one hundred calories from a high-fat food.

Examine the following "fat-storing" days and ask yourself if you've *ever* eaten 2,000 or more calories in a day.

EATING OUT DAY			NIBBLE DAY		
		FG/CAL			FG/CAL
Breakfast : Sausage and Egg			**Breakfast:**	5 oz. M &M's	30/720
Biscuit	35/529		**Lunch:**	9 Ritz & Butter	
Lunch : Cheese Potato and				Sandwiches	71/898
Diet Cola	34/590		**Snack:**	1 lg. Chocolate Malt	25/1060
Dinner: Taco Salad with			**Dinner:**	1 Apple Fritter	37/580
Ranch Dressing	87/1167				
Total: 61% fat	156/2286		**Total:**	45% fat	163/3258

Many dieters and meal-skippers eat between 600 and 1,200 calories on Monday through Friday. Then, the weekend comes, and their cravings for fats and sweets hit the roof because of their week-long starvation. But rather than eat everything in sight, they "restrain" themselves and eat "just a little bit" of the foods they're craving. If only they knew about the fat content in that "little bit" of food! Eat *a lot,* and be moderate with fat. You'll lose the cravings!

Overcoming Your Fear of Eating
Lean & Free 2000 Plus Compared to the Four Basic Food Groups and the USDA Eating Right Pyramid

Lean & Free 2000 Plus is a revolutionary program founded on old-fashioned common sense and the latest research into health, fat loss, and nutrition.

The Lean & Free 2000 Plus lifestyle isn't based on hypothetical theories or guesswork. It has evolved directly from years of public and private research and study.

As a youngster, you were told about the Four Food Groups—milk, meat, fruits and vegetables, and grains. Lately, you may have heard about the Eating Right Pyramid developed by the United States Department of Agriculture.

The Eating Right Pyramid is an outline of what to eat each day.

The Eating Right Pyramid
A Guide to Daily Food Choices

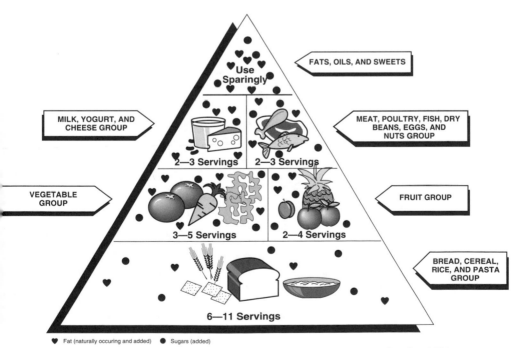

This is the USDA Eating Right Pyramid based on *Consumer Reports*, October 1991.

As you can see, the pyramid calls for eating a variety of foods for the maintenance of good health. The pyramid also focuses on reducing dietary fat because most American's diets are too high in fat, especially saturated fat.

The following chart represents the similarities and differences between the Four Food Groups, the Pyramid, and the LEAN & FREE 2000 PLUS LIFESTYLE.

The 2000 PLUS eating guidelines place a heavier emphasis on generous quantities of whole grains, legumes, vegetables, and fruits, supplemented by moderate amounts of lowfat dairy products and lean meats. Notice that recommended amounts of animal protein are not less than recommended by the Four Food Groups or the Pyramid. However, *complex-carbohydrate*, high-fiber servings are *increased*. In other words you'll be eating *more* of the foods you crave— whole-grain breads, potatoes, pasta, chili, enchiladas, and so on, and the *same* amount of dairy products and meat you're used to eating following the Four Food Groups. (You can eat less animal protein and more whole-grain–legume combinations if you desire—a very healthy choice.)

	Four Food Groups	USDA Eating Right Pyramid	LEAN & FREE 2000 PLUS Five Fingers of Balance
Grains	4 servings	6-11 servings	8-12+ servings
Fruits and vegetables	4 servings (fruits and vegetables are combined into one group)	3-5 vegetables 2-4 fruits (fruits and vegetables are separate groups)	6+ vegetables 4+ fruits (fruits and vegetables are separate groups
Milk (or other dairy products) and meat	2-4 servings milk 2-3 servings meat (milk and meat are separate groups)	2-3 servings milk 2-3 servings meat (milk and meat are separate groups)	2-4 servings milk 2-3 servings meat Emphasis on legumes (milk and meat are combined groups)
Fats and sweets	"Use sparingly" (non-specific)	"Use sparingly" (non-specific)	FATS: Approx. 20% of *total* calories (30% maximum if not dealing with high cholesterol or obesity; 10% min.) SWEETS: 0-5% of *total* daily calories

While the Eating Right Pyramid is significantly simpler than the Basic Four Food Groups, the LEAN & FREE 2000 PLUS nutrition is even simpler because you have your visual reminder with you at all times, your "fingers." As a result, balancing your meals couldn't be easier. (To review the concept of "balancing," re-read chapter 4 which introduced you to the "Five Fingers of Balance.")

As you can see, the LEAN & FREE 2000 PLUS program is a revolutionary step in the evolution of healthy eating and excess fat loss, and its rules are the *same* for a person who is under-fat, overly-fat, or just right.

Healthy people all around the world eat balanced diets that conform to the basic principles in the LEAN AND FREE 2000 PLUS program. But whatever your ethnic background, you can easily select familiar foods that will help make you lean and healthy. If you eat complex carbohydrates as the main part of each meal and are moderate with your intake of animal proteins, fats, and sweets, you may dramatically reduce your body fat and your susceptibility to heart disease, stroke, diabetes, and many types of cancer.

The Pima Indians of Arizona are a prime example of the effects of a low-fat, low-animal protein diet. For hundreds of years they consumed many foods high in complex carbohydrates, and they were exceptionally healthy. Now, with their recent changes to a high-fat "Americanized" diet, more than 50 percent of the adults over thirty-five are diabetic.[1]

It is also interesting to note that Japanese people who consume an "American-ized" diet have four times the incidence of diabetes compared to those eating a traditional Japanese diet (complex grains, vegetables, fruits, and moderate animal protein intake).[2] Throughout the world we see the same patterns. Those who eat good, nutritious, balanced foods are healthier and leaner than those who do not. The LEAN & FREE 2000 PLUS program provides you with the knowledge you need to eat healthily—no matter what your background. And whether you love Mexican, Italian, Chinese, or American cooking, you'll find it in the LEAN & FREE menus and in your ability to *healthify* your own favorite recipes.

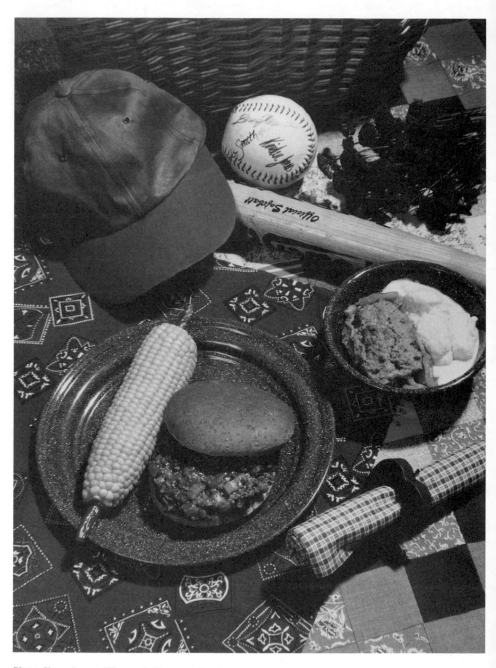

Photo: Sloppy Joes p. 287 served with corn on the cob
Instant Blueberry and Peach Ice Cream p. 278

LEAN&FREE 2000 PLUS*™

SCIENTIFIC,
NUTRITION,
FITNESS,
AND WELLNESS

REFERENCES

* Your LEAN & FREE COOKBOOK SAMPLER begins on page 240.

REFERENCES

Introduction

1. Melby, CL; Schmidt, W; Daniel, CD. Resting metabolic rate in weight-cycling collegiate wrestlers compared with physically active, noncycling control subjects. American Society for Clinical Nutrition. 1990; 52:409-14.
2. Moore, T J. The hospital diet scandal. *Family Circle.* February 1, 1992; pp. 50-57.
3. Department of Physical Education, University of California, Davis. Impact of energy intake and exercise on resting metabolic rate. *Sports Medicine,* August 1990; 10:72-87.
4. Poehlman, ET; Melby, CL; Goran, MI. The impact of exercise and diet restriction on daily energy expenditure. *Sports Medicine* (Auckland), Feburary 1991; 11 (2) 78-101.
5. Ballor, DL; Tommerup, LJ; Thomas, DP; Smith, DB; Keesey, RE. Exercise training attenuates diet-induced reduction in metabolic rate. *Journal of Applied Physiology* (Bethesda, Md.), June 1990; 68 (6) 2612-17.
6. Dulloo, A.G; Girardier, L. Adaptive changes in energy expenditure during refeeding following low-calorie intake; evidence for a specific metabolic component favoring fat storage. *American Journal of Clinical Nutrition,* September 1990; 52 (3) pp. 415-20.
7. Rumpler, WV; Seale, JL; Miles, CW; Bodwell, CE. Energy-intake restriction and diet-composition effects on energy expenditure in men. *American Journal of Clinical Nutrition,* February 1991; 53 (2) 430-36.
8. Stefanik, P. Caloric intake in relation to energy output of obese and nonobese adolescent boys. *American Journal of Clinical Nutrition,* 1959; 7:55-62.
9. Schwartz, R. Increase of adipose-tissue lipoprotein lipase activity with weight loss. *Journal of Clinical Investigation,* 1981; 67:1425-30.
10. Blackburn, G. Weight Cycling: The experience of human dieters. *American Journal of Clinical Nutrition,* 1989; 49:1105-9.
11. Tuschi, R. Energy expenditure and everyday eating behavior in healthy young women. *American Journal of Clinical Nutrition,* 1990; 52:81-86.
12. Poehlman, ET. The impact of food intake and exercise on energy expenditure. *Nutrition Reveiw,* May 1989; 47 (5) 129-37.
13. Poehlman, ET; Melby, CL; Goran, MI. The impact of exercise and diet restriction on daily energy expenditure. *Sports Medicine* (Auckland), February 1991; 11 (2) 78-101.
14. Ballor, DL; Tommerup, LJ; Thomas, DP; Smith, DB; Keesey, RE. Exercise training attenuates diet-induced reduction in metabolic rate. *Journal of Applied Physiology* (Bethesda, Md.), June 1990, 68 (6) 2612-17.
15. Dulloo, AG; Girardier, L. Adaptive changes in energy expenditure during refeeding following low-calorie intake; evidence for a specific metabolic component favoring fat storage. *American Journal of Clinical Nutrition,* September 1990; 52 (3) 415-20.

Chapter 1

1. Brewerton, Hefferman and Rosenthal, 1986.
2. Poehlman, ET. The impact of food intake and exercise on energy expenditure. *Nutrition Review,* May 1989; 47 (5) 129-37.
3. Poehlman, ET; Melby, CL; Goran, MI. The impact of exercise and diet restriction on daily energy expenditure. *Sports Medicine* (Auckland), February 1991; 11 (2) 78-101.
4. Ballor, D L; Tommerup, LJ; Thomas, DP; Smith, DB; Keesey, RE. Exercise training attenuates diet-induced reduction in metabolic rate. *Journal of Applied Physiology* (Bethesda, Md.), June 1990; 68 (6) 2612-17.

5. Dulloo, AG; Girardier, L. Adaptive changes in energy expenditure during refeeding following low-calorie intake; evidence for a specific metabolic component favoring fat storage. *American Journal of Clinial Nutrition*, Sept 1990; 52 (3), 415-20.
6. Tuschl, R. Energy expenditure and everyday eating behavior in healthy young women. *American Journal of Clinical Nutrition*, 1990; 52:81-86.
7. Cryer, A. Tissue lipoprotein lipase activity and its action in lipoprotein metabolism. *International Journal of Biochemistry*, 1981; 13:525-41.
8. Eckel, R. Lipoprotein lipase. A multifunctional enzyme relevant to common metabolic diseases. *New England Journal of Medicine*, 1989; 320:1060-68.
9. Schwartz, R. Increase of adipose-tissue lipoprotein lipase activity with weight loss. *Journal of Clinical Investigation*, 1981; 67:1425-30.
10. George, V; Tremblay, Q; Despres, J; Further Evidence for the presence of small eaters and large eaters among women. *American Journal of Clinical Nutrition*, February 1991; 53:425-29.
11. Frank, A. *Washington Post*; reprinted in *Houston Chronicle*, December 8, 1980.
12. Hamilton, E: Whitney, E; and Sizer, F. Water and Minerals. *Nutrition Concepts and Controversies*, 5th ed., St. Paul, West Publishing Co., 1991; 242-44.
13. Guyton, A. *Textbook of Medical Physiology*, 6th ed., Philadelphia: W. B. Saunders, publisher, 1981; 857-58.
14. Hamilton E; Whitney, E; Sizer, F. *Nutrition Concepts and Controversies*, 5th ed. St. Paul, West Publishing Co., 1991; 124.
15. Horstra, G. Influence of dietary fat on platelet function in men. *Lancet*, 1973; 1:1155-57.
16. Hamilton, E; Whitney, E; Sizer, F. *Nutrition Concepts and Controversies*, 5th ed. St. Paul, West Publishing Co., 1991; 128-29.
17 Ibid., 121.
18. Carrol, K. Experimental evidence of dietary factors and hormone-dependent cancers. *Cancer Research*, 1975; 35:3374-83.
19. Hamilton, E; Whitney, E; Sizer, F. *Nutrition Concepts and Controversies*, 5th ed. St. Paul, West Publishing Co., 1991; 136.
20. Flatt, JP. The difference in the storage capacities for carbohydrate and for fat, and its implications in the regulation of body weight. *Anal New York Academy of Science*, 1987; 499:104-31.
21. O'Brien, J. Acute platelet changes after large meals of saturated fats. *Lancet*, 1976; 1:878-80.
22. Simpson, H. Hypertriglyceridemia and hypercoagulability. *Lancet*, 1983; 1:786-89.
23. Mendis, S. The effects of replacing coconut oil with corn oil or human serum lipid profiles and platelet derived factors active in atherogenesis. *Nutrition Reports International*, 1989; 40:773-82.
24. Reddy, B. Effect of a diet with high levels of protein and fat on colon carcinogenesis in 344 rats treated with 1,2 dimethylhydrazine. *National Cancer Institute Journal*, 1976; 57:567-69.
25. Dyerberg, J. Hemostatic function and platelet polyunsaturated fatty acids in Eskimos. *Lancet*, 1979; 2:433-35.
26. Sanders, T. Cod-liver Oil, platelet fatty acids, and bleeding time [letter]. *Lancet*, 1980; 1:1189.
27. Sanders, T. Effect on blood lipids and hemostases of a supplement of cod-liver oil, rich in eico-sap-entaenoic and docosadheraenoic acids, in healthy young men. *Clinical Science*, 1981; 61:317-24.
28. Gannon, MA.; and Mitchell, JE. Subjective evaluation of treatment methods by

patients treated for bulimia. *Journal of the American Dietetic Association,* 1986; 86:520-21.

29. Hamilton, E; Whitney, E; Sizer, F. Controversy for sugar: Is it bad for you? *Nutrition Concepts and Controversies,* 5th ed. St. Paul, West Publications. Co., 1991; 112.

30. Hallfrisch, J; Reiser, S; and Prather, ES. Blood lipid distribution of hyperinsulinemic men consuming three levels of fructose, *American Journal of Clinical Nutrition,* 1983; 37:740-48.

31. Wallace, JF.; and Wallace, MJ. The effects of excessive consumption of refined sugar on learning skills, behavior attitudes and/or physical condition in school-aged children (a booklet available from Parents for Better Nutrition, 33 North Central, Room 200, Medford, OR 97501). Buchannan, S. The most ubiquitous toxin, *American Psychology,* November 1984, 1327-328, as cited by R. Milich, S. Lindgren, and M. Wolraich, The behavioral effects of sugar: a comment on Buchanan, *American Psychology,* February 1986; 218-20.

32. Garn, SM; Solomon, MA; and Schaefer, A. Internal validation of sugar-food intakes in obese adolescents (letter to the editor), *American Journal of Clinical Nutrition,* 1980; 33:1890.

33. Hamilton, E; Whitney, E; Sizer, F. Controversy for Sugar: Is it bad for you? *Nutrition Concepts and Controversies,* 5th ed. West Publishing Co., 1991; 115.

34. Glinsmann, Irausquin and Park, 1986.

35. Flatt, JP. The difference in the storage capacities for carbohydrate and for fat, and its implications in the regulation of body weight. *Anal of New York Academy of Science,* 1987; 499:104-31.

36. Hamilton, E; Whitney, E; Sizer, F. *Nutrition Concepts and Controversies,* 5th ed. St. Paul, West Publishing Co., 1991; 90.

37. Brewer, J; Williams, C; Patton, A. The influence of high carbohydrate diets on endurance running performance. *European Journal of Applied Physiology and Occupational Physiology* (Berling, FRG), July 1988; 57 (6) 698-706.

38. Wurtman, J J. Disorders of food intake: Excessive carbohydrate snack intake among a class of obese people. *Anal of New York Academy Science,* 1987 June; 499:197-202.

39. Hamilton, E; Whitney, E; Sizer, F. *Nutrition Concepts and Controversies,* 5th ed. St. Paul, West Publications. Co., 1991; 90.

40. Ibid., 136

41. Ibid., 90

42. Ibid.

43. Chen, WJL; and Anderson, WJ; Hypocholesterolemic effects of soluble fiber, *Dietary Fiber,* 1986; p. 275-86.

44. Swain, JF; et al. Comparison of the effects of oat bran and low-fiber wheat on serum lipoprotein levels and blood pressure. *New England Journal of Medicine,* 1990; 322:147-52.

45. Anderson, JW. Dietary fiber in nutrition management of diabetes, *Dietary Fiber,* 1986; 343-60.

46. Saheen, SM; Fleming, SE. High-fiber foods at breakfast: Influence on plasma glucose and insulin responses to lunch, *American Journal of Clinical Nutrition,* 1987; 46:804-11.

47. Hamilton, E; Whitney, E; Sizer, F. The proteins and amino acids. *Nutrition Concepts and Controversies,* 5th ed. St. Paul, West Publishing Co., 1991; 162.

48. Ibid., 163.

49. Ibid., 164
50. Ibid.
51. Ibid., 166.
52. Ibid.
53. Ibid., 173-74.
54. Carroll, KK. Dietary protein and heart disease, *Nutrition and the M. D.,* June 1986; 1.
55. Hamilton, E; Whitney, E; Sizer, F. The proteins and amino acids. *Nutrition Concepts and Controversies,* 5th ed. St. Paul, West Publishing Co., 1991; 173-74.
56. Sherman, AR; Helyar, L; Wolinsky, I. Effects of dietary protein concentration on trace minerals in rat tissues at different ages. *Journal of Nutrition,* 1985; 115:607-14.
57. Sandstead, HH. Zinc: Essentiality for brain development and function, *Nutrition Today,* November/December 1984; 26-30. B. Worthington—Roberts, Nutrition and maternal health, *Nutrition Today,* November/December 1984; 6-19.
58. Politt, E; Lewis, N. Nutritional educational achievement, *Food and Nutrition Bulletin 2,* 1980; 33-37, as cited by C. G. Neumann and E. F. P. Jelliffe, Effects of infant feeding, 529-74 in E. F. P. Jelliffe and D. B. Jelliffe, eds, *Adverse Effects of Foods,* New York: Plenum Press, 1982; 549.
59. Alfin-Slater, RB. Vit B_6 and coronary heart disease, *Nutrition and the Medical Doctor,* March 1983; 4.
60. Hamilton, E; Whitney, E; Sizer, F. The proteins and amino acids. *Nutrition Concepts and Controversies,* 5th ed. West Publishing Co., 1991; 173-74.
61. Holl, MG; Allen, LH. Comparative effects of meals high in protein, sucrose, or starch or human mineral metabolism and insulin secretion, *American Journal of Clinical Nutrition,* 1988; 48:1219-225. Zemel, MB. Calcium utilization: Effects of varying level and source of dietary protein, *American Journal Clinical Nutrition,* 1988; 48:880-83.
62. Hamilton, E; Whitney, E; Sizer, F. The proteins and amino acids. *Nutrition Concepts and Controversies,* 5th ed. St. Paul, West Publishing Co., 1991; 175.
63. Ibid., 250-51.
64. Remington, D. *The Bitter Truth About Artificial Sweeteners. Provo, Utah:* Vitality House International, Publishers, 1987; 78-79.
65. Schildkraut, JJ. The catecholamine hypothesis of affective disorders: a review of supporting evidence. *American Journal of Psychiatry,* 1965; 122:509-22.
66. Bunney, WE, Jr.; Davis, JM. Norepinephrine in depressive reactions. A review. *Archives General Psychiatry,* 1965; 13:483-94.
67. Hanin, I; Frazer, J; et al. Depression: implications of clinical studies for basic research. *Fed. Proc.,* 1985; 44/1(1): 85-90.
68. Evaluation of consumer complaints related to aspartame use. *Morb Mortal Weekly Report,* 1984; 33:243-49.
69. Wurtman, RJ. Possible relationship between aspartame (NutraSweet) consumption, seizures, and other CNS abnormalities. Introductory comments presented to the Food and Drug Administration, April 21, 1986.
70. Walton, RGW. Seizures and mania after high intake of aspartame. *Psychosomatics,* April 1986; 218-219.
71. Wurtman, RJ. Aspartame: possible effect on seizure susceptibility. *Lancet,* May 9, 1985, 1060.
72. Pinto, JMB; Maher, T. High dose aspartame lowers the seizure threshold to subcutaneous pentylenetetrazol in mice. *Pharmacologist,* 1986; 28:201.
73. Personal communication with Dr. Richard Wurtman.
74. Johns, DR. Migraine provoked by aspartame. *New England Journal of Medicine,* 1986; 315-456.

75. Clinical symptoms attributed to aspartame by Dr. H. J. Roberts (A clinician's adventures in medicine: Is aspartame safe? *On Call* (the official publication of the Palm Beach Country Medical Society) January 1987; 16-20.

76. _____. Aspartame alert. *Flying Safety,* May 1992.

77. Intersalt Cooperative Research Group. Intersalt: An international study of electrolyte excretion and blood pressure. Results for 24-hour urinary sodium and potassium excretion. *British Medical Journal,* 1988; 297:319-28.

78. Kaelber, C. Symposium on alcohol and cardiovascular diseases. *Circulation,* 1981; 64, supplement III:1-84.

79. Sorenson, M. Matters of the heart. *Mega Health,* 1992; 145.

80. Shultz, J. National Centers for Disease Control. Quoted in the *Flagstaff Sun*, Sunday, March 25, 1990; 4.

81. Saville, P. Changes in bone mass with age and alcoholism. *Journal of Bone Joint Surgery,* 1965; 47A:492-98.

82. Getting pickled. *Scientific American,* April 1985; 76.

83. Hamilton, E; Whitney, E; Sizer F. Lifecycle nutrition: Mother and Infant. *Nutrition Concepts and Controversies,*

84. Ibid., 433.

85. Leonard, TK; Watson, RR; and Mohs, ME. The effects of caffeine on various body systems: A review. *Journal of the American Dietetic Association,* 1987; 87:1048-53.

86. Watson, P. Caffeine: Is it dangerous to health? *American Journal of Health Promotion,* Spring 1988; 3-22.

87. Tufts University Diet and Nutrition Letter, February 1990; 3-6.

88. Wilcox, A. Caffeinated beverages and decreased fertility, *Lancet,* December 1988; 24/31:1453-55.

89. Joesoef, MR. et al. Are caffeinated beverages risk factors for delayed conception? *Lancet,* 1990; 335:136-37.

90. Sasaki, H. Effects of sucrose or caffeine ingestion on running performance and biochemical responses to endurance running. *International Journal of Sports Medicine* (Stuttgart), June 1987; 8 (3) 203-7.

91. Gilbert, R. Caffeine—the most popular stimulant. *Encyclopedia of Psychoacitive Drugs.* New York Chelsea House, 33.

92. McDougall, J. Getting the kitchen set up. *The McDougall Plan.* E. Orange, N.I., New Century Publishers, Inc., 1983; 220.

93. Heaney, R. Effects of nitrogen, phosphorous and caffeine on calcium balance in women. *Journal of Laboratory Clinical Medicine,* 1982; 99:46-55.

94. Hamilton, E; Whitney, E; Sizer, F. Nutrition and Disease Prevention. *Nutrition Concepts and Controversies,* 5th ed. St. Paul, West Publishing Co., 1991; 387.

94.5 Fehily, AM; Phillips, KM; Yarnell, JWG. Diet, smoking, social class and body mass index in the Caterphilly Heart Disease Study, *American Journal of Clinical Nutrition,* 1984; 40:827-33.

95. Morris, J. Incidence and prediction of ischemic heart disease in London busmen. *Lancet,* 1966; 2:553-59.

95.5 Keeler, E. The external costs of a sedentary life-style. *American Journal of Public Health,* 1989; 79:978-81.

96. Ibid.

97. Adams, T; Fisher, A.; Yanowitz, FG. Guidelines for better sleep. *Maintaining the Miracle*. Vitality House International, 1991; 149.

98. Ibid., 150.

Chapter 4

1. Sims, EAH. Studies in human hyperphagia. In. *Treatment and Management of Obesity.* Eds: Bray, G; Bethune, J. New York, NY: Harper and Row, 1974; 29.
2. Sims, EAH; Horton, ES. Endocrine and metabolic adaptation to obesity and starvation. *American Jounral of Clinical Nutrition,* 1986; 21:1455-70.
3. Campbell, T. A study on diet, nutrition and disease in the People's Republic of China. Division of Nutritional Science, Cornell University, Ithaca, New York 1989; 1-9.
4. Hamilton, E; Whitney, E; Sizer, F. The proteins and amino acids. *Nutrition Concepts and Controversies,* 5th ed. St. Paul, West Publishing Co., 1991; 164.
5. Ibid., 173-174.
6. Carroll, KK. Dietary protein and heart disease, *Nutrition and the Medical Doctor,* June 1986; 1.
7. Hamilton, E; Whitney, E; Sizer, F. The proteins and amino acids. *Nutrition Concepts and Controversies,* 5th ed. St. Paul, West Publishers Co., 1991; 173-174.
8. Sherman, AR; Helyar, L; Wolinsky, I. Effects of dietary protein concentration on trace minerals in rat tissues at different ages, *Journal of Nutrition,* 1985; 115:607-14.
9. Sandstead, HH. Zinc: Essentiality for brain development and function, *Nutrition Today,* November/December 1984; 26-30. B. Worthington—Roberts, Nutrition and maternal health, *Nutrition Today,* November/December 1984; 6-19.
10. Politt, E.; Lewis, N. Nutritional educational achievement, *Food and Nutrition Bulletin 2,* 1980; 33-37, as cited by C. G. Neumann and E. F. P. Jelliffe, Effects of infant feeding, in E. F. P. Jelliffe and D. B. Jelliffe, eds, *Adverse Effects of Foods,* New York: Plenum Press, 1982; 549.
11. Alfin-Slater, RB. Vit B_6 and coronary heart disease, *Nutrition and the Medical Doctor,* March 1983; 4.
12. Hamilton, E; Whitney, E; Sizer, F. The proteins and amino acids. *Nutrition Concepts and Controversies,* 5th ed. St. Paul, West Publishing Co., 1991; 173-174.
13. Holl, MG; Allen, LH. Comparative effects of meals high in protein, sucrose, or starch or human mineral metabolism and insulin secretion, *American Journal of Clinical Nutrition,* 1988; 48:1219-25. Zemel, MB. Calcium utilization: Effects of varying level and source of dietary protein, *American Journal of Clinical Nutrition,* 1988; 48:880-83.
14. Hamilton, E; Whitney, E; Sizer, F. The proteins and amino acids. *Nutrition Concepts and Controversies,* 5th ed. St. Paul, West Publishing Co., 1991; 175.

Chapter 5

1. Poehlman, ET. The impact of food intake and exercise on energy expenditure. *Nutrition Review,* May 1989; 47 (5) 129-37.
2. Pavlou, KN; Steffee, WP; Lerman, RH; Burrsues, BA. Effects of dieting and exercise on lean body mass, oxygen uptake, and strength. *Medicine and Science in Sports and Exercise* (Indianapolis, Ind.), Aug 1985; 17 (4) 466-71.
3. Tremblay, A. The effects of exercise-training on energy balance and adipose tissue morphology and metabolism. *Sports Medicine* (Auckland), May/June 1985; 223-2 (3) 233.
4. Larsen, J, DSW. Exercise Benefits Summary, article, 1.
5. Sobloski, J. Protection against ischemic heart disease in the Belgian physical fitness study: Physical fitness rather than physical activity? *American Journal of Epidemiology,* 1987; 125:601-10.

6. American College of Sports Medicine Position Stand. The recommended quality of exercise for developing and maintaining cardiorespiratory and muscular fitness in healthy adults. *Medical Science Sports Exercise,* 1990; 22 (2) 265-74.

7. Herz, Kreislauf, Funktion, Cardiovascular function, physique and the basic motor function capacity of male prisoners in a penal establishment and the effects of a 10-week training program. Deutsche Zeitschrift feur Sportmedizin (Cologne), July 1985; 36 (7) 209-14.

8. Pavlou, K; Steffee, WP; Lerman, RH; Burrsues, BA. Effects of dieting and exercise on lean body mass, oxygen uptake, and strength. *Medicine and Science in Sports and Exercise* (Indianapolis, Ind.), August 1985; 17 (4) 466-71.

9. Poehlman, ET. The impact of food intake and exercise on energy expenditure. *Nutrition Review,* May 1989; 47 (5) 129-37.

10. Galbo, H. Thyroid and testicular hormone responses to graded and prolonged exercise in man. *European Journal of Applied Physiology,* January 14 1977; 36 (2) 101-6, ISSN 0301-5548.

11. Report of the U. S. Preventive Services Task Force. Exercise counseling. In *Guide to Clinical Preventive Services.* Health and Human Services, prepublication copy 1989, 198-202.

12. Harris, SS; Casperson, CJ; DeFriese, GH; et al. Physical activity counseling for healthy adults as primary preventive intervention in the clinical setting: Report of the U. S. Preventive Services Task Force. *Journal of the American Medical Association,* 1898; 261:3590-98.

13. Shephard, RJ. Nutritional benefits of exercise. *Journal Sports Medicine and Physical Fitness* (Turin), May 1989; 29 (1) 83-90.

14. Dalsky, G. Weight-bearing exercise training and lumbar bone-mineral content in postmenopausal women. *Annual Internal Medicine,* 1988; 108:824-28.

15. Chow, R. Effect of two randomized programs on bone mass of healthy postmenopausal women. *British Medical Journal,* 1987; 295:1441-1444.

16. Richter, E. Diabetes and exercise. *American Journal of Medicine,* 1984; 70:201-9.

17. Kohl, H. Physical activity and cancer: An epidemiological perspective. *Sports Medicine,* 1988; 6:222-37.

18. Blair, S. Physical fitness and incidence of hypertension in nonmotensive men and women. *Journal of the American Medical Association,* 1984; 252:487-90.

19. Blair, S. Changes in coronary heart-disease risk factors associated with increased treadmill time in 753 men. *American Journal of Epidemiology,* 1983; 118:352-59.

20. Hagan, RD. The effects of aerobic conditioning and/or caloric restriction in overweight men and women. *Medicine and Science in Sports and Exercise* (Indianapolis), February 1986; 18 (1) 87-94.

21. Paffenbarger, R. Work activity and coronary heart mortality. *New England Journal of Medicine,* 1975; 292:545-50.

22. Blair, S. Physical fitness and all cause mortality. A prospective study of healthy men and women. *Journal of the American Medical Association,* 1989; 262:2395-401.

23. Stoller, J. Letter. *New England Journal of Medicine,* 1990; 318:708-9.

24. Pate, RR. Dietary intake of women runners. *International Journal of Sports and Medicine* (Stuttgart, FRG), December 1990; 11 (6) 461-66.

24.5 Quinn, F. Paper presented at the American College of Sports Medicine—Annual Meeting; University of New Hampshire, Exercise Physiology Lab; Durham, New Hampshire, May 1992.

25. Brewer, J. The influence of high carbohydrate diets on endurance running performance. *European Journal of Applied Physiology and Occuppational Physiology* (Berlin,), July 1988; 57 (6) 698-706.

Question and Answer
Fat-Storing Stressors

1. Hamilton, E; Whitney, E; Sizer, F. Lifecycle nutrition: Medicines, other drugs and nutrition. *Nutrition Concepts and Controversies,* 5th ed. St. Paul, West Publishing Co., 1991; 434-35.
2. Rossignol, A. and coauthors. Tea and premenstrual syndrome in the People's Republic of China, *American Journal of Public Health,* 1989; 79:67-69.
3. McDougall, J. Getting the kitchen set up. *The McDougall Plan.* New Century Publishers, Inc. 1983; 221.

How Often Should I Eat?

1. Verboeket-van de Venne, WP; Weterterp, KR. Influence of the feeding frequency on nutrient utilization in man: consequences for energy metabolism. *European Journal of Clinical Nutrition,* Department of Human Biology, University of Limburg, Mastricht, the Netherlands. *European Journal of Clinical Nutrition,* March 1991; 45 (3) 161-69.
2. Antoine, JM; Rohr, R; Gagey, MJ; Bleyer, RE; Debry, G. Feeding frequency and nitrogen balance in weight-reducing obese women. *The Human Nutrition of Clinical Nutrition,* January 1984; 38 (1) 31-38.
3. Garrow, JS; Durrant, M; Blaza, S; Wilkins, D; Royston, P; Sunkin, S. The effect of meal frequency and protein concentration on the composition of the weight lost by obese subjects. *British Journal of Nutrition,* January 1981; 45 (1) 5-15.
4. van Gent, CM.; Pagano, Mirani-Oostdijk, C.; van Reine, PH.; Frolich, M.; Hessel, LW.; Terpstra, J. Influence of meal frequency on diurnal [daily] lipid, glucose and insulin levels in normal subjects on a high fat diet; comparison with data obtained on a high carbohydrate diet. *European Journal of Clinical Investments,* December 1979; 9 (6) 443-46.
5. Jenkins, DJ; Solever, TM; Vuksan, V; Brighenti, F; Cunnane, SC; Rao, AF; Jenkins, AL; Buckley, G; Patten, R; Singer, W; et. al. Nibbling versus gorging: metabolic advantages of increased meal frequency. *New England Journal of Medicine,* October 5, 1989; 321 (14) 929-34.
6. Elmadfa, L; Seelbach, D. Nutrition and capacity for concentration in automobile drivers. *Fortschritte der Medicinischen,* March 10, 1983; 101 (9) 349-54.

The Devastation of Dieting

1. Melby, CL; Schmidt, WD; Corrigan, D. Resting metabolic rate in weight-cycling collegiate wrestlers compared with physically active, noncycling control subjects. *American Journal of Clinical Nutrition,* 1990; 52:409-14.
1.5 Tukaski, HC; Crash dieting could lead to cruncled bones. Study presented at American Society for Clinical Nutrition in Baltimore, Mass.; *Reported in Salt Lake City Deseret News,* May 7-8, 1992.
2. Johnson, ML; Burke, BS; Mayer, J. The prevalence and incidence of obesity in a cross-section of elementary school children. *American Journal of Clinical Nutrition,* 1956; 4:231-38.
3. Stefanik, PA; Heald, FP, Jr.; Mayer, J. Caloric intake in relation to energy output of obese and non-obese adolescent boys. *American Journal of Clinical Nutrition,* 1959; 7:55-62.
4. Braitman, LE; Adlin, EV; Stanton, JL, Jr. Obesity and caloric intake: The national health and nutrition examination survey of 1971-75 (HANES 1). *Journal of Chronic Diseases,* 1985; 38:727-32.

5. Keys, A; Brozek, J; et. al. *The Biology of Human Starvation.* Minneapolis: University of Minnesota Press, 1950; 819-918.
6. Sims, EAH. Studies in human hyperphagia. In *Treatment and Management of Obesity.* Edited by: Bray G, Bethune, J. New York: Harper and Row, 1974; 29.
7. Neuman, RO. Experimentelle Beitrage zurLehre von dem Taglichen Nahrungsbedarf des Menschen unter besonderer Berucksichtigung der notwendigen Eiwiessmenge. *Archives fur Hygiene,* 1902; 45:1-87.
8. Reminton, D; Fisher, G; Parent, E. *How to Lower Your Fat Thermostat,* Provo, Utah: Vitality House International, 1983; p. 69.
8.5 Moore, TJ. The Hospital Diet Scandal. *Family Circle,* February 1, 1992; pp. 50-57.
9. Kaw, KT; Barret-Conner, E. Dietary potassium, and stroke-associated mortality; A 12-year prospective population study. *New England Journal of Medicine,* 316:235-40
10. Garcia-Palmieri, MR; Sorlie, P; et al. Relationship of dietary intake to subsequent coronary heart disease incidence. *American Journal of Clinical Nutrition,* 1980; 33:1818-27
11. McCarron, DA; Morris, CD; et al. Blood pressure and nutrient intake in the United States. *Science,* 1984; 224:1392-98.
12. Yano, K; Rhoads, GG; Kagan, A; Tillotson, J. Dietary intake and the risk of coronary heart disease in Japanese men living in Hawaii. *American Journal of Clinical Nutrition,* 1978; 31:1270-79.
13. Morris, N; Marr, JW; Clayton, DG. Diet and heart: A postscript. *British Medical Journal,* 1977; 2:1307-14.
14. Remington, D; Higa, B. *The Bitter Truth about Artificial Sweeteners.* Provo, Utah:Vitality House International, 1987; 42.
15. Ogura, M; Ogura, H; Ikehara, S; Good, RA. Influence of dietary energy restriction on the numbers and proportions of Ly-1+ B lymphocytes in autoimmunity-prone mice. *Processed National Academy Science.* 86 (11) 4225-5229.
16. Department of Physical Education, University of California, Davis. Impact of energy intake and exercise on resting metabolic rate. *Sports Medicine,* August 1990; 10: 72-87.
17. Poehlman, ET; Melby, CL; Goran, MI. The impact of exrcise and diet restriction on daily energy expenditure. *Sports Medicine* (Auckland), February 1991; 11 (2) 78-101.
18. Ballor, DL; Tommerup, LJ; Thomas, DP; Smith, DB; Keesey, RE. Exercise training attenuates diet-induced reduction in metabolic rate. *Journal of Applied Physiology* (Bethesda, Md.), June 1990; 68 (6) 2612-17.
19. Dulloo, AG; Girardier, L. Adaptive changes in energy expenditure during refeeding following low-calorie intake; evidence for a specific metabolic component favoring fat storage. *American Journal of Clinical Nutrition,* September 1990; 52 (3) 415-20.
20. Atomi, Y; Miyashita, M. Influences of weight reduction on aerobic power and body composition of middle-aged women. *Journal of Sports Medicine and Physical Fitness* (Torino, Italy), December 1987; 27 (4) 501-9.
21. Walberg, JL. Aerobic exercise and resistance weight-training during weight reduction: implications for obese persons and athletes. *Sports Medicine* (Auckland), June 1989; 7 (6) 343-56.
22. Rock, CL; Coulsston, AM. Weight-control approaches: A review by the California Dietetic Association. *Journal of American Dietetic Association,* January 1988; 88 (1) 44-48.

23. Baecke, JA; van Staverern, WA; Burema, J. Food consumption, habitual physical activity, and body fatness in young Dutch adults. *American Journal of Clinical Nutrition*, February 1983; 37 (2) 278-86.
24. King, AC; Tribble, DL. The role of exercise in weight regulation in exercise. *Sports Medicine* (Auckland), May 1990; 11 (5) 331-49.
25. Rumpler, WV; Seale, JL; Miles, CW; Bodwell, CE. Energy-intake restriction and diet-composition effects on energy expenditure in men. *American Journal of Clinical Nutrition*, February 1991; 53 (2) 430-36.
26. McCarty, MF. The unique merits of a low-fat diet for weight control. *Medical Hypotheses*, June 1986; 20 (2) 183-97.
27. Lissner, L; Habicht, JP; Strupp, BJ; Levitsky, DA; Haas, JD; Roe, DA. Body composition and energy intake: Do overweight women overeat and underreport? *American Journal of Clinical Nutrition*, February 1989; 49 (2) 320-25.
28. Forbes, GB. Lean Body mass-body fat interrelationships in humans. *Nutrition Reviews*, August 1987; 45 (8) 225-31.
29. Prewitt, TE; Schmeisser, D; Bowen, PE; Aye, P; Dolecek, TA; Langenberg, P; Cole, T; Brace, L. Changes in body weight, body composition, and energy intake in women fed high- and low-fat diets. *American Journal of Clinical Nutrition*, 1991; 54:304-10.

Cultural Cuisine Comparison

1. Nabhan, G. Native Seeds Search Information Packet, Tucson, Arizona, 1990.
2. Hamilton, E; Whitney, E; Sizer, F. *Nutrition Concepts and Conroversies,* 5th ed. St. Paul, West Publishing Co., 1991; 59.

Low-Calorie Dieting

1. Hamilton, E; Whitney, E; and Sizer, F. *Nutrition Concepts and Controversies,* 5th ed. 1991; St. Paul, West Publishing Co., 83.
2. Dreon, D. Dietary fat: Carbohydrate ratio and obesity in middle-aged men. *American Journal of Clinical Nutrition*, 1988; 47:995-1000.
3. Johnson, M. Relative importance of inactivity and overeating in the energy balance of obese high school girls. *American Journal of Clinical Nutrition*, 1956; 4:37-44.
4. Sorenson, M. *Mega Health,* 1992; 45.
5. Dullo, A. Adaptive changes in energy expenditure during refeeding following low-calorie intake: Evidence for a specific metabolic component favoring fat storage. *American Journal of Clinical Nutrition*, 1990; 52:415-20.
6. Allon, N. The stigma of overweight in everyday life. In Wolman, B. *Psychological Aspects of Obesity.* New York Van Nostrand Reinhold, 1982.
7. Foryet, J. Limitations of behavioral treatment of obesity: Review and analysis. *Journal of Behavial Medicine,* 1981; 4:159-73.
8. Keys, A. *The Biology of Human Starvation.* University of Minnesota Press, 1950; 819-918.
9. Higa, B. Staying—or Getting—Well. *This People,* fall 1989; 18.
10. Sorenson, M. *Mega Health,* 1992; 24.

Excess Fat and Cholesterol or
Insufficient Fat Intake

1. New Way to Lose Weight: Let's Get Tall. *Washington Post,* October 1990.
2. Hibscher, J. Obesity, dieting and the expression of "obese" characteristics. *Journal of Comparitive Psychology,* 1977; 2:374-80.

3. Bray, G. Obesity: A serious symptom. *Annual International Medicine*, 1972; 77:779-805.
4. Stunkard, A. Dieting and depression reexamined. *Annuals of Internal Medicine*, 1974; 81:526-33.
5. Ernsberger, P. The death of dieting. *American Health*, 1985; 4:29-33.
6. Lissner, L. Variability of body weight and health outcomes in the Framingham population. *New England Journal of Medicine*, 1991; 324:1839-1844.
7. Polivy, J. *Breaking the Diet Habit*. Basic Books, 1983.
8. Rothblum, E. Women and weight: Fad and fiction. *Journal of Psychology*, 1990; 124:5-24.
9. *Obesity Update*, July/August 1991, 1.
10. Andres, R. Effect of obesity on total mortality. *International Jouranl of Obesity*, 1980; 4:381-86.
11. Gittleman, A. *Beyond Pritikin: The Monounsaturates and Saturates Among Us*, Bantam Books, 1988; 51-59.
12. Jackson, T. Influence of polyunsaturated and saturated fats on plasma lipids and lipoproteins in man. *American Journal of Clinical Nutrition*, 1984; 39:589-97.
13. Paul, R. On the mechanism of hypocholestserollemic effects of polyunsaturated lipids. *Advances in Lipid Research*, 1979; 17:155-71.
14. Goodnight, S. Polyunsaturated fatty acids, hyperlipidemia and thrombosis. Arterio-sclerosis, 1982; 2:87-113.
15. Shepherd, J. Effect of saturated and polyunsaturated fat diets on the chemical composition and metabolism of low-density lipoproteins in man. *Journal of Lipid Research*, 1980; 21:91-99.
16. Turner, J. Effect of changing dietary fat saturation on low-density lipoprotein metabolism in man. *American Journal of Physiology*, 1981; 241:E57-E63.
17. Lewis, B. Towards an improved lipid-lowering diet: Additive effects of changes in nutrient intake. *Lancet*, 1981; 2:1310-3.
18. Vega, G. Influence of polyunsaturated fats on composition of plasma lipoprotein and apolipoprotein. *Journal of Lipid Research*, 1982; 23:811-22.
19. Artzenuis, A. Diet, lipoproteins and the progression of coronary atherosclerosis. *New England Journal of Medicine*, 1985; 312:805-11.
20. Grundy, S. Comparison of monounsaturated fatty acids and carbohydrates for lowering plasma cholesterol. *New England Journal of Medicine*, 1986; 314:745-48.
21. Ibid.
22. Hamilton, E.; Whitney, E.; Sizer, F. The Lipids: Fats and Oils, *Nutrition Concepts and Controversies*, 5th ed. St. Paul, West Publishing Co., 1991; 127.
23. Leaf, A; Weber, PC. Cardiovascular effects of n-3 fatty acids, *New England Journal of Medicine*, 1988; 318:549-55.
24. Hamilton, E.; Whitney, E.; Sizer, F. *Nutrition Concepts and Controversies*, 5th ed. St. Paul, West Publishing Co., 1991; 29.
25. Ibid., 131.
26. Corbett, SW; Stern, JS; Keesey, RE. Energy expenditure in rats with diet-induced obesity, *American Journal of Clinical Nutrition*, 1986; 44:173-80.
27. Lipid Research Clinics Program, The Lipid Research Clinics coronary primary prevention trial results: I. Reduction in incidence of coronary heart disease. *Journal of American Medical Association*, 1984; 251:351-64.
28. Hamilton, E; Whitney, E; Sizer, F. *Nutrition Concepts and Controversies*, 5th ed. St. Paul, West Publishing Co., 1991, 135.

Nutrition

1. Wicks, A. Insulinopenic diabetes in Africa. *British Medical Journal*, 1973; 1:773-76.
2. Trowell, H. Dietary-fiber hypothesis of the etiology of diabetes mellitus. *Diabetes*, 1975; 24:762-65.
3. Trowell, H. Definition of dietary fiber and hypotheses that it is a protective factor in certain diseases. *American Journal of Clinical Nutrition*, 1976; 29:417-27.
4. Tsunehara, C. Diet of second generation Japanese-American men with and without non-insulin dependent diabetes. *American Journal of Clinical Nutrition*, 1980; 52:731-38.

Alcohol and Certain Drugs, Artificial Sweeteners, Caffeine, and Excessive Refined Carbohydrates, or Insufficient Complex Carbohydrates

1. Handa, K. Alcohol consumption, serum lipids and severity of angiographically determined coronary artery disease. *American Journal of Cardiology*, 1990; 65:287-89.
2. NOMSG, National Organization Mobilized to Stop Glutamate, P. O. Box 367, Santa Fe, New Mexico, 87504.
3. Hamilton, E; Whitney, E.; Sizer, F. Lifecycle Nutrition: *Nutrition Concepts and Controversies*, 5th ed. St. Paul, West Publishing Co., 1991; 211.
4. Marut, EL. Oral Contraceptives—who, which, when, and why? *Postgraduate Medicine*, 1987; 82:66-70.
5. Ibid.
6. Miller, LT. Do oral contraceptive agents affect nutrient requirements—vitamin B_6? *Journal of Nutrition*, 1986; 116:1344-45.
7. Shephard, BD. Oral contraceptives—An overview, *Journal of the Florida Medical Association*, 1986; 73:763-67.
8. Sorenson, M. A terrible Trio. *Mega Health*, 1992; 363.
9. Remington, D. *The Bitter Truth about Artificial Sweeteners*, Provo, Utah:Vitality House International, 25.
10. Roberts, H. *Aspartame (Nutrasweet): Is It Safe?* Philadelphia: Charles Press, 1990; 1, 10-15.
11. Remington, D. *The Bitter Truth about Artificial Sweeteners*. Provo, Utah: Vitality House International, 1987;
12. American Cancer Society. Cancer Prevention Study II, An epidemiological study of lifestyles and environments. *CPS II Newsletter*, spring 1986; 4/1:3.
13. McCann, MB; Trulson, MF; Stubb, SC. Non-caloric sweeteners and weight reduction. *Journal of American Dietary Association*, 1956; 32:327-30.
14. Roseman, K. Benefits of saccharin: A review. *Environmental Research*, 1989; 15:70-81.
15. Stare, FJ. Sugar and sugar substitutes in preventative medicine and nutrition. *Nutrition Metabolism*, 1975; 18:133-42.
16. Millar, W. Diet composition, energy intake, and exercise in relation to body fat in men and women. *American Journal of Clinical Nutrition*, 1990; 52:426-30.
17. Story, M; Brown, JE. Do young children instinctively know what to eat? *New England Journal of Medicine*, 1987; 316:103-6.
18. Cowart, BJ. Development of taste perception in humans: Sensitivity and preference throughout the life span. *Psychological Bulletin*, 1981; 90:43-73.
19. Sclafini, A. Feeding inhibition and death produced by glucose ingestion in the rat. *Physiological Behavior*, 1973; 11:595-601.

20. American Cancer Society. Cancer Prevention Study II, An epidemiological study of lifestyles and environments. *CPS II Newsletter,* spring 1986; 4/1:3.
21. Hamilton, E; Whitney, E; Sizer, F. *Nutrition Concepts and Controversies,* 5th ed. St. Paul, West Publishing Co., 1991; 434-35.
22. Rossignol, A. and coauthors. Tea and premenstrual syndrome in the People's Republic of China, *American Journal of Public Health,* 1989; 79:67-69.
23. McDougall, J. Getting the kitchen set up. *The McDougall Plan.* E. Orange, New Century Publishers, 1983; 221.
24. Lecos, C. Our insatiable sweet tooth. *FDA Consumer,* October 1985; 25.
25. Hamilton, E.; Whitney, E.; Sizer, F. *Nutrition Concepts and Controversies,* 5th ed. St. Paul, West Publishing Co., 1991; 111.
26. Ibid., 116.
27. Kane, J. Studies of carbohydrate metabolism in idiopathic hyper-triglyceridemia. *Metabolism,* 1965; 14:471-86.
28. Ibid.
29. Leslie, P. Effect of optimal glycemia control with continuous subcutaneous insulin infusion on energy expenditure in type 1 diabetes mellitus. *British Medical Journal,* 1986; 293:1121-26.
30. Jenkins, D. Dietary fibres, fibre analogues and glucose tolerance. Importance of viscosity. *British Journal of Medicine,* 1987; 1:1392-94.
31. Albrink, M. Effect of high and low-fiber diets on plasma lipids and insulin. *American Journal of Clinical Nutrition,* 1979; 32:1486-91.
32. Ashby, P. Effects on insulin, gluco-corticoids and adrenalin on the activity of rat adipose tissue lipoprotein lipase. *Biochemical Journal,* 1980; 188:185-192.
33. Lohman, D. Diminished insulin response in highly trained athletes. *Metabolism,* 1978; 27:521-24.
34. Bjorntorp, P. The effect of physical training on insulin production in obesity. *Metabolism,* 1970; 19:631-38.
35. Hamilton, E; Whitney, E; Sizer, F. *Nutrition Concepts and Controversies,* 5th ed. St. Paul, West Publishing Co., 1991; 93.
36. Ibid., 94.
37. Hekkens, WTJM. Feeding weight and obesity abstracts. Lab. Gastssroenterol, Acad. Ziekenhuis, Leiden, Netherlands. 1976; 37 (4) 192-200.

Protein Imbalance and Stress

1. Hamilton, E; Whitney, E; Sizer, F. *Nutrition Concepts and Controversies,* 5th ed. St. Paul, West Publishing Co., 1991; 176-78.
2. Blair, S. Physical activity leads to fitness and pays off. *Physician Sports Medicine,* 1985; 13:153-57.
3. Koplan, J. Physical activity, physical fitness and health: Time to act. *Journal of the American Medical Association,* 1989; 262:2347.
4. Keeler, E. The external costs of a sedentary life-style. *American Journal of Public Health,* 1989; 79:978-81.
5. Ornish, D. *Stress, Diet and Your Heart.* New York: Holt, Rinehart, and Winston, 1982.
6. Warning: Hostility can be Dangerous to Your Health. University of Texas, *Lifetime Health Letter,* October 1989, p. 1.
7. Hamilton, E; Whitney, .; Sizer, F. *Nutrition Concepts and Controversies,* 5th ed. St. Paul, West Publishing Co., 1991; 444-45.

8. Atkins, RM. The basis of immediate hypersensitivity reactions to foods, *Nutrition Reviews,* 1983; 41:229-34.
9. May, CD. Food allergy: Perspective, principles, practical management, *Nutrition Today,* November/December 1980; 28-31.
10. Hamilton, E.; Whitney, E.; Sizer, F. *Nutrition Concepts and Controversies,* Fifth Edition. St. Paul, West Pub. Co., 1991; p. 102.
11. Ibid., 307.

Exercise

1. Atomi, Y; Miyashita, M. Influences of weight reduction on aerobic power and body composition of middle-aged women. *Journal of Sports Medicine and Physical Fitness,* December 1987; 27 (4) 501-9.
2. Warwick, PM; Garrow, JS. The effect of addition of exercise to a regime of dietary restriction on weight loss, nitrogen balance, resting metabolic rate and spontaneous physical activity in three obese women in a metabolic ward. *International Journal of Obesity,* 1981; 5 (1) 25-32.
3. Astrand, PO. Exercise physiology and its role in disease prevention and in rehabilitation. *Archives of Physical Medical Rehabilitation,* 1987; 68:305-9.
4. Tipton CM; Vailas AC; Matthes RD. Experimental studies on the influences of physical activity on ligaments, tendons, and joints: A brief review. In Astrand P-O, Grimby G, (eds). *Physical Activity in Health and Disease.* Acta Med Scand Symposium Series no 2. Stockholm: Almquist and Wiksell International, 1986; 157-68.
5. Paffenbarger, R. Physical activity, all cause mortality, and longevity of college alumni. *New England Journal of Medicine,* 1986; 314, 605-13.
6. Askew, EW. Role of fat metabolism in exercise. *Clinical Sports Medicine* (United States), July 1984; 3 (3) 605-21, ISSN 0278-5919.
7. Leon, Leisure-time physical activity levels and risk of coronary heart disease and death. *Journal of the American Medical Association,* 1987; 258:2388-95.
8. Dalsky, G. Weight-bearing exercise training and lumbar bone-mineral content in postmenopausal women. *Annual International Medicine,* 1988; 108:824-828.
9. Beverly, M. Local bone-mineral response to brief exercise that stresses the skeleton. *British Medical Journal,* 1989; 299:233-35.
10. Cooper, K. The aerobic Point System—Quantifying Your Effort. In *The New Aerobics For Women,* New York: Bantam Books, 1988; 33.
11. Adams, T; Fisher, G; Yanowitz, F. Daily health check #1, physical activity programs. Provo, Utah: Vitality House International, 1991; 42.
12. Tremblay, A. Diminished dietary thermogenesis in exercise-trained human subjects. *European Journal of Applied Physiology and Occupational Physiology,* November 1983; 5 (1) 1-4.
13. Oleshansky, MA. The influence of fitness on neuroendocrine responses to exhaustive treadmill exercise. *European Journal of Applied Physiology and Occupational Physiology* (Berlin), January 1990; 59 (6) 405-10.
14. The Centers for Disease Control. Progress toward achieving the 1990 national objectives for physical fitness and exercise. *Morb Mortal Weekly Report,* 1989; 38:449-53.
15. American College of Sports Medicine Position Stand. The recommended quantity and quality of exercise for developing and maintaining cardiorespiratory and

muscular fitness in healthy adults. *Medical Science of Sports Exercise,* 1990; 22 (2) 265-274.

16. Dickson, P. Effects of a short-term exercise program on caloric consumption. *Journal of Health-Physiology,* 1985; 4 (5) 437-48.

17. Hagan, D. Physiologic and performance responses to arm, leg and combined arm and leg work on the Schwinn Air-Dyne Ergometer. In Cooper, K., *The New Aerobics for Women.* New York: Bantam Books, 988; 111.

18. Centers for Disease Control. Protective effects of physical activity on coronary heart disease: Progress in chronic disease prevention. *Morb Mortal Weekly Report,* 1987; 36 (26) 426-30.

19. Gwinup, G. Weight loss without dietary restriction: efficacy of different forms of aerobic exercise. *American Journal of Sports Medicine* (Columbus, Ga.), May/June 1987; 15 (3) 275-79.

20. Jang, KT. Energy balance in competitive swimmers and runners. *Journal of Swimming Research* (Fort Lauderdale, Fl.), spring 1987; 3 (1) 19-23.

21. A.M. Exercisers stay with it. *Aviation Medical Bulletin,* December 1990; 1.

22. Sharma, VM. Differential effects of hot-humid and hot-dry environments. International Archives of Occupational Environmental Health, 1983; 52 (4) 315-27.

23. Brouns, F. Metabolic changes induced by sustained exhaustive cycling and diet manipulation. *International Journal of Sports Medicine,* May 1989; 10 Suppl 1:S49-62.

24. Highet, R. Ahtletic amenorrhoea: An update on aetiology, complications and management. *Sports Medicine* (Auckland), February 1989; 7 (2) 82-108.

25. Sasaki, H. Effects of sucrose or caffeine ingestion on running performance and biochemical responses to endurance running. *International Journal of Sports Medicine* (Stuttgart), June 1987; 8 (3) 230-207.

26. Janssen, GM. Food intake and body composition in novice athletes during a training period to run a marathon. *International Journal of Sports Medicine* (Stuttgart,), May 1989; 10, Supl 1, S17-S21.

27. Van Erp Beart, AM. Carbohydrate, protein, and fat intake. *International Journal of Sports Medicine* (Stuttgart), May 1989; 10, Suppl 1, S3-S10.

28. Saris, WH. Study on food intake and energy expenditure during extreme sustained exercise. *International Journal of Sports Medicine* (Stuttgart), May 1989; 10, Suppl 1, S26-S31.

29 Brewer, J. The influence of high carbohydrate diets on endurance running performance. *European Journal of Applied Physiology and Occupatioanl Physiology* (Berlin), July 1988; 57 (6) 698-706.

30. Sorenson, M. *Eat More, Move More, Lose More.* Publishers Press, 1985; 54.

LEAN&FREE 2000 PLUS™

DAILY SUCCESS MENU

Date:____

			FG/CAL
Breakfast	Water		
	Grain		
	Protein		
	Fruit		
Snack	Water		
	Veggie+		
Lunch	Water		
	Vegetable		
	Grain		
	Protein		
	Fruit		
Snack	Water		
	Veggie+		
Dinner	Water		
	Vegetable		
	Grain		
	Protein		
	Fruit		
Snack	Water		
	Veggie+		

DAY'S TOTAL ▶

Calories: _____
Fat Grams: _____
Percent Fat: _____

At the back of this book, you'll find more Daily Success Menu sheets.

© Dana Thornock 1994

237

LEAN&FREE 2000 PLUS™

THE LEFT-BRAIN PLANNER

NAME: _____ DATE: _____

1. KNOWLEDGE
2. COMMITMENT
3. NURTURING
4. NOURISHMENT
5. MOTION
6. SERVICE
7. PLAN   8. ACTION

	Points		
PLAN	5__	Breakfast	
		Lunch	
		Dinner	
		Snacks	
		Exercise	
		Failure Avoidance	Today, I foresee and resolve any problem that could cause me to fail.*

KNOWLEDGE	5__	Knowledge	Today I studied or reinforced LEAN&FREE . principles. This knowledge empowers my success.*
COMMITMENT	5__	Commitment	Today I am realizing and enjoying signs of success and feel a passion to be LEAN&FREE.*
NURTURING	5__	Nurturing	I am practicing positive body talk. I am a friend and partner with my body.*

				FG/Cal
NOURISHMENT	5__	Comfortable Satisfaction	**BREAKFAST**	
	1__	Water		XXXXX
	1__	Grain		
	1__	Protein		
	1__	Fruit		
	2__	Water & Snack		
	5__	Comfortable Satisfaction	**LUNCH**	XXXXX
	1__	Water		XXXXX
	1__	Vegetable		
	1__	Grain		
	1__	Protein		
	1__	Fruit		
	2__	Water & Snack		
	5__	Comfortable Satisfaction	**DINNER**	XXXXX
	1__	Water		XXXXX
	1__	Vegetable		
	1__	Grain		
	1__	Protein		
	1__	Fruit		
	2__	Water & Snack		
	5__	Fat Grams	Score 5 points if fat grams are about 20% of total calories. (Record calories once a week.) Total FG/Cal ▶	

	10__	Stressors*	Score 10 points for avoiding ALL of the following fat-storing stressors—0 points otherwise.
		A.	Alcohol, unnecessary drugs (smoking & caffeine), and artificial sweeteners.
		B.	Excessive amounts of refined flour, sugar, and salt.
		C.	Desserts and sweets, except after comfortable satisfaction on W.V.G.P.F.
		D.	Extreme anger with self or others.

TYPE (Non-stop aerobic)	MINUTES (Goal 30 - 60)	PULSE (110 - 180 per minute)

MOTION	15__	Exercise	Score 15 points for meeting your exercise goal and recording your exercise
	5__	Adequate sleep	pulse*. Score 5 points for receiving adequate sleep. (Hours slept:_____)
SERVICE	10__	Personal Service	Today, I used my increased health and energy in service to myself and others.*
ACTION		Do It Now!	Action enables you to feel LEAN&FREE success daily and get on with living a happy, fulfilled life. Take it just ONE DAY at a time. Get Excited! Go for it!
DAILY SCORE	100 Total	Scoring	"A" Day = 90 to 100 pts. = Superior day for physical and mental health. "B" Day = 80 TO 89 pts. = Very good "coasting" day. "A" Week = 630 to 700 pts. "B" Week = 560 to 629 pts.

Permission granted to enlarge and copy this page.   © Dana Thornock 1994

URGENT! YOU MUST READ THIS!

Before you turn another page, read this journal entry. The following MIX & MATCH MENUS range between about 2,000 and 4,000 calories. You *must adjust* these calories to your own personal hunger and metabolic needs. If you have a 1,000 calorie metabolism today, you will not have a 2,000 calorie metabolism by tomorrow. Your metabolism will increase gradually. So how do you adjust the menus to your personal metabolic needs? Start by writing down exactly what you ate today (or on any "average" day) on page 237. Then add up your fat grams and calories by referring to the fat gram/calorie charts in this book.

This is absolutely essential for the prevention of unnecessary body-fat gain because, if you are a dieter or a meal skipper, you must *increase your calories gradually* from where you are right now. You should never feel miserably stuffed; you should feel comfortably satisfied. Start by eating six small meals and gradually increase as your metabolism and lean muscle tissue increase.

If you look at a 3,000-calorie menu and you normally eat 1,500 calories, simply cut the portion sizes in half and gradually increase them as your hunger and energy gradually increases.

If you look at a 2,000-calorie menu, and you normally eat 1,000 calories, simply cut each portion size in half. But if you normally eat 4,000 calories, you may want to double each portion size to meet your metabolic needs. And make certain not to exclude one food and double up on another. The balance is essential!

If you do not increase your calories and your high-fiber foods gradually, you may place unnecessary "fat-storing" stress on your body, so please –*listen to your body*! You should get hungry for your next meal, not be stuffed all day long and your calorie needs will vary from day to day. Mine range between about 2,000 and 3,500 calories on different days. I simply listen to my body. Beginners often range between about 1,400 and 2,000 calories. And if you think 2,000 calories is an unheard of amount to eat, refer to page 216 for some fascinating information.

Also, remember that you can mix and match your meals and the foods at your meals as long as you include water, vegetable, grain, protein, and fruit at each meal. (Exception: breakfast vegetable. Refer to the Nourishment chapter for more information.)

Relax — At last you can *eat and enjoy real, normal food*! This is truly not a diet. It's a delicious, easy, abundant way of life.

Dana's
LEAN&FREE

14 DAY
COOKBOOK
SAMPLER

Featuring

- **Grab 'n' Go Menus**
- **Budget Menus**
- **Mix & Match Menus**
- **Detailed Shopping Lists**
- **Fast, Delicious Recipes**
- **Fat Gram/Calorie Charts**
- **Fast Food and Restaurant Food Recommendations**

 Don't read another page until you've read page 239.

LEAN & FREE IS NOT A DIET!

My definition of a diet is: any dietary plan that cuts your calories or makes you eat weird food. This is *lots* of *normal,* delicious food and it's *so easy!* Just follow the Five Fingers of Balance:

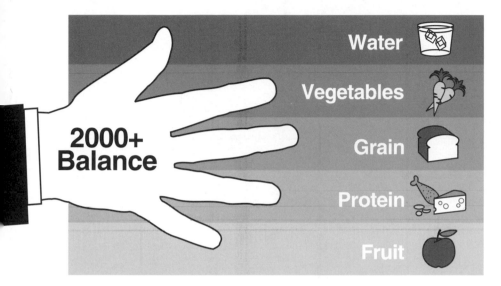

The following menus each contain a little gold mine of information to guide you to optimal health and leanness. Each menu contains the Five Fingers of Balance and *all* the essential elements discussed in the nourishment chapter beginning on page 54. These menus and their companion shopping lists *must* be adjusted to your personal needs. Carefully study the menu on the next page.

PERSONALIZE THESE DELICIOUS MENUS

This *Grab "n" Go* menu can be easily adjusted to your personal:
1. Time schedule
2. Budget needs
3. Special health needs (allergies, diabetes, etc.)
4. Family needs and tastes (whether you're single or cook for a large family)
5. Calorie and fiber needs (increase fiber and calories *very* gradually)

LEAN&FREE 2000 PLUS™

GRAB 'N' GO DAILY SUCCESS MENU

			FG/CAL
Breakfast	**Water**	12 oz.	
	Grain	1 1/2 cups Kellogg's Just Right Cereal	2/280
Quick & Easy	**Protein**	1 1/2 cups skim milk	t/129
	Fruit	(in cereal)	
Snack	**Water**	8 oz.	
	Veggie+	6 baby carrots	0/35
Lunch	**Water**	8 oz.	
	Vegetable	1/2 foot-long Seafood Sandwich with extra veggies and no dressings	7/343
	Grain	(whole-grain bun)	
Fast Food Subway	**Protein**	(seafood and cheese)	
	Fruit	1 large orange (from home)	t/62
Snack	**Water**	8 oz.	
	Veggie+	1/2 leftover foot-long sandwich	7/343
Dinner	**Water**	8 oz.	
	Vegetable	1 cup Quick, Delicious Beef Stew* p. 287	8/302
	Grain	1 slice whole-grain bread with 1 Tb. All Fruit Jam* p. 275	t/158
Quick & Easy	**Protein**	(in beef stew)	
	Fruit	1 apple	t/81
Snack	**Water**	8 oz.	
	Veggie+	1 cup leftover stew	8/302

32 fat grams x 9 calories = 288 calories from fat 288 + 2,035 + 14%	Total: 32/2,035

How to Personalize These Menus for Your Real Life!

1. TIME SCHEDULE: If you hate to cook or simply never have time, this Grab "n" Go menu is already adjusted to your needs. You can't get much faster than cold cereal, pre-cut (at the grocery store) vegetables, fast-food sandwiches, fruits, and canned stew and vegetables. This is deliciously fast and easy the LEAN & FREE way!

2. BUDGET NEEDS: Oatmeal or cracked wheat with honey and bananas makes a much cheaper breakfast . A homemade sandwich for lunch and homemade stew for dinner make very frugal choices. Make extra stew and freeze it to help save money and time too! Buy fruits and vegetables in season.

3. SPECIAL HEALTH NEEDS: (allergies, diabetes, etc.) A small amount of diluted non-dairy coffee creamer works well on cereal when milk isn't tolerated well, and leave the cheese off your sandwich. If you're allergic to wheat, try wheat-free breads, cereals, muffins, and pasta. Use corn tortillas for sandwiches.

The only change you might make on this menu, if you suffer from diabetes, is to pick a cold cereal with three grams of sugar or less per serving. Try mixing corn flakes, Shredded Wheat, and Grapenuts. Enjoy sliced bananas for added sweetness.

4. FAMILY NEEDS AND TASTES: Adjust your shopping lists to fit the size of your family. Include a lot of their old favorites while you gradually introduce these new, easy, delicious foods. Don't *make* them change. Let it be totally *their decision.*

5. CALORIE AND FIBER NEEDS: Don't focus on calories. Just eat until you are *comfortable.* Eat at least three times a day. People who eat *six* times a day may lose body fat *twice* as fast because of thermogenesis (increased heat production and metabolism that occur when you digest food). *Start out by eating six little meals* and very gradually increase as your hunger increases along with your metabolism. (It's normal for hunger to fluctuate from day to day.) Start out with more canned fruits and vegetables rather than all fresh. Also, use some white and some whole-wheat flour. This may be much easier on your system. Too much fiber and too many calories added too quickly can make you sick, stress your body, and encourage excess body fat gain.

Remember that leftovers from your meal make great snacks. Also, remember to mix and match the breakfasts, lunches, and dinners that best meet your individual needs.

PLANNING: The planning chapter on page 110 contains a marvelous plan that implements all eight steps of the LEAN & FREE LIFESTYLE. It is easy to complete, and following it gives you a very thorough wellness education. However, if you're used to drinking two diet shakes and eating a frozen dinner in the evening, you may initially be overwhelmed by even the thought of pouring milk on cold cereal. So follow an even simpler plan, illustrated on the following page, if you want it ultra simple!

This plan does three things. It teaches you to eat, exercise, and be kind to yourself and others. You'll learn to eat more vegetables, grains, and fruits and to be moderate, but not excessively low in animal protein and fat.

All you do is follow the LEAN & FREE MENUS and check off the boxes. It's just that simple!

THE PERFECTLY SIMPLE LEAN & FREE PLAN
THE RIGHT-BRAIN PLANNER

Simply follow the LEAN & FREE MENUS and check each completed box. Boxes vary in size according to the foods you should be eating the most of. If you miss a food at a meal, just include it with your next snack and check it off. Snacks are not essential, but are very helpful for increasing metabolism.

BREAKFAST

WATER: ☐

GRAIN: ☐

PROTEIN: ☐

FRUIT: ☐

SNACK

WATER: ☐

(VEGGIE + ☐)

LUNCH

WATER: ☐

VEGGIE + ☐

GRAIN: ☐

PROTEIN: ☐

FRUIT: ☐

SNACK

WATER: ☐

(VEGGIE+ ☐)

Today I exercised aerobically (nonstop, entire-body, rhythmic movement) for:

(CHECK ONE)

15 minutes: ☐

30 minutes: ☐

45 minutes ☐

60 minutes: ☐

DINNER

WATER: ☐

VEGGIE + ☐

GRAIN: ☐

PROTEIN: ☐

FRUIT: ☐

SNACK

WATER: ☐

(VEGGIE+ ☐)

Today I practiced positive body talk. I like myself today!

YES ☐

NO ☐

All Appropriate Boxes Checked = A+, Healthy, High-Energy, Fat-Burning Habits

---

Permission granted to enlarge and copy this page.   © Dana Thornock 1994

244

Grab 'n' Go Menu Sampler

DAY #1

BREAKFAST

 Water

 Kellogg's Crispix Cereal *(or another low sugar, lowfat whole-grain cereal)*

 Skim or 1% milk *(or a milk substitute if you have a dairy allergy)*

 Orange *(or another citrus fruit)*

LUNCH

 Water

 Sliced cucumber *(or other green or yellow vegetables with lowfat or nonfat dip)*

 Whole-grain toast with fat free cream cheese

 Potato-Corn Soup* p. 291

 Apple *(or another in-season fruit)*

DINNER

 Water

 Quick, Delicious Beef Stew* p. 287 in a bun *(Purchase large wheat or white soup buns at bakery and hollow out center. Fill with stew and top with bread lid. Or have regular whole-grain* bread or rolls.)*

 Red or green grapes

SNACKS

 Water

 Veggies, soup, stew, etc.

If you are not hungry, but have time to snack in between meals, snack mainly on veggies. If you are hungry, snack on veggies and other nutritious foods.

* *Go with part whole-grain breads or rolls if you are accustomed to eating mainly white bread.*

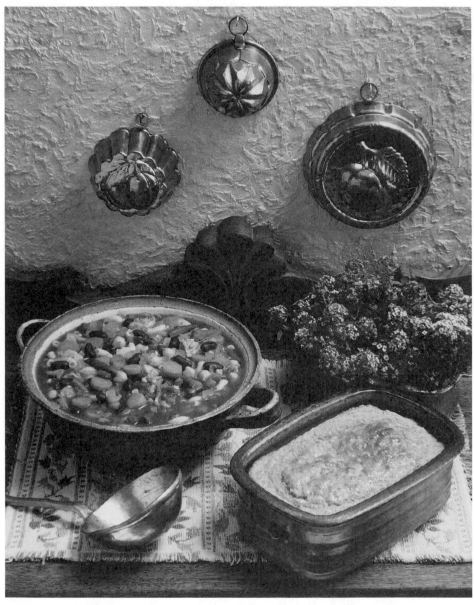

Photo: Country Corn Bread p. 272
Creamy Bean & Ham Soup p. 290

DAY #7

BREAKFAST

 Water

 Breakfast Shake* p. 275

 Whole-grain toast with fat free cream cheese

LUNCH

 Water

 Chick-Fil-A Hearty Breast of Chicken Soup

 Chick-Fil-A Carrot-Raisin Salad

DINNER

 Water

 Chilighetti *(Serve chicken chili or lowfat beef chili over*

cooked spaghetti or macaroni noodles.)

 Instant Blueberry Ice Cream* p. 278

SNACKS

 Water

 Veggies, veggie soup, veggie salad, a few

 whole grains *(if hungry)*, etc.

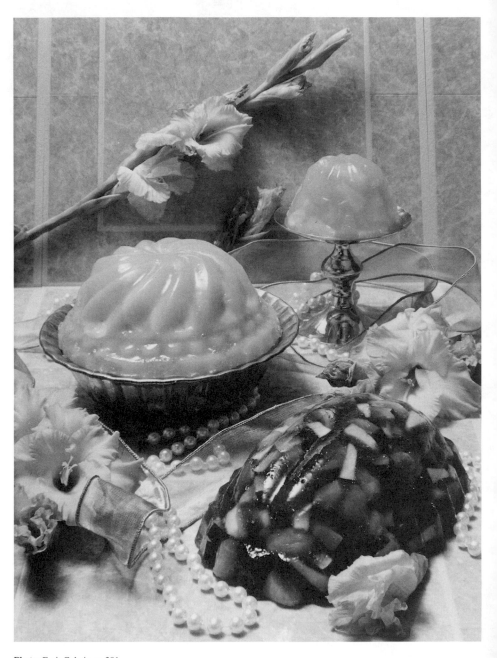

Photo: Fruit Gelatin p. 281

DAY #22

BREAKFAST

 Water

 Whole or part whole-grain bagels topped with fat free
strawberry cream cheese

 Nonfat fruit yogurt

 Grapefruit, kiwifruit, strawberries *(or another
in-season, high-vitamin C fruit)*

LUNCH

 Water

 Blimpie's Veggie & Cheese Pita Pockets without
oil and mayonnaise *(or a Blimpie turkey, tuna, or
seafood sandwich with a whole-grain bun, extra
veggies, and no oil or mayonnaise)*

 Pears (or other fruit from home)

DINNER

 Water

 La Choy Chicken Chow Mein with plenty of quick
brown or white rice *(Brown rice is the more
nutritious, high-fiber choice, but white rice is also fine.)*

 Whole-grain bread or rolls with fat free cream cheese

 Dole Tropical Fruit Mix (or other fruit)

SNACKS

 Water

 Veggies, leftover veggie pockets, leftover chow mein
with rice, etc.

249

BUDGET MENU SAMPLER

Day #1

BREAKFAST

 Water

 Oatmeal (*Mix with a small amount of honey, cinnamon, brown sugar, sugar, maple syrup, fructose, apple-juice concentrate, or All-Fruit Jam* p. 275.*)

 Skim or 1% milk (*Mix equal parts of regular milk with prepared powdered milk to save money.*)

 Grapefruit (*or another in-season or on-special fruit that's high in vitamin C*)

LUNCH

 Water

Tuna Sandwiches* p. 288

 Apple or applesauce (*or another in-season fresh fruit or canned fruit in extra-light syrup or fruit juice*)

DINNER

 Water

 Chicken Fajitas* p. 284

 Peaches (*fresh or canned in extra-light syrup or fruit juice; or another fruit of your choice*)

SNACK

 Water

 Veggies, Tuna Sandwiches, Chicken Fajitas, etc.

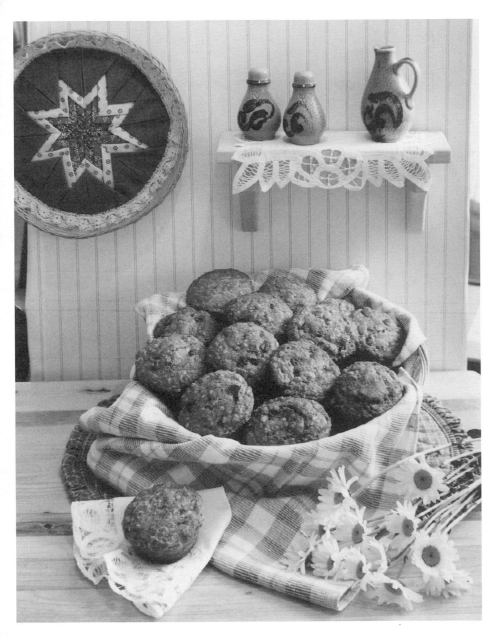

Photo: Marvelous Muffins p. 272

Day #9

BREAKFAST

 Water

 French Toast* p. 277 *(Top with a small amount of bulk maple syrup or nonfat fruit yogurt and All Fruit Jam* p. 275. Make your own bread to save money.)*

 Skim or 1% milk

 Orange *(or another citrus fruit)*

LUNCH

 Water

 Leftovers from last night's dinner

(Leftovers are an excellent time and money saver. Make certain to include veggies, grain, protein, and fruit.)

DINNER

 Water

 Easy Chicken 'n' Dumplings* p. 285

(Make extra and freeze to save time and money. Use your own garden veggies to save more money.)

 Apricots *(Or another fresh or canned fruit in extra-light syrup or fruit juice; or choose in-season or on-special fruit)*

SNACKS

 Water

 Veggies, leftover Chicken 'n' Dumplings, etc.

252

Day #22

BREAKFAST

 Water

 Super Cinnamon Rolls* p. 273 or Cracked Wheat,
Raisin, and Honey Cereal* p. 276

 Skim or 1% milk

 Kiwi slices *(or another high-vitamin C fruit)*

LUNCH

 Water

 Chili Stuffed Baked Potato *(Stuff with lowfat chili
and fat free sour cream or plain, nonfat yogurt.)*

 Celery *(or another green or yellow vegetable)*

 Bananas *(or another fruit that is on special)*

DINNER

 Water

 Creamy Bean & Ham Soup* p. 290

 Tossed Salad* p. 292 with Buttermilk
Dressing* p. 280

 Perfect Whole-Wheat Bread* p. 273

 Plums *(or another on-special, fresh or canned fruit)*

 Chocolate Chip Cookies *("B" Choice)* p. 277*

SNACKS

 Water

 Veggies, leftover Chili-Stuffed Potato, leftover soup,
leftover salad, etc.

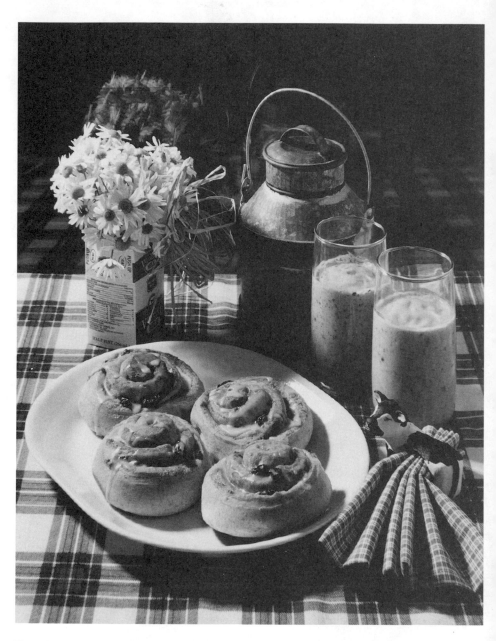

Photo: Tropical Fruit Ice p. 280
Super Cinnamon Rolls p. 273

MIX & MATCH MENU SAMPLER

🕐 *This clock indicates that the meal takes between about 2 and 15 minutes to prepare.*

DAY 1

🕐 *Quick & Easy*	**Breakfast**	fg/cal
Water	8 oz.	
Grain	1 cup Kellogg's Strawberry Fruit Wheats	0/180
Protein	1 cup 1% milk	3/102
Fruit	1 large banana, sliced, on cereal	0/105
Water/Snack	12 oz. water/ 1 cup Fruit Wheats/ 1 cup 1% milk	3/282

🕐 *Quick & Easy*	**Lunch**	
Water	8 oz.	
Vegetable	1/2 can Campbell's Chunky Bean & Ham Soup	8/250
Grain	2 slices whole or cracked-wheat toast with 1 Tb. All Fruit Jam* p. 275	1/174
Protein	(ham, beans, and bread combined)	
Fruit	1 cup green grapes	t/108
Water/Snack	8 oz. water/ 1 cup steamed veggies	t/76

🕐 *Quick & Easy*	**Dinner**	
Water	8 oz.	
Vegetable	2 Pizza Wheels* p. 286 (1 vegetable and 1 Canadian bacon, pineapple, and mushroom)	14/439
Grain	(pizza buns)	
Protein	(pizza meat and cheese)	
Fruit	1 cup Instant Peach Ice Cream* p. 278	t/117
Water/Snack	12 oz. water/ 1 leftover Veggie Pizza Wheel	6/200

> Total: 35/2033
> 35 fat grams x 9 calories = 315 calories from fat
> 315 ÷ 2033 = 15% fat

To avoid fat-storing stress on your body, it is essential that you increase your calories and fiber gradually. Eat each meal and snack until you are comfortably full, not stuffed! If this is too much food for your comfortable satisfaction, decrease the amounts but keep the balance and eat often!

MIX & MATCH MENUS

MIX & MATCH MENUS

DAY 2

	Breakfast	fg/cal
Easy		
Water	12 oz.	
Grain	1 large piece Country Corn Bread* p. 272 with 1 Tb. Smucker's Simply Fruit Spread	5/249
Protein	3/4 to 1 cup Egg Scramble (2 egg whites and 1 whole egg scrambled with a small amount of part-skim mozzarella cheese)	10/254
Fruit	1/2 large grapefruit	0/50
Water/Snack	8 oz./ 6 baby carrots	0/20

	Lunch	
Easy		
Water	12 oz.	
Vegetable	1 cup Short-cut Tossed Salad* p. 291, with 2 Tb. Buttemilk Dressing* p. 280	1/142±
Grain	1 Blueberry Muffin* p. 271	3/151
Protein	1/2 large Chili Stuffed Baked Potato (stuff with lowfat chili)	6/357
Fruit	1 large slice watermelon	t/50
Water/Snack	8 oz./ 1 Big Soft Pretzel* p. 271	1/52
	8 oz. skim milk	t/86
	1 cup mixed, raw vegetables	t/50±

	Dinner	
Water	8 oz.	
Vegetable	3/4 cup Au Gratin Potatoes* p. 290	9/418
	2 cups steamed broccoli	0/48
Grain	1 slice Perfect Whole-Wheat Bread* p. 273	1/88
Protein	1 - 5 oz. Parmesan Halibut Steak* p. 285	8/245
Fruit	1 cup strawberries, fresh*	1/45
Water/Snack	12 oz./ 1 cup mixed, raw veggies	t/50±

> Total: 45/2355
> 45 fat grams x 9 calories = 405 calories from fat
> 405 ÷ 2355 = 17% fat

Purchase fruits in season.

Remember, this is not a diet! You do not have to eat everything on this page. Just do a little mixing and matching and make sure you keep your meals balanced. A cheaper, faster breakfast may include oatmeal and honey with bananas and skim or 1% milk. A faster dinner might include a tuna fish or turkey sandwich stuffed with veggies and a bowl of peaches. Simply delicious!

DAY 3

		fg/cal
⏱ *Quick & Easy*	**Breakfast**	
Water	8 oz.	
Grain	2 French Toast* p. 277 slices with	
	4 Tb. syrup	1/191
Protein	(egg in French Toast), 8 oz. skim milk	t/86
Fruit	1 cup mixed fresh fruit	t/100±
Water/Snack	12 oz./ 1 cup steamed veggies	t/76
⏱ *Quick & Easy*	**Lunch**	
Water	12 oz.	
Vegetable	(lettuce, tomatoes, onions, and taco sauce)	
Grain	(corn taco shells)	
Protein	2 large Tempting Tacos* p. 288	16/578
Fruit	1 cup sliced apples in lemon water	t/81
Water/Snack	8 oz./ 1 lg. Tempting	
	Taco leftover from lunch	8/289
Easy	**Dinner**	
Water	12 oz.	
Vegetable	1 cup Tossed Salad* p. 292 with 2 Tb.	
	lowfat or fat free dressing	1/142±
Grain	(noodles)	
Protein	1 cup Beef Stroganoff* p. 282	5/253
Fruit	3/4 cup Fruit Gelatin (cherry)* p. 281	0/75
Water/Snack	8 oz./1-1/2 cups leftover Tossed Salad	
	with 2 Tb. lowfat dressing	1/192±

Total:	32/2063

32 fat grams x 9 calories = 288 calories from fat
288 ÷ 2063 = 14% fat

My kids love this menu. The French Toast is a favorite, along with the Tempting Tacos. They especially love the Beef Stroganoff and Fruit Gelatin.

DAY 4

🕐 *Quick & Easy*	**Breakfast**	fg/cal
Water	8 oz.	
Grain	1 Super Cinnamon Roll* p. 273	
	(make ahead to save time)	5/218
Protein	1 cup skim milk	0/86
Fruit	1 cup cantaloup chunks	t/57
Water/Snack	12 oz./ 1 cup mixed	
	vegetable chunks	t/50±

Golden Corral Restaurant	**Lunch**	
Water	8 oz.	
Vegetable	1/2 baked potato with	
	4 Tb. cottage cheese	1/160
	2 cups salad bar	
	vegetables with 1/2 cup cottage cheese	2/300±
Grain	1 order Texas Toast	6/170
Protein	1 order Sirloin Tips with onions and	
	peppers	13/290
Fruit	1 cup fresh fruit	
	(from salad bar)	t/100±
Water/Snack	12 oz./ leftover half of baked potato	t/110

🕐 *Quick & Easy*	**Dinner**	
Water	8 oz.	
Vegetable	(in salad)	
Grain	1 large slice Zucchini Pineapple-Nut	
	Bread* p. 274	6/230
Protein	1 cup Veggie-Tuna Pasta Salad* p. 289	1/215
Fruit	3 sliced kiwifruit	t/138
Water/Snack	8 oz. 1 sliced cucumber	t/39

Total: 34/2163

34 fat grams x 9 calories = 306 calories from fat

306 ÷ 2163 = 14% fat

If you aren't accustomed to eating whole-grain breads, fruits, and raw vegetables, go with part whole-grains, such as cracked-wheat breads and rolls, and eat steamed or canned vegetables and fruits.

ADJUST TO YOUR NEEDS SHOPPING LISTS
FOR THE "MIX & MATCH" MENU SAMPLER

> ### YOU MUST READ THIS!
> *These shopping lists are for families of four adult size people eating approximately 2,000 to 3,000 calories each. Adjust them to your family size or single needs and your own personal taste, budget, time schedule, calorie needs, and food allergies. I generally buy food for seven to ten people. I find that a **four day** shopping list, adjusted to my family's size, **usually lasts us seven days** because of leftovers and unplanned eating-out exursions. It looks expensive to plan ahead like this, but you may actually save a lot of money, especially on junk food and doctor bills. But remember, you must adjust these shopping lists to meet **your** individual needs!*

Stock your kitchen with the following master list items. You will use these items often and will not need to purchase them weekly.

MASTER LIST

BAKING

baking powder	rice
baking soda	rolled oats
brown sugar	unflavored gelatin
cocoa powder	vegetable oil
corn meal	white flour
cornstarch	white sugar
honey	whole wheat
powdered egg	(kernels)
whites	whole-wheat flour
powdered sugar	yeast

CONDIMENTS

all-fruit jams or jellies,	lemon juice
(fruit-juice sweetened)	maple syrup
fat free mayonnaise	mustard
fat free miracle whip	parmesan cheese
fat free or lowfat salad	vinegar
dressings	Worcestershire
ketchup	Sauce

SPICES AND SEASONINGS

allspice	ginger
almond extract	Italian Seasoning
basil leaves	mapleine
barbecue spices	minced garlic
beef bouillon	minced onion
chicken bouillon	nutmeg
chilli powder	oregano
cinnamon	paprika
cloves	seasoned salt
cream of tartar	soy sauce
curry powder	taco seasoning
dill weed	tarrogon leaves
dried parsley flakes	thyme
dry mustard	rosemary
garlic	vanilla
garlic salt	

SPECIAL REMINDER:
You must *adjust* these menus to your individual:

1. **Time schedule**
2. **Budget needs**
3. **Special health needs** (allergies, diabetes, etc.)
4. **Family needs and tastes** (whether you're single or cook for a large family)
5. **Calorie and fiber needs** (increase fiber and calories *very* gradually)

And remember to buy fruits and vegetables that are in season and to take advantage of in-store specials. (Buy foods in bulk quantities, if this meets your needs.)

Two separate families of four purchased the foods on the first shopping list (after the master list). The first family spent $79. The second family spent $24. (They used bulk items they had in storage as well.) These shopping lists are *very* flexible.

259

SHOPPING LIST / DAYS 1 – 4

This four day shopping list may actually last a family of four up to seven days because of leftovers and unplanned eating-out excursions.

BREAD / CEREAL / GRAINS

bread, whole wheat, 1 loaf
cereal, Kellogg's Strawberry Fruit Wheats, 1 box
hamburger buns, whole wheat, 1 doz.
noodles, whole grain (or white), 12 oz.
pasta, whole grain (or white), corkscrew 12 oz.
taco shells, corn, (12 jumbo taco shells or 24 mini taco shells)

FRUITS AND VEGETABLES

apples, 5
bananas, 4
cantaloupe, 11
grapefruit, 2
grapes, 4 cups
kiwifruit, 6
strawberries, 1 quart
watermelon, 1 half

broccoli, 3 bunches
carrots, 5 lbs.
baby carrots, 1 sm. bag
cauliflower, 1 head
cherry tomatoes, 10
cucumbers, 3
lettuce, 2 heads
mushrooms, 2 cups
onions, green, 1 bunch
onions, yellow, 3
peppers, green, 2
potatoes, baking, 16
tomatoes, salad, 6
vegetables, mixed (broccoli, pea pods, onions, carrots), 2 lg. bags
zucchini, 2 medium

MEAT AND DAIRY*

bacon, Canadian, 4 oz.
beef, extra lean stew, 1 lb.
fish, halibut, 4 steaks

butter, 1/2 lb.
buttermilk, 1 pint
cheese, cheddar, 4 oz.

cheese, mozzarella, part-skim, 1 1/2 lbs.
cheese, parmesan, 3 oz.
cream cheese, nonfat, 1 pkg.
eggs*, 3 dozen (or 1 dozen fresh and 2 dozen powdered egg whites–you will use mostly whites)
milk, 1%, 1 quart
milk, skim, 1 gallon
sour cream, fat free, 1 pint
yogurt, plain, nonfat, 1 pint

CANNED GOODS

applesauce, one 16 oz. can
beans, refried (no fat), two 16 oz. cans
chili, chicken, four 15 oz. cans
corn, cream style, one 16 oz. can
fruit cocktail (own juice), one 16 oz. can
milk, evaporated skim, one 12 oz. can
mushrooms, one 8 oz. can
pineapple, chunks (own juice), one 15 oz. can
pineapple, crushed (own juice), one 15 oz. can
Pizza Quick Sauce, two 15 oz. cans
soup, Campbell's chunky Bean & Ham, two 19 1/4 oz. cans
tuna (white or regular, water packed), two 6 1/2 oz. cans

FROZEN

blueberries, 1 cup
juice, Dole Mountain Cherry concentrate, one 12 oz. can
juice, apple concentrate, one 12 oz. can
juice, Dole Orchard Peach concentrate, one 12 oz. can peaches, 4 cups

MISCELLANEOUS

dressing, ranch, nonfat, 1 bottle
salsa, one 16 oz. jar
taco seasoning mix, 1 package
walnuts, 1/2 cup
wheat gluten, 1/2 cup

*Meat and dairy products are used in great moderation. Egg whites, which are fat free, generally replace the whole egg. Small amounts of butter replace margarine and shortening because butter is a highly saturated "natural" fat rather than a man-made, "heat-damaged," partially saturated fat. Be very moderate with its use.

If you choose to buy many of your bread items already made, such as bread, muffins, cinnamon rolls, etc., you will need to purchase fewer eggs and less butter.

MIX & MATCH MENUS

DAY 53

		fg/cal
⏱ *Quick & Easy*	**Breakfast**	
Water	12 oz.	
Grain	1 cup Cinnamon-Maple Oatmeal* p. 276	3/278
Protein	1 cup skim milk	t/86
Fruit	1 large sliced orange	t/62
Water/Snack	8 oz./ 1 cup leftover oatmeal and milk	3/278
	1 cup purple cabbage slices	t/20

⏱ *Quick & Easy*	**Lunch**	
Water	8 oz.	
Vegetable	1/2 can Campbell's Old Fashioned Vegetable Beef Soup	5/160
Grain	2 Marvelous Muffins* p. 272 (make ahead)	6/296
Protein	1 cup nonfat fruit yogurt	0/200
Fruit	2 cups honeydew melon chunks	t/120
Water/Snack	12 oz./ 8 baby carrots	0/35

Easy	**Dinner**	
Water	8 oz.	
Vegetable	2 cups Easy Cabbage Dinner* p. 284	9/620
Grain	1 Marvelous Muffin left over from lunch	3/148
Protein	(in cabbage dinner)	
Fruit	1 2-1/2" by 2" square Peach Cobbler* p. 279 ("B+" Choice)	6/316
Water/Snack	12 oz./ 1 cup purple cabbage slices	t/20

> Total: 35/2639
> 35 fat grams x 9 calories = 315 calories from fat
> 315 ÷ 2639 = 12% fat

This is what I call a "cabbage day". Even people who formerly didn't like cabbage love this Easy Cabbage Dinner.

DAY 54

		fg/cal
Easy	**Breakfast**	
Water	12 oz.	
Grain	2 slices Zucchini-Pineapple-Nut Bread* p. 274 (make ahead)	6/230
Protein	1 cup nonfat fruit yogurt	0/200
Fruit		
Water/Snack	8 oz./ 1 cup mixed fresh vegetables/ 4 Tb. Ranch Dip* p. 281	1/120±

Subway	**Lunch**	
Sandwiches		
Water	12 oz.	
Vegetable	1 foot-long turkey sandwich on whole wheat (no oil or mayonnaise, add extra vegetables)	10/624
Grain	(crust)	
Protein	(cheese)	
Fruit	1 apple (from home)	t/81
	5 oz. TCBY Frozen Yogurt ("B" choice)	3/160±
Water/Snack	8 oz./ 2 slices leftover Zucchini-Pineapple-Nut Bread	6/230

Easy	**Dinner**	
Water	8 oz./ 1-1/4 cups Saucy Green Beans and Almonds* p. 291	7/139
Vegetable	1 large baked potato/ 6 Tb. Ranch Dip left over from snack	1.5/325
Grain	2 Marvelous Muffins* left over from Day 53	6/296
Protein	1 BBQ Chicken Breast* p. 282	6/236
Fruit	12 oz. Dole Country Raspberry Juice mixed with 1/2 cup Sprite or 7-Up	0/221
Water/Snack	12 oz./ 1 sliced cucumber	t/39

Total: 46.5/3001

46.5 fat grams x 9 calories = 418.5 calories
from fat   418.5 ÷ 3001 = 14% fat

*You could turn this day into an "all quick and easy" day by having cold cereal for breakfast and leftovers for dinner. And remember, **you** may be eating only **half** this much food. Listen to your body and adjust accordingly.*

DAY 55

		fg/cal
⏱ *Quick & Easy*	**Breakfast**	
Water	12 oz.	
Grain	1-1/2 cups corn flakes mixed with 1/2 cup Post Grapenuts	0/385
Protein	1-1/2 cups 1% milk	4.5/153
Fruit	1 sliced banana (on cereal)	t/105
Water/Snack	8 oz./ 1-1/2 cup Total cereal/ 1 cup 1% milk	4.5/252
	8 baby carrots	0/35

⏱ *Quick & Easy*	**Lunch**	
Water	12 oz.	
Vegetable	11 oz. La Choy Fresh and Lite Beef Broccoli	7/290
Grain	1/2 cup Chow Mein Noodles	5/228
Protein	1-1/2 cups LaChoy Sweet and Sour Oriental with Chicken	4/480
Fruit	1-1/2 cups Tropical Fruit Ice*p. 280	1/228
Water/Snack	8 oz./ 2 slices Zucchini-Pineapple-Nut Bread left over from Day 54	6/230

⏱ *Quick & Easy*	**Dinner**	
Water	8 oz.	
Vegetable	1-1/2 cups Tossed Salad* p. 292 with 6 Tb. Buttermilk Dressing* p. 280	3/276±
Grain	(2 whole-grain hamburger buns)	
Protein	2 Sloppy Joes* p. 287	26/824
Fruit	1 cup green grapes	t/72
	Dessert: 1-1/2 cups root beer float (1 cup root beer with 1/2 cup vanilla ice milk = "B" Choice)	2/270
Water/Snack	12 oz./ 1 cup leftover Tossed Salad with 4 Tb. Buttermilk Dressing	2/184±

> Total: 65/4012
> 65 fat grams x 9 calories = 585 calories from fat
> 585 ÷ 4012 = 15% fat

My teenage boys eat more than this menu illustrates. I sometimes eat this much if I'm exercising a lot (hiking, etc.) or nursing a baby. Less than half this much may fill you up, so make certain to adjust this menu to your individual needs. Success is a feeling, not a number! If you're a stuffer, lighten up your meals a little. Go heavier on the veggies and lighter on the grains. Enjoy the freedom to feel energized, not miserable after a meal. And, only snack on veggies, (unless you're really hungry) especially in the evening.

263

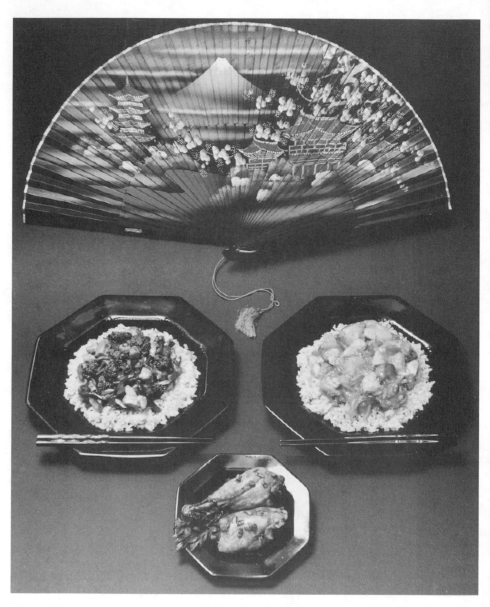

Photo: La Choy Fresh and Lite Beef Broccoli and Chicken Chow Mein served over brown rice with baked chicken—quick and easy!

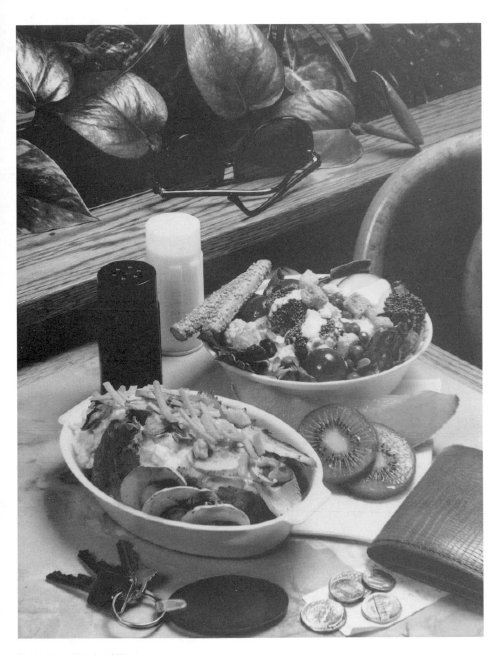

Photo: Tossed Salad p. 292
Baked potato stuffed with veggies, fat free sour cream, lowfat cottage cheese,
and a small amount of part-skim mozzarella cheese.

DAY 56

		fg/cal
🕐 **Quick & Easy**	**Breakfast**	
Water		
Grain	1 3" square Country Corn Bread* p. 272	5/201
	with 1 Tb. honey butter (or All Fruit Jam*	
	p. 275)	6/80
Protein	1-1/2 cups Breakfast Shake* p. 275	0/244
Fruit	(in shake)	
Water/Snack	12 oz./ 1 sliced zucchini	t/18

🕐 **Quick & Easy**	**Lunch**	
Water	8 oz.	
Vegetable	1 cup fresh carrot and celery sticks/ 6 Tb.	
	Ranch Dip left over from Day 54	2/145
Grain	15 oz. Franco-American PizzO's	
	("B+" choice)	4/340
Protein	(in PizzO's and cottage cheese)	
Fruit	1 cup Pineapple and Cottage Cheese	
	Salad* p. 281	2/202
Water/Snack	12 oz./ 1 sliced cucumber	t/39

Easy	**Dinner**	
Water	8 oz.	
Vegetable	2 cups Zucchini Casserole* p. 289	12/366
Grain	(stuffing in casserole)	
Protein	(in casserole and cottage cheese)	
Fruit	1 cup Pineapple and Cottage Cheese Salad	
	left over from lunch	2/202
Water/Snack	12 oz./ 1 cup Kellogg's Crispix Cereal	0/110
	with 3/4 cup 1% milk	2/76
	1 sliced green pepper	t/26

Total:	35/2049

35 fat grams x 9 calories = 315 calories from fat

315 ÷ 2049= 15% fat

This menu contains 35 fat grams and is 15 percent fat. Day 55 contains 65 fat grams and is 15 percent fat. How could this be? Day 55 contains 4012 calories and Day 56 has 2,049 calories, so it takes about twice as many fat grams to give the first day the same fat percentage as the second day. Your hunger and energy needs may easily vary 500 or more calories on any given day. I average between about 2,000 and 3,500 calories a day. In hot weather hunger lessens. With more activity hunger increases. LISTEN to your body!

SHOPPING LIST / DAYS 53 – 56

These shopping lists are very detailed. Some people thoroughly enjoy following them. Others prefer less stucture and follow the Grab 'n' Go or Budget Menus. They plan ahead two or three days at a time.

BREAD / CEREAL / GRAINS

buns, hamburger, (whole grain or white), one-8 count package
cereal, cornflakes, 1 box
cereal, Post Grapenuts, 1 box

FRUIT AND VEGETABLES

apples, 4
bananas, 8
grapefruit, 4
grapes, 4 lbs.
melon, honeydew, 1
oranges, 4
peaches, 6
pineapple, 1

cabbage, green, 1 head
cabbage, purple, 1 head
carrots, 5 lbs.
carrots, baby, 1 medium bag
celery, 1 bunch
cucumbers, 8
lettuce, 1 head
onions, 4
peppers, green, 5
potatoes, baking, 12
tomatoes, salad, 2
zuchini, 14

MEAT / DAIRY

beef, extra-lean ground, 1/2 lb.
chicken, breasts (boneless, skinless), 8

butter, 1/2 lb.
buttermilk, 12 pint
cheese, cheddar, 4 oz.
cottage cheese, lowfat, 32 oz.
eggs, 18 (you'll use mostly whites)
milk, 1% (or skim), 1 gallon

milk, skim, 1 gallon
yogurt, fruit, nonfat, 32 oz.
yogurt, plain, nonfat, 16 oz.

CANNED GOODS

applesauce, two 16 oz. cans
beans, green (French cut), two 16 oz. cans
corn, one 17 oz. can
corn, cream style, one 16 oz. can
Franco American PizzO's, four 15 oz.
LaChoy Fresh and Lite Beef and Broccoli, 2 43 1/2 oz. cans
milk, evaporated skim, one 12 oz. can
noodles, chow mein, one 5 oz. can
oranges, mandarin, two 11 oz. cans
pineapple, crushed (own juice), one 20 oz. can
LaChoy Sweet and Sour Chicken, soup, Campbell's Old Fashioned Vegetable Beef, two 19 oz. cans
soup, cream of chicken, lowfat, one 10 3/4 oz. can
soup, cream of mushroom, lowfat, one 10 3/4 oz. can
soup, tomato, two 10 3/4 oz. cans
tomato sauce, one 8 oz. can

FROZEN

juice, apple concentrate, one 12 oz. can
juice, Dole Country Raspberry concentrate, one 12 oz. can
juice, Dole Orchard Peach concentrate, one 12 oz. can
juice, orange concentrate, one 12 oz. can
juice, pineapple concentrate, one 12 oz. can
strawberries, 64 oz.

MISCELLANEOUS

almonds, slivered, 4 oz.
ice milk, vanilla, 1/2 gallon
root beer, 2 liters
salad dressing, Hidden Valley Lite Ranch, 1 envelope
7-Up, 2 liters
walnuts, 2 oz.

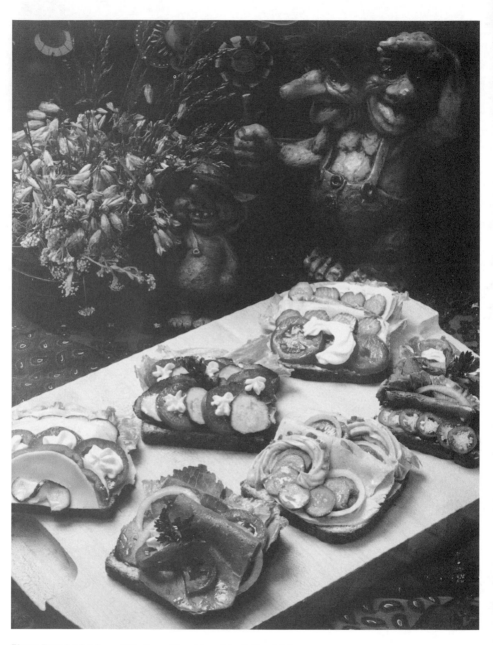

Photo: *Tuna Sandwich — p. 288, along with a wide variety of other delicious sandwiches featured in Dana's LEAN & FREE 2000 PLUS COOKBOOK*

Dana's

LEAN&FREE

Recipe Sampler

Normal!
Delicious!
Exceptionally Fast!

"A" Choices = Nutritional fat-loss choices when combined with other good foods.

"B" Choices = Good coasting or maintenance choices. Some people see optimal fat loss with a few "B" choices added into their "A" days. Others have more resistant bodies and see much more success with all "A" choices.

Listen to **your** body and adjust to your needs.

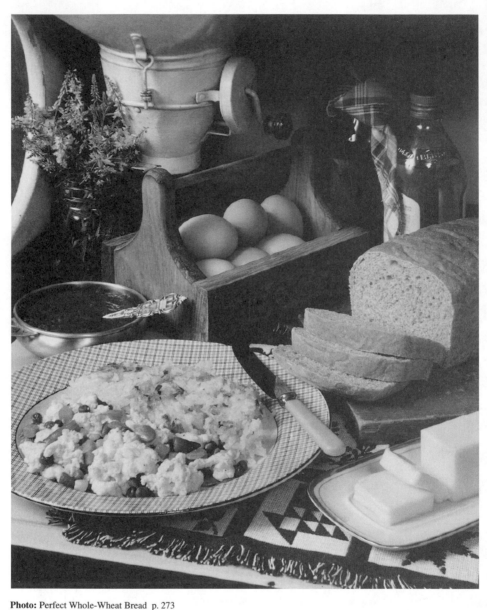

Photo: Perfect Whole-Wheat Bread p. 273
Hash Brown Potatoes served with the
delicious Veggie and Cheese Egg Scramble
featured in Dana's LEAN & FREE 2000 PLUS COOKBOOK

270

BREADS AND MUFFINS

Big Soft Pretzels ("A" Choice)

1	cup whole-wheat flour
1/2	cup unbleached flour
2	teaspoons baking powder
1	teaspoon sugar
1/2	teaspoon salt
2/3	cup skim milk
2	tablespoons soft butter

1	egg white
	coarse salt

Big Soft Pretzels

Calories per serving:	52
Fat grams per serving:	1
Number of servings:	16
Serving size:	1

Mix flours, baking powder, sugar, and salt in bowl. Add milk and soft butter. Mix with fork to make a soft dough. Knead 10 times. Divide dough in half. Roll half of dough into rectangle 12" x 8". Cut lengthwise into 8 1-inch strips. Fold each strip in half lengthwise and pinch edges to seal. Twist each strip into pretzel shape. Place seam-side down on greased baking sheet. Repeat with remaining half of dough. Beat egg white in small bowl with fork. Brush pretzels with egg and sprinkle lightly with coarse salt. Bake at 400 degrees 16-20 minutes or until golden brown. Makes 16 large pretzels. Remove with wide pancake turner and place on rack to cool.

Blueberry Muffins ("A" Choice)

11/2	cups whole-wheat flour (white wheat)
3/4	cup rolled oats
1	teaspoon soda
1	teaspoon baking powder
1/4	teaspoon salt
2	slightly beaten egg whites
3/4	cup skim milk
2	tablespoons "good" oil (see page 165)
1/2	cup honey or 2/3 cup sugar
1/2	cup applesauce

1/2	cup honey or 2/3 cup sugar
1/2	cup applesauce
3/4	cup fresh or frozen blueberries

Blueberry Muffins

Calories per serving:	151
Fat grams per serving:	3
Number of servings:	12
Serving size:	1 muffin

If you are diabetic or have a sugar allergy, replace the 1/3 cup honey with 1/4 cup frozen concentrated apple juice and 1/4 cup frozen concentrated pineapple juice and decrease the milk to 2/3 cup.

In a mixing bowl combine flour, oats, soda, baking powder, and salt. Make a well in the center. Combine egg whites, milk, oil, honey, and applesauce in a separate bowl; add all at once to well in flour mixture. Stir just until moist, allowing batter to be lumpy. Gently fold 3/4 cup fresh or frozen blueberries into muffin batter. Line muffin tin with paper baking cups. Fill 2/3 full. Bake at 375 degrees for 15 to 20 minutes or until lightly browned. Remove from pans and serve warm. Makes 10 to 12 muffins.

271

Country Corn Bread ("A" Choice)

1/2   cup whole-wheat flour
1/2   cup white flour
1   cup cornmeal
1/2   teaspoon salt
4   teaspoons baking powder
4   egg whites
2   whole eggs
1/4   cup fat free dairy sour cream
1   can (16 oz.) cream-style corn
       (blended)
2   tablespoons "good" oil (see page 165)

Country Corn Bread	
Calories per serving:	201
Fat grams per serving:	5
Number of servings:	9
Serving size:	3" square

Sift dry ingredients and set aside. Beat whole eggs and egg whites until frothy and light. Add sour cream, corn, and oil. Gradually stir in dry ingredients and beat well. Pour into a 9 x 9 pan that has been thoroughly sprayed with nonstick cooking spray. Bake at 400 degrees for 30 minutes. (This recipe can be made into muffins—bake 15-20 minutes at 400 degrees.)

Marvelous Muffins ("A" Choice)

11/2   cups whole-wheat flour
       (white wheat)
3/4   cup rolled oats
1   teaspoon soda
1   teaspoon baking powder
1/4   teaspoon salt
2   slightly beaten egg whites
3/4   cup skim milk
2   tablespoons "good" oil (see page 165)
1/2   cup honey or 2/3 cup sugar
1/2   cup applesauce

1/2   cup honey or 2/3 cup sugar
1/2   cup applesauce

Marvelous Muffins	
Calories per serving:	148
Fat grams per serving:	3
Number of servings:	12
Serving size:	1 muffin

If you are diabetic or have a sugar allergy, replace the 1/3 cup honey with 1/4 cup frozen concentrated apple juice and 1/4 cup frozen concentrated pineapple juice and decrease the milk to 2/3 cup.

In a mixing bowl combine flour, oats, soda, baking powder, and salt. Make a well in the center. Combine egg whites, milk, oil, honey, and applesauce in a separate bowl; add all at once to well in flour mixture. Stir just until moist, allowing batter to be lumpy. Line muffin tin with paper baking cups. Fill 2/3 full. Bake at 375 degrees for 15 to 20 minutes or until lightly browned. Remove from pans and serve warm. Makes 10 to 12 muffins.

Perfect Whole-Wheat Bread ("A" Choice)

10 to 12 cups whole-wheat flour
2   tablespoons dry yeast
1/2 cup wheat gluten
4   cups warm water (120-130 degrees)
1/3 cup "good" oil (see page 165)
1/3 cup honey
1   tablespoon salt

Perfect Whole Wheat Bread	
Calories per serving:	88
Fat grams per serving:	1
Number of servings:	approximately 16 slices
Serving size:	1 slice

Place 6 cups flour into mixer bowl with kneading arm. Add dry yeast and gluten; mix well. Add water and mix for 1 minute. Cover and let dough sit for 10 minutes. This makes the bread lighter. Add oil, honey, and salt. Turn on mixer and quickly add remaining flour, 1 cup at a time, until dough forms a ball and cleans the sides of the bowl. Knead 7 to 10 minutes; by hand 12 to 15 minutes. Dough should be smooth and elastic.

Preheat oven to 150 degrees. Lightly oil hands. Divide dough into four equal portions. Shape and place in greased bread pans. Place into warm oven and let rise about 15 to 20 minutes. When almost double in bulk, turn oven to 350 degrees and bake about 25 minutes or until golden brown. Turn out of pans onto a wire cooling rack immediately. When cool, store bread in plastic bags in the freezer. Makes 4 1-pound loaves.

Super Cinnamon Rolls ("A–" Choice)

1   can nonfat evaporated milk
11/2 cups warm water
11/2 tablespoons yeast
1/2 cup "good" oil (see page 165)
1   tablespoon lemon juice, freshly squeezed
3/4 cup honey
1   egg white
1   teaspoon salt
11/2 teaspoons baking powder

8   cups whole-wheat flour (may use half white and half whole-wheat flour)
raisins (optional)

Super Cinnamon Rolls	
Calories per serving:	218
Fat grams per serving:	5
Number of servings:	24
Serving size:	1 large roll

Warm the milk and add warm water. Dissolve the yeast in the liquid mixture. Mix the remaining ingredients into the liquid and add just enough flour to make a soft dough. (If you want light rolls, make sure the dough is soft and not stiff. The flour is the ingredient that determines the dough texture.) Knead the dough for 10 minutes and let it relax for 15 minutes. Take half of the dough and roll it out with a rolling pin to 1/4 to 1/2 inch thickness. Brush the surface lightly with melted butter and sprinkle with cinnamon and a thin amount of brown sugar. Roll up the dough like a jelly roll and cut into 1" slices. Put them on nonstick cooking-sprayed cookie sheets and allow them to rise until they are double in bulk. Bake at 350 degrees for 20 minutes or until lightly brown. Remove and eat as is, or frost lightly with powdered sugar and water or skim milk mixed.

Finely ground "white wheat" flour (a new variety of whole wheat) makes delectable cinnamon rolls.

For faster raising, place in oven set at 150 degrees for 15 minutes; then bake.

These are excellent with diced apples in the filling.

Zucchini-Pineapple-Nut Bread ("A–" Choice)

6 egg whites
1/2 cup "good" oil (see page 165)
2 cups sugar
2 cups zucchini, grated
1 cup crushed pineapple, well drained
1/2 cup chopped walnuts or pecans
3 teaspoons vanilla
3 cups whole-wheat flour
1/2 teaspoon salt
3 teaspoons cinnamon
11/2 teaspoons baking powder
11/2 teaspoons baking soda

Zucchini-Pineapple-Nut Bread	
Calories per serving:	115
Fat grams per serving:	3
Number of servings:	34
Serving size:	1/2" slice or 1" slice mini loaf

Mix together egg whites, oil, and sugar. Add zucchini, pineapple, nuts, and vanilla, and stir into the mixture. In a seperate bowl, sift together flour, salt, cinnamon, baking powder, and baking soda; blend well. Stir dry mixture into wet mixture. Blend well.

Pour into small, nonstick cooking-sprayed pans. Bake for 60 minutes at 325 degrees. (This bread freezes well.) For cupcakes, bake 30 minutes at 325 degrees.

BREAD SPREADS

All Fruit Jam ("A" Choice)

2   envelopes unflavored gelatin
1/2   cup frozen unsweetened apple-
      juice concentrate, thawed
1/2   cup frozen unsweetened Dole
      Mountain Cherry juice
      concentrate, thawed
11/2 quarts fresh strawberries, washed,
      hulled, and mashed
3   cups very ripe mashed bananas
1   tablespoon lemon juice

All Fruit Jam	
Calories per serving:	32
Fat grams per serving:	trace
Number of servings:	48
Serving size:	2 tablespoons

Sprinkle gelatin over 1/2 cup apple-juice concentrate and set aside. Combine 1/2 cup cherry-juice concentrate, strawberries, bananas, and lemon juice in heavy saucepan. Cook over medium-low heat for 10 to 15 minutes, stirring constantly.

Remove from heat and add softened gelatin mixture, stirring constantly until gelatin is completely dissolved. Cool at room temperature. Store in refrigerator. Makes approximately 6 cups.

Bread Spread Suggestions: Store-brought all-fruit jams; Fat free cream cheeses; Very small amounts of real butter

BREAKFAST FOODS

Breakfast Shake ("A" Choice)

3/4 cup skim milk
1/2 cup nonfat yogurt, any flavor
1   ripe banana, peeled and frozen
1/4 cup sliced fruit, frozen (any type
      of fruit you would like)
1/4 cup orange juice

Breakfast Shake	
Calories per serving:	244
Fat grams per serving:	0
Number of servings:	2
Serving size:	1 cup

Blend ingredients together in blender. Delicious! Be creative and try a variety of fruits combined with juices.

To freeze bananas: remove peel, cut in half, wrap each piece in plastic, and freeze. Never throw away overripe bananas. Always freeze them for breakfast shakes. Over-ripe bananas are very sweet.

Cinnamon-Maple Oatmeal ("A" Choice)

regular oatmeal
cinnamon
maple syrup*

Cinnamon-Maple Oatmeal	
Calories per serving:	417
Fat grams per serving:	3
Serving size:	1 1/2 cups

Prepare oatmeal according to package directions. Add cinnamon and maple syrup to taste. (Go for lightly sweet, not heavily sweetened cereal.)
If you are diabetic, omit syrup and use All Fruit Jam.

Cracked Wheat, Raisin, and Honey Cereal ("A+" Choice)

11/2 cups cracked wheat (cracked in blender)
6   cups boiling water
1/2 teaspoon salt
1/4 cup raisins
1/4 to 1/2 cup honey*

Cracked Wheat Raisin and Honey Cereal	
Calories per serving:	450
Fat grams per serving:	1
Number of servings:	5 to 6
Serving size:	approximately 1 cup

Add salt to boiling water. Stir in wheat and cook on warm for 10 to 25 minutes, covered. (Cooking time depends on how crunchy you like your cereal.) Stir in raisins and honey. Serve with skim, 1%, or evaporated skim milk.
* If you are diabetic, sweeten with All Fruit Jam.*

French Toast ("A" Choice)

6   slices whole-grain bread
4   egg whites, lightly beaten
1/4 teaspoon salt
1/2 cup skim milk
1/4 teaspoon vanilla
1/8 teaspoon ground cinnamon

French Toast	
Calories per serving:	191
Fat grams per serving:	1
Number of servings:	3
Serving size:	2 slices

In a shallow bowl, beat together egg whites, salt, milk, vanilla, and cinnamon. Dip bread into egg mixture, coating both sides. Do not drench.

Heat skillet on medium heat until water droplets scatter. Spray with nonstick cooking spray. Cook bread on both sides until golden brown. Serve with syrup, fruit sauces, or fresh fruit and vanilla yogurt.

DESSERTS

Chocolate Chip Cookies ("B" Choice)

2/3 cup applesauce
1/3 cup butter*
2/3 cup sugar
2/3 cup brown sugar
4   egg whites
2   teaspoons vanilla
3   cups whole-wheat flour
1   teaspoon soda
1   teaspoon salt
1   package (6 oz.) chocolate chips

Chocolate Chip Cookies	
Calories per serving:	86
Fat grams per serving:	2 1/2
Number of servings:	48
Serving size:	1 cookie

Heat oven to 375 degrees. Mix apple-sauce, butter, sugars, egg whites, and vanilla. Stir in remaining ingredients. Drop dough by rounded teaspoons 2 inches apart onto ungreased baking sheet. Bake 8 to 10 minutes or until light brown. Cool slightly before removing from baking sheet.

Because butter is naturally saturated instead of heat-damaged and partially saturated (as in margarine or shortening), I consider butter the best choice. But be very moderate with it as it is a highly-saturated, 100 percent fat choice. These cookies contain only 2 1/2 fat grams each.

SAMPLER RECIPES

277

Instant Blueberry Ice Cream
("A" Choice)

1   cup skim milk or evaporated
       skim milk
2   cups frozen blueberries
1/4   cup frozen pineapple-juice
       concentrate
1/4   cup frozen apple slices

Instant Blueberry Ice Cream	
Calories per serving:	224
Fat grams per serving	trace
Number of servings:	2
Serving size:	1 1/2 cups

Blend all ingredients in blender until smooth. Serve in parfait glasses.

Other variations:

Try any combination of frozen fruit and fruit-juice concentrate mixed with skim or 1% milk. Be sure to break the fruit into little chunks to aid in the blending process.

You can also use water in place of milk if you have dairy-product intolerance or if you prefer a fruit "ice" instead of a fruit "ice cream." For milk-shake thickness, use 2 cups skim milk.

Instant Peach Ice Cream
("A" Choice)

1   cup skim milk (or 1%)
2   cups frozen peaches
       (broken apart)
1/2   cup Dole frozen Orchard Peach
       juice concentrate, sweeten
       to taste

Instant Peach Ice Cream	
Calories per serving:	176
Fat grams per serving:	trace
Number of servings:	2
Serving size:	1 1/2 cups

Blend all ingredients in blender until smooth. Serve in parfait glasses. You can use canned peaches. Drain and spread on cookie sheet in separate pieces. Freeze and then use.

SAMPLER RECIPES

Peach Cobbler ("B+" Choice)

Peach Filling:

6	cups sliced peaches
1/3	cup sugar
3	tablespoons Dole Orchard Peach frozen juice concentrate, thawed
1	tablespoon lemon juice
2	tablespoons cold water
1	tablespoon cornstarch

Peach Cobbler	
Calories per serving:	316
Fat grams per serving:	6
Number of servings:	6
Serving size:	2 1/2" x 2"

Cook and stir 6 cups sliced peaches with the sugar, thawed Dole Orchard Peach juice concentrate concentrate, and lemon juice. Stir until boiling; reduce heat. Cover and simmer for 5 minutes, stirring occasionally until fruit is almost tender. Combine 2 tablespoons cold water and 1 tablespoon cornstarch; add to filling, cooking and stirring until thick and bubbly. Keep hot.

For topping:

1	cup whole-wheat flour	3	tablespoons butter
1/4	cup sugar	2	egg whites, beaten
1	teaspoon baking powder	3	tablespoons skim milk
1/2	teaspoon ground cinnamon		

Mix flour, sugar, baking powder, and cinnamon. Cut in butter until mixture looks like course crumbs. Combine egg and milk. Add to flour mixture. Stir just until moist.

Pour apple filling into an 8 x 8 x 2 baking dish. Drop topping into 6 equally spaced mounds on top of the filling. Bake at 400 degrees for 20 to 25 minutes or until toothpick comes out clean. Top with ice milk.

Tropical Fruit Ice ("A" Choice)

2	bananas, chunked and frozen on cookie sheet
2	large cans drained mandarin oranges frozen on cookie sheet
1	quart strawberries, topped, halved, and frozen on cookie sheet
1/3	cup frozen pineapple-juice concentrate
1/3	cup frozen apple-juice concentrate
1	cup evaporated skim milk (or regular skim milk)
	nonfat vanilla yogurt

Tropical Fruit ice	
Calories per serving:	228
Fat grams per serving:	1
Number of servings:	4
Serving size:	1 1/2 cups

Blend all ingredients except yogurt in blender, adding more or less milk to achieve desired consistency and more or less juice concentrate to achieve desired sweetness. Top with nonfat vanilla yogurt and a tiny oriental umbrella.

Note: Water can replace milk for a more "icy" treat or in the case of a dairy allergy.

DIPS & DRESSINGS

Buttermilk Dressing ("A" Choice)
This is delicious!

1/2	cup nonfat mayonnaise
1/4	cup nonfat salad dressing
1/2	cup buttermilk
1	teaspoon dried parsley flakes
1/2	teaspoon instant minced onion
1/2	to 1 clove crushed garlic
1/2	teaspoon salt
	dash of pepper

Buttermilk Dressing	
Calories per serving:	42
Fat grams per serving:	1
Number of servings:	8
Serving size:	2 Tb.

Shake all ingredients together in a covered container and refrigerate 2 or 3 hours. Shake and serve. If dressing is thick, use additional buttermilk to thin to desired consistency.

Ranch Dip ("A" Choice)

1/4   cup skim milk
1   small carton (16 oz.) lowfat
     cottage cheese
1   envelope Hidden Valley Lite
     Ranch Dressing

Ranch Dip	
Calories per serving:	35
Fat grams per serving:	.5
Number of servings:	16
Serving size:	2 tablespoons

Blend all ingredients in blender until smooth. Great for vegetables and lowfat crackers.

FRUIT

Fruit Gelatin ("A" Choice)

2   envelopes unflavored gelatin
1 1/2   cups boiling water
1   cup frozen unsweetened apple-
     juice concentrate, thawed
1   cup frozen unsweetened Dole
     Mountain Cherry juice
     concentrate, thawed
1   can packed-in fruit-juice
     fruit cocktail, drained
1   red apple, diced

Fruit Gelatin	
Calories per serving:	75
Fat grams per serving:	0
Number of servings:	6
Serving size:	3/4 cup

In a large bowl pour boiling water over gelatin and let sit about 2 or 3 minutes. Stir until dissolved completely. Add fruit-juice concentrates. Refrigerate until mixture is half set. Add fruit; mix in well. Refrigerate until firm. (Dole Country Raspberry Juice is also delicious in this recipe.)

Pineapple and Cottage Cheese Salad ("A" Choice)

1   can crushed pineapple in its own
     juice, drained
2   cups lowfat cottage cheese
1   teaspoon cinnamon

Pineapple and Cottage Cheese Salad	
Calories per serving:	303
Fat grams per serving:	4
Number of servings:	2
Serving size:	1 1/2 cups

Mix together all ingredients. Chill. Serve on a crisp lettuce leaf. Top with a maraschino cherry, if desired.

MAIN DISHES

BBQ Chicken ("A" Choice)

1	medium onion, chopped
2	tablespoons butter
2	tablespoons vinegar
2	tablespoons brown sugar
1	cup ketchup
3	tablespoons Worcestershire sauce
1	teaspoon mustard
1	cup water
11/2	teaspoons chili powder
	salt and pepper to taste
8	skinless, boneless chicken breasts

BBQ Chicken	
Calories per serving:	236
Fat grams per serving:	6
Number of servings:	8
Serving size:	1 piece

In a medium sauce-pan saute onion in butter. Then stir in vinegar, brown sugar, ketchup, Worcestershire sauce, mustard, water, chili powder, salt, and pepper. Cook for 10 to 15 minutes. Then pour sauce over chicken breasts.

Bake for 1 hour and 15 minutes at 350 degrees. These are also delicious when cooked on the grill. Serve on whole-grain hamburger buns, with all the lowfat trimmings, if desired.

Beef Stroganoff ("A" Choice)

1	pound extra-lean beef stew meat cut into thin strips*
1	tablespoon butter
21/4	cups beef broth
2	tablespoons ketchup
2	teaspoons instant minced garlic
1	teaspoon salt
1	cup sliced mushrooms
1/2	cup chopped onion
2	cups chopped carrots
3	tablespoons whole-wheat flour
1	cup nonfat plain yogurt or fat free sour cream
5	cups hot, cooked whole-wheat noodles** or regular noodles

Beef Stroganoff	
Calories per serving:	505
Fat grams per serving:	10
Number of servings:	6
Serving size:	2 cups

Cook beef in 1 tablespoon butter in a large nonstick skillet over low heat until brown. Reserve 1 cup of the broth. Stir remaining broth, ketchup, garlic, and salt into skillet. Heat until boiling. Reduce heat; cover and simmer until beef is tender, about 1 to 1 1/2 hours.

Boil and stir 1 minute. Then reduce heat and stir in yogurt. Heat thoroughly. Serve beef mixture over the hot noodles.

Stir in mushrooms, onions, and carrots. Cover and simmer for about 10 minutes or until tender. Shake reserved bouillon and the flour in a tightly covered container. Then stir gradually into beef mixture. Heat to boiling, stirring constantly.

*Beef is easier to slice thin if partially frozen.

**Use white or preferably artichoke noodles if your family rebels against whole-wheat noodles.

Chicken Bake ("A" Choice)

2 1/2   pounds skinless, boneless
        chicken breasts
1   can (10 3/4 oz.) condensed lowfat
        cream of mushroom soup
1/2   envelope onion soup mix

Chicken Bake	
Calories per serving:	225
Fat grams per serving:	5
Number of servings:	10
Serving size:	1 chicken breast 4 to 5 oz.

Heat oven to 375°. Arrange chicken in baking pan sprayed with cooking spray. Mix mushroom soup and dry onion soup mix. Pour over chicken. Cover tightly with foil and bake for 30 minutes. Uncover and bake 45 minutes longer or until done.

Chicken-Chili Enchiladas ("A" Choice)

12   whole-wheat tortillas
1   large can (31 oz.) refried
        beans (no fat added)
2   cans (15 oz. each) lowfat
        chicken chili
2   cups picante sauce; mild,
        medium, or hot
2   cups canned spaghetti sauce,
        lowfat
1   cup diced green peppers,
        optional
1   cup diced onion, optional

1   cup tomato, optional
11/2   cups grated part-skim
        mozzarella cheese

Chicken-Chili Enchiladas	
Calories per serving:	516
Fat grams per serving:	11 1/2
Number of servings:	6
Serving size:	2 enchiladas

Combine refried beans and chicken chili in a large bowl. Set aside. Mix together picante sauce and spaghetti sauce in separate bowl. Blend 1/2 cup sauce into bean mixture. Place about 1/3 cup of bean mixture in center of each tortilla from end to end. Sprinkle with diced green pepper, onion, and tomato, if desired, and roll up. Place side by side in a large oblong glass cake dish that has been thoroughly sprayed with nonstick cooking spray.

Top with 2 to 2 1/2 cups remaining sauce, cheese, remaining green peppers, onions, and tomatoes. Place 3 green-pepper rings in the center.

Bake in a 375 degree oven for 25-35 minutes. Serve with a fresh-fruit platter.

Beef Fajitas ("A" Choice)
or turkey or chicken

2	whole-wheat flour tortillas
3	oz. extra-lean round steak, or skinless turkey or chicken breast, thinly sliced
1/2	package taco mix
1/2	clove garlic
1	onion
2	green peppers
1	red pepper
	lettuce

	tomato
2	tablespoons part-skim mozzarella cheese, grated

Beef Fajitas	
Calories per serving:	275
Fat grams per serving:	6
Number of servings:	2
Serving size:	1 fajita

Pan-fry the meat until brown. Then add about 1/4 cup water and steam for a few minutes. While steaming add a little diced garlic and 1/2 package of taco mix for flavor.

Slice vegetables into 1/2-inch wedges. When meat is done, add vegetables and stir-fry until tender.

Roll mixture inside whole-wheat, soft tortillas and garnish with shredded lettuce, tomato, and a tablespoon of grated cheese.

Easy Cabbage Dinner ("A" Choice)

7	potatoes, cubed
1/2	head green cabbage
1	medium onion
1	can whole-kernel corn, drained
1/2	pound extra-lean ground beef, cooked
	salt and pepper to taste

Easy Cabbage Dinner	
Calories per serving:	310
Fat grams per serving:	4 1/2
Number of servings:	8
Serving size:	1 cup

Boil potatoes in small amount of water in skillet for 5 minutes. Add cabbage and onion, cooking until tender. Add remaining ingredients and warm through.

Easy Chicken 'n' Dumplings
("A" Choice)

2	cups cooked white, skinless chicken or turkey, cubed	1/2	teaspoon salt
1	can (16 oz.) whole onions, with liquid	1/4	teaspoon thyme
			dumpling dough (Bisquick)
1	can (16 oz.) sliced carrots, with liquid		
1	can (16 oz.) cut-up green beans, with liquid		
1	can (16 oz.) corn, with liquid (optional)		
2	cups canned chicken broth		
1 1/2	teaspoons barbecue spice or seasoning packet		

Easy Chicken 'n' Dumplings

Calories per serving:	277
Fat grams per serving:	5
Number of servings:	6
Serving size:	1 1/2 cups chicken mixture with 2 dumplings

In a large pot combine chicken, onions, carrots, green beans, corn, chicken broth, barbecue spice, salt, and thyme. Heat to boiling, stirring occasionally.

Mix dumpling dough according to Bisquick package directions. Drop dough by tablespoonfuls onto hot vegetables and chicken.* Cook uncovered for 10 minutes. Then cover and cook 10 more minutes. Liquid should gently bubble.

Serve in soup bowls. A bowl of peaches or cut-up melons goes nicely with this dish.

You could cook the biscuits on a pancake grill in a small amount of butter.

Parmesan Halibut Steaks
("A–" Choice)

4	5 oz. halibut steaks, about 3/4 inch thick	1/3	cup grated parmesan cheese, freshly grated (Check in the deli section of your supermarket.)
1/4	teaspoon salt		
1/8	teaspoon pepper	3	green onions, chopped
3/4	cup fat free dairy sour cream	10	cherry tomato halves, optional
1/4	cup dry whole-wheat bread crumbs		
1/4	teaspoon garlic salt		
1 1/2	teaspoons chopped chives		
1	teaspoon paprika		
1/8	teaspoon dried tarragon leaves, optional		

Parmesan Halibut Steaks

Calories per serving:	245
Fat grams per serving:	8
Number of servings:	4
Serving size:	one 5 oz. fillet

Place steaks close together in a shallow, baking dish coated with cooking spray. Sprinkle with salt and pepper. Mix sour cream, bread crumbs, garlic salt, chives, and dried tarragon leaves together; spread over steaks and sprinkle with parmesan cheese and paprika. Bake uncovered at 400 degrees for 15 to 20 minutes until fish is firm and flaky. Garnish with onions and cherry tomato halves.

285

Pizza Wheels ("A" & "B" Choices)

8	whole-wheat hamburger buns 16 halves), homemade or grocery-store variety. Sometimes you can't find 100% whole wheat, so get as close as possible.
2	15 1/2 oz. bottles pizza sauce
1	cup mixed fresh broccoli, pea pods, onions, and carrot slivers
4	3-inch round thin slices Canadian bacon
1/2	cup pineapple tidbits (own juice)
1/2	cup fresh, sliced mushrooms
12	1 1/2 inch round thin slices pepperoni
3	cups grated part-skim mozzarella cheese

Pizza Wheels

Calories per serving:

Vegetable	200 / round
Bacon, etc.	239 / round
Pepperoni	301 / round
Cheese:	185 / round

Fat grams per serving:

Vegetable	6 fg / round
Bacon, etc.	8 fg / round
Pepperoni	12 fg / round
Cheese:	6 fg / round
Number of servings:	4
Serving size:	4 rounds each

Place pizza rounds on 2 cookie sheets sprayed lightly with cooking spray. Bake each sheet for 7 to 10 minutes at 375 degrees.

Pizza Variations

Veggie Pizza Rounds: Spread 3 tablespoons pizza sauce on each of 4 bun halves. Place 1/4 cup mixed vegetables and 3 tablespoons cheese on top of each half.

Canadian Bacon, Pineapple, and Mushroom Pizza Rounds: Spread 3 tablespoons pizza sauce on each of 4 bun halves. Place one slice Canadian bacon, 2 tablespoons pineapple tidbits, 2 tablespoons sliced mushrooms, and 3 tablespoons cheese on top of each half.

Pepperoni Pizza Rounds: Spread 3 tablespoons pizza sauce on each of 4 bun halves. Place 3 pepperoni slices and 3 tablespoons cheese on top of each half.

Cheese Only Pizza Rounds: Spread 3 tablespoons pizza sauce on each of 4 bun halves. Sprinkle with 3 tablespoons cheese.

Special Note: Kids love to help make these. Set up an ingredient assembly line and let them help!

A fresh-fruit plate with nonfat vanilla yogurt on the side goes perfectly with this delicious, novel meal.

Quick, Delicious Beef Stew ("A" Choice)

1   can (40 oz.) Nalley's Big Chunk
       Beef Stew (or another brand
       with
       moderate fat content)

2   cans (17 oz. each) Campbell's
       Chunky Beef and Vegetable
       Soup

1   can (15 oz.) kidney or pinto
       beans, drained

1   can (17 oz.) corn, drained

1   can (17 oz.) green beans, drained

Quick, Delicious Beef Stew	
Calories per serving:	302
Fat grams per serving:	8
Number of servings:	8
Serving size:	1 cup

Mix all ingredients together in a large pot or kettle. Heat on medium heat, stirring frequently and scraping bottom, until stew is hot. Serve with whole-grain toast and fruit.

Sloppy Joes ("A–" to "B+" Choice)

1   pound extra lean ground beef*
11/2 cups celery, chopped
11/2 cups onion, chopped
1   can (8 oz.) tomato sauce
1   can tomato soup
1   teaspoon salt
1/4 teaspoon chili powder
      few drops tabasco
6   whole-wheat hamburger bun
      (White will do if you can't
      find wheat.)

Sloppy Joes	
Calories per serving:	412
Fat grams per serving:	13
Number of servings:	6
Serving size:	1/2 cup plus 1 bun

Brown meat in large skillet. Drain meat well. Add celery and onion; cook until tender. Add remaining ingredients. Simmer uncovered 20 minutes. For best flavor, cool and reheat before serving on whole-wheat hamburger buns.

Occasionally I eat one or two Sloppy Joes with lots of fruits and veggies on the side. Remember to be moderate with dairy prducts and meats—especially red meats.

Tempting Tacos ("A" Choice)

8   jumbo corn taco shells
         (regular will do)
24   mini taco shells
1   envelope taco seasoning mix (dry)
2   large cans (30 oz.) refried beans
         (no fat added—lowfat will do)
         shredded cheddar cheese
         or taco-flavored cheese
         shredded lettuce
         diced tomatoes
         diced onions
         taco salsa or picante sauce

Tempting Tacos

Calories per serving:	
Jumbo taco	289
Mini taco	265
Fat grams per serving:	
Jumbo taco	8
Mini taco (per 3 tacos)	7
Number of servings:	16
Serving size:	1 large or
	3 mini

Heat all taco shells in a 250-degree oven while heating refried beans in a saucepan. After beans are thoroughly heated, season to taste with taco seasoning mix. Fill each taco shell about 1/4 to 1/3 full of beans. Then add 2 tablespoons cheese to large tacos and 2 teaspoons cheese to small tacos. Finish with lettuce, tomato, onion, salsa or picante sauce, and fat free sour cream. Both kids and adults love these.

Note: You may also decide to use extra- lean ground beef or extra-lean ground turkey in place of the beans. Or, you may choose to mix the beans with equal parts of extra-lean ground meat and season to taste. I prefer the taste of all beans. I like extra fat grams from the cheese, not the meat. Choose what *you* like best.

Homemade Tuna Sandwich ("A" Choice)

Place the following ingredients on whole-wheat or other multi-grain breads. Dressings include fat free or light mayo, salad dressing, mustard, and lowfat buttermilk dressing.

Mix 3 oz. tuna (in water, drained) with fat free mayonnaise and salad dressing—add green peppers, onions, lettuce, and tomatoes.

Homemade Tuna Sandwich

Tuna Sandwich	2/400

Veggie-Tuna Pasta Salad ("A" Choice)

13/4 cups corkscrew vegetable pasta, whole-wheat, corn, artichoke pasta, or white pasta (or a mixture)
1 cup (8 oz.) fat free cream cheese
1 cup nonfat bottled ranch dressing
1 cup skim milk
1 teaspoon dried dill weed
2 cans (61/2 oz.) solid white tuna, drained (you can use regular tuna)

1 medium tomato, seeded and chopped
1 cucumber, diced
4 green onions, chopped

Veggie-Tuna Pasta Salad	
Calories per serving:	215
Fat grams per serving:	1
Number of servings:	8
Serving size:	approximately 1 cup

Cook pasta according to package directions. Drain. Transfer hot pasta immediately to a large bowl. Blend cream cheese and ranch dressing; add to pasta. Toss until completely blended. Stir in milk and dill weed. Add tuna, tomato, cucumber, and green onion. Toss lightly. Cover and chill for 4 or more hours.

Zucchini Casserole ("B+" Choice)

2 pounds or 6 cups cubed zucchini
1/4 cup chopped onion
1 can lowfat cream of chicken soup
1/2 cup fat free sour cream
1/2 cup plain, nonfat yogurt
1 cup shredded carrots
1 package lowfat stuffing mix (cornbread is great)
1/4 cup butter*, melted
4 tablespoons water

Zucchini Casserole	
Calories per serving:	183
Fat grams per serving:	6
Number of servings:	10
Serving size:	1 cup

Boil sliced squash and onion 5 minutes only. Drain very well. Combine soup, yogurt, and sour cream, Sir in carrots. Combine dry stuffing, seasonings, butter, and water. Spread half of dressing mixture in 12 x 71/2 x 2 baking dish. Spoon in zucchini mixture; pour soup mixture over the top and sprinkle rest of dressing mixture on the top. Bake at 350 degrees for 30 minutes. Note: Make certain zucchini is well drained. Serves 10.

Butter is high in naturally saturated fat and is used sparingly in this "B+" choice recipe.

SIDE DISHES

Au Gratin Potatoes ("A"choice)

12	medium potatoes—boiled
	with skin on; peel after cooking
4	tablespoons butter*
6	tablespoons whole-wheat flour
3	teaspoons salt
	pepper to taste
4	cups heated skim milk
11/2	cups grated, loosely packed,
	part-skim mozzarella cheese

Au Gratin Potatoes

Calories per serving:	418
Fat grams per serving:	9
Number of servings:	8
Serving size:	3/4 cup

Dice cooked potatoes. Melt butter in saucepan and stir in flour, salt, and pepper. Heat and stir constantly until mixture bubbles. Gradually add milk and cook over low heat, stirring constantly until sauce boils and thickens. Stir in 3/4 cup cheese and diced potatoes. Pour into baking dish and top with rest of cheese. Bake at 375 degrees for 15 minutes or until cheese melts and browns.

Even with 4 tablespoons of butter, this recipe is still under 20% fat! And according to recent media reports, butter may be more healthful than margarine.

SOUPS

Creamy Bean and Ham Soup ("A" Choice)

1	can (8 oz.) tomato sauce
1	up water
1	cup cooked extra-lean ham, cubed
1	cup onion, chopped
1	teaspoon instant beef bouillon
1	teaspoon salt
1/2	teaspoon pepper
1	clove garlic, crushed
	medium stalks celery cut into
	1/2 inch pieces
2	cans (15 oz.) undrained navy or
	great northern beans

2	cans sliced carrots, drained
2	cups mashed potatoes (you can
	use instant)

Creamy Bean and Ham Soup

Calories per serving:	365
Fat grams per serving:	1
Number of servings:	6
Serving size:	1 1/2 cups

Heat tomato sauce, water, ham, onion, bouillon, salt, pepper, garlic, and celery in a large kettle. Heat to boiling; reduce heat, cover, and simmer for 15 to 20 minutes until celery is tender. Stir in beans, carrots, and potatoes. Heat to boiling. Reduce heat, cover, and simmer for 10 to 15 minutes to blend flavors. If soup is too thick, add skim or evaporated skim milk until desired consistency is achieved.

SAMPLER RECIPES

290

Potato, Corn, and Cheese Soup
(with cheese = "B+" Choice
without cheese = "A" Choice)

2   cans cream of potato soup
1/2   soup can skim milk
1   can creamed corn
1   cup grated sharp cheddar cheese,
      optional

Potato, Corn, and Cheese Soup	
Calories per serving with cheese:	201
Calories per serving w/o cheese:	128
Fat grams per serving with cheese:	8 1/2
Fat grams per serving w/o cheese:	3
Number of servings:	6
Serving size:	1 cup

Blend together all ingredients in saucepan. Heat on medium, stirring constantly until bubbly and cheese is melted. For thinner soup, add more milk. Delicious!

VEGETABLES

Saucy Green Beans
and Almonds ("B+" Choice)

2   cans (15 oz. each) French-cut
      green beans, drained
1   can lowfat cream of mushroom
      soup
1/4   cup slivered almonds
1/4   cup cheddar cheese

Saucy Green Beans and Almonds	
Calories per serving:	136
Fat grams per serving:	9
Number of servings:	6
Serving size:	1 cup

Mix together beans, soup, and almonds. Heat thoroughly in 350-degree oven or microwave. Top with cheese.

(Short-cut) Tossed Salad
Colorful—Nutritious—Easy!
("A+" Choice)

Mix together:
1   bag prepared tossed salad
1   package fresh stir-fry vegetables
     (carrot slivers, onions, pea pods,
     broccoli, cauliflower)
1   carton cherry tomatoes

Short-Cut Tossed Salad	
Calories per serving:	50 to 150±
Fat grams per serving:	trace
Serving size:	1 cup

Tossed Salad or Homestyle
Salad Bar ("A+" Choice)

All vegetables are very low in fat and high in nutrients and fiber. Eat an abundance of a good variety and enjoy! Use color—mix and match!

Be creative. Enjoy a variety of any of the following colorful vegetables:

Lettuce (iceberg, endive, leaf, etc.), purple or yellow or green cabbage, slivered carrots, diced green or yellow or red peppers, tomatoes, cauliflower, broccoli, celery, onions, cucumbers, radishes, jicama, corn, peas, sprouts, beets, mushrooms, etc. Pineapple, apples, raisins, mandarin oranges, and cottage cheese mix well with a beautiful array of veggies.

Tossed Salad	
Calories per serving:	50 to 150±
Fat grams per serving:	trace
Serving size:	1 cup

Fat Gram/Calorie Evaluation Charts

Study These Charts Very Carefully — They Will Give You a Marvelous Education. They Hold Exciting Surprises!

	Serving Size	Fat Grams	Calories
ALFALFA			
Sprouts	1 cup	tr	40
ALMONDS			
Blanched, slivered, whole or sliced	1 oz	15	170
APPLES			
CANNED			
Applesauce, sweetened	1/2 cup	tr	97
Applesauce, unsweetened	1/2 cup	tr	53
FRESH			
Apple, medium	1	tr	81
JUICE			
Apple (Tree Top)	6 oz	0	90
Apple, frozen; not prepared	6 oz	1	349
APRICOTS			
CANNED			
Apricots, with skin & light syrup	3 hlvs	tr	54
FRESH			
Apricots	3	tr	51
ASPARAGUS			
FRESH			
Asparagus, cooked	1/2 cup	tr	22
AVOCADOS			
Avocado	1/2	14	153
BACON			
(see also BACON SUBSTITUTES)			
Oscar Mayer; cooked	1 strip (6g)	3	35
Turkey Bacon (Butterball)	1 strip	2	30
Canadian bacon	2 sl	4	86
BACON SUBSTITUTES			
Breakfast Strips			
Lean 'n Tasty Pork; cooked (Oscar Mayer)	1 strip	5	54
Sizzlean	1 strip	4	50
BAGELS			
Cinnamon & Raisin (Sara Lee)	1	2	240
BAKING POWDER			
Calumet	1 tsp	tr	3
BAKING SODA			
Arm & Hammer	1 tsp	0	0
BAMBOO SHOOTS			
Bamboo shoots; sliced	1 cup	1	25
BANANAS			
FRESH			
Banana	1	tr	105
BEANS			
Barbecue Beans (Campbell's)	7 7/8 oz	4	250
Cut green beans	1/2 cup	0	20

	Serving Size	Fat Grams	Calories
Four Bean Salad (Hanover)	1/2 cup	0	80
Kidney beans	1/2 cup	0	120
Pork & beans in tomato sauce	8 oz	3	240
Refried Beans	1/2 cup	2	43
BEEF			
CANNED			
Corned beef	1 sl (21 g)	3	53
Chuck arm pot roast, lean only, choice; braised	3 oz	9	199
Ground, extra-lean; cooked medium	3 oz	14	213
Ground, regular; cooked medium	3 oz	18	244
T-bone steak, choice, raw	4 oz	30	348
BEEF DISHES			
CANNED			
Stew with vegetables	1 cup	7	186
Quick & Delicious Beef Stew (LEAN & FREE)	1 cup	4	238
BEETS			
CANNED			
Diced (Libby)	1/2 cup	0	35
BLUEBERRIES			
FRESH			
Blueberries	1 cup	1	82
BREAD			
(See also BAGLES, MUFFINS)			
Whole Wheat	1 sl	tr	71
Cracked Wheat (Pepperidge Farm)	1 sl	1	70
Honey Wheat Berry (Roman Meal)	1 sl	1	66
Pita, whole wheat, regular size	1 pkg (2 oz)	2	150
Rye, Jewish, seeded	1 sl	1	80
White	1 sl	1	70
Whole wheat 100%	1 sl	1	75
BROCCOLI			
FRESH			
Broccoli, raw; chopped	1/2 cup	tr	12
Broccoli, whole; cooked	1/2 cup	tr	23
BRUSSEL SPROUTS			
FRESH			
Brussels sprouts; cooked	1/2 cup	tr	30
BUTTER			
(see also BUTTER BLENDS, BUTTER SUBSTITUTES, MARGARINE)			

BUTTER BLENDS   **CLAMS**

	Serving Size	Fat Grams	Calories
REGULAR	1 Tbsp	11	100
Butter (1 pat)	1 tsp	4	36
Butter (1 stick)	4 oz	92	813
Butter, whipped	1 tsp	3	27
BUTTER BLENDS			
Honey-Butter	1 Tbsp	5	34
BUTTER SUBSTITUTES			
(see also *BUTTER BLENDS, MARGARINE*)			
Butter Buds	1 oz	0	12
Butter Buds Sprinkles	1/2 tsp	0	4
Molly McButter All Natural Butter Flavor Sprinkles	1/2 tsp	0	4
Molly McButter Natural Sour Cream & Butter Flavor Sprinkles	1/2 tsp	0	4
CABBAGE			
FRESH			
Green, shredded, raw	1/2 cup	tr	8
Red, shredded, raw	1/2 cup	tr	10
Red, shredded; cooked	1/2 cup	tr	16
CANADIAN BACON			
Oscar Mayer	1 sl	1	35
CANTALOUPE			
Cantaloupe	1/2	1	94
Cubed	1 cup	tr	57
CARROTS			
CANNED	1/2 cup	0	20
Sliced,			
FRESH	1/2 cup	0	35
Fresh, cooked	1	0	35
Raw			
CASHEWS			
Dry roasted	1 oz	13	160
CAULIFLOWER			
FRESH			
Fresh, cooked	1/2 cup	tr	15
Raw	1/2 cup	tr	12
CELERY			
Diced; cooked	1/2 cup	tr	11
Raw	1 stalk	tr	6
CEREAL			
(Cereals are listed in A, B, C, D, and F categories on pages 363 through 366)			
CHEESE (4 oz. grated, "loosely packed" cheese = 1 cup (see also *COTTAGE CHEESE, CREAM CHEESE*)			
Cheddar	1 oz	9	110
Colby	1 oz	9	110
Monterey Jack	1 oz	9	110
Mozzarella, low moisture, part-skim	1 oz	5	79
Mozzarella, whole milk	1 oz	6	90
Parmesan, grated	2 Tbsp	3	46
Provolone	1 oz	7	100

	Serving Size	Fat Grams	Calories
Ricotta, part skim	1 oz	2	32
Swiss	1 oz	8	110
CHERRIES			
CANNED			
Sweet, in water	1/2 cup	tr	57
Juice, Mountain Cherry Pure & Light	6 oz	tr	87
CHESTNUTS			
Roasted	1 oz	tr	70
Roasted	1 cup	3	350
CHICKEN			
(see also *CHICKEN DISHES*)			
CANNED			
Chunk Premium, White (Swanson)	2.5 oz	2	90
Chunk White & Dark (Swanson)	2.5 oz	4	100
FRESH			
Breast, meat only, roasted	1/2 breast (3 0z)	3	142
Dark meat with skin; roasted	(5.9 oz)	26	423
Dark meat without skin; roasted	1 cup	14	286
Light meat with skin; roasted	1/2 chicken (4.6 oz)	14	293
Light meat without skin; roasted	1 cup	6	242
CHICKEN DISHES			
CANNED			
Chicken Stew (Chef Boy.ar.dee)	7 oz	5	140
CHILI			
Chicken Chili (Hormel)	7.5 oz	3	200
Mixed Vegetarian with beans (Health Valley)	4 oz	6	120
CHIPS			
(see also *POPCORN, PRETZELS, SNACKS*)			
Corn Chips (Health Valley)	1 oz	11	160
Potato	10 chips	7	105
Tortilla:			
Doritos, Cool Ranch	1 oz	7	140
Doritos, Nacho Cheese	1 oz	7	140
Doritos, Nacho Cheese, Light	1 oz	4	120
CHOCOLATE			
(see also *COCOA, ICE CREAM TOPPINGS*)			
Chocolate Flavored Chips (Bakers)	1/4 cup	9	196
Real Semi-Sweet Chocolate Chips (Bakers)	1/4 cup	14	201
CLAMS			
CANNED			

294

COCOA

	Serving Size	Fat Grams	Calories
Meat only	1 cup	3	236
COCOA			
(see also *CHOCOLATE*)			
MIX			
Hershey's Cocoa	1/3 cup	4	120
Cocoa mix	1 oz.	1	102
COCONUT			
Angel Flake, Bag			
(Bakers)	1/3 cup	8	116
CORN			
CANNED			
Cream Style (Libby)	1/2 cup	0	80
Whole Kernel (Libby)	1/2 cup	1	80
FROZEN			
On the cob; cooked	1 ear (2.2 oz)	tr	59
CORNSTARCH			
Argo	1 Tbsp	tr	30
COTTAGE CHEESE			
LOWFAT			
Land O'Lakes,	4 oz	2	100
Regular	1/2 cup	5	109
CRAB			
CANNED			
Blue	1 cup	2	133
CRACKERS			
Grahams (Nabisco)	2	1	60
Wheat Thins (Nabisco)	8	3	70
CRANBERRIES			
CANNED			
Cranberry Sauce			
Jellied, Old Fashioned,			
(S&W)	1/4 cup	0	90
Cranberries; chopped	1 cup	tr	54
CREAM			
(see also *SOUR CREAM, SUBSTITUTES, WHIPPED TOPPING*)			
Half & Half	1 Tbsp	2	20
Half & Half	1 cup	28	315
Heavy whipping	1 Tbsp	6	52
Light whipping	1 Tbsp	5	44
WHIPPED			
Whipped, heavy whipping	1 cup	44	411
Whipped, light whipping	1 cup	37	345
CREAM CHEESE			
LIGHT REDUCED FAT			
Philadelphia Brand Light			
Cream Cheese Product	1 oz	5	60
REGULAR			
Philadelphia Brand	1 oz	10	100
Philadelphia Brand			
with chives & onion	1 oz (2 Tbsp)	9	100
Philadelphia Brand			
with strawberries	1 oz	8	90

FISH

	Serving Size	Fat Grams	Calories
Philadelphia Brand			
with pineapple	1 oz	8	90
CROUTONS			
Croutettes (Kellogg's)	1 cup	tr	144
CUCUMBERS			
Raw	1	tr	39
DATES			
DRIED			
Chopped	1 cup	1	489
DIPS			
Creamy Onion Dip (LEAN & FREE)	2 Tbsp	1	40
Delicious Dill Dip (LEAN & FREE)	2 Tbsp	1	40
Ranch Dip (LEAN & FREE)	2 Tbsp	1/2	35
Sour Cream Fruit Dip (LEAN & FREE)	2 Tbsp	1	52
Spinach-Vegetable Dip			
(LEAN & FREE)	1/2 cup	tr	87
EGGS			
(see also *EGG DISHES*)			
Lowered Cholesterol			
(Full Spectrum Farms)	11g	1	60
Fried with butter	1	6.4	83
Raw	1	5.6	79
White only	1	tr	16
Yoke only	1	5.6	63
EGG DISHES			
(See also *EGGS*)			
Omelets (LEAN & FREE)	5"x6"	10	254
Egg Scramble, (LEAN & FREE)	1 cup	10	289
FAT			
(see also *BUTTER, BUTTER BLENDS, BUTTER SUBSTITUTES, MARGARINE, AND OIL*)			
Crisco	1 Tbsp	12	110
Beef fat; cooked	1 oz	20	193
Chicken fat, raw	1 oz	22	201
Lard	1 Tbsp	13	115
Pork fat	1 oz	21	200
Shortening, lard, &			
vegetable oil	1 Tbsp	13	115
Turkey fat	1 Tbsp	13	115
FISH			
(see also *INDIVIDUAL NAMES*)			
FROZEN			
Light Recipe Lightly			
Breaded Fish Fillets			
(Gorton's)	1 fillet	7	170
Today's Catch Fish Fillets			
(Van De Kamp's)	5 oz	4	100

Many types of fish contain omega 3 fatty acids, which help to increase HDL levels (good cholesterol) and decrease LDL levels (bad cholesterol). Make certain to avoid deep-fried fish choices, which can be high in fats that can increase not only body fat but also triglyceride and LDL levels. Enjoy baked, broiled, and canned fish choices.

FLOUR

	Serving Size	Fat Grams	Calories
Value Pack Fish Sticks (Gorton's)	4 sticks	11	210
FLOUR			
All-Purpose (Gold Medal)	1 cup	1	400
Medium Rye (Pillsbury Best)	1 cup	2	400
Whole Wheat (Gold Medal)	1 cup	2	390
FRENCH TOAST			
French Toast (LEAN & FREE)	2 sl	1	191
French toast (regular)	1 sl	14	270
FRUIT DRINKS			
Frozen: White Grape Juice; As prepared (Seneca)	6 oz	0	110
Ready-To-Use: Grape	6 oz	0	94
Ready-To-Use: Orange	6 oz	0	94
FRUIT, MIXED			
(See also *INDIVIDUAL NAMES*)			
CANNED			
Fruit Cocktail in Juice (Dole)	1/2 cup	tr	56
Tropical Fruit Salad in Juice (Dole)	1/2 cup	tr	62
FRUIT JUICES			
Cherry, Mountain Cherry (Dole)	6 oz	0	87
Orange	6 oz	0	90
Orange-Grapefruit	1 cup	tr	107
Peach, Orchard Peach (Dole)	6 oz	0	90
Pineapple Pink Grapefruit (Dole)	6 oz	tr	101
Pineapple-Orange-Banana (Dole)	6 oz	tr	90
Raspberry, Country Raspberry (Dole)	6 oz	0	87
GELATIN			
MIX			
Dry, unsweetened	1 Tbsp	tr	23
GRAPES			
Grapes, fresh	10	tr	36
GRAPEFRUIT			
Grapefruit, Fresh	1/2 med	0	50
GRAVY			
CANNED			
Beef (Franco-American)	2 oz.	1	25
Chicken Giblet (Franco-American)	2 oz.	2	30
Mushroom (Franco-American)	2 oz.	1	25
Turkey (Franco-American)	2 oz.	2	30
DRY:			
Brown; as prepared	1/4 cup	0	15
Home Style; as prepared	1/4 cup	0	15
GREEN BEANS			
CANNED			
Cut Premium Blue Lake (S&W)	1/2 cup	0	20

ICE CREAM TOPPINGS

	Serving Size	Fat Grams	Calories
French Natural Pack (Libby)	1/2 cup	1	20
HADDOCK			
FROZEN			
Today's Catch, Haddock (Van De Kamp's)	5 oz	0	110
HALIBUT			
FRESH			
Atlantic & Pacific; cooked	3 oz	4	199
HAM			
(see also *LUNCHEON MEATS AND COLD CUTS*)			
Boneless	1 oz	1	33
Oscar Mayer Breakfast Ham, water added	1 sl(43g)	2	52
HAMBURGER (see BEEF, Ground)			
HONEY	1 Tbsp	0	60
HONEYDEW MELON	1 cup	tr	60
Cubed			
ICE CREAM AND FROZEN DESSERT			
Chocolate Ice Milk (Borden)	1/2 cup	2	100
Cookies 'n Cream on a stick	1 bar	15	220
Instant Peach Ice Cream (LEAN & FREE)	1 1/2 cups	3	176
Instant Blueberry Ice Cream (LEAN & FREE)	1 1/2 cups	3	224
Orange Sherbet	1/2 cup	1	110
Peach Fruit & Cream (Chiquita)	1 bar	1	80
Pina Colada Fruit 'n Juice Bars (Dole)	1 bar	tr	90
Pineapple Sorbet (Dole)	4 oz	tr	120
Raspberry Fruit & Yogurt Bars	4 oz	tr	70
Strawberry Banana Fruit & Cream	1 bar	2	80
Strawberry Banana Fruit & Juice Bars	1 bar(2oz)	1	50
Vanilla Ice Cream (Land O'Lakes)	1/2 cup	7	140
Vanilla Ice Milk (Borden)	1/2 cup	2	90
Vanilla Ice Milk, soft serve	1 cup	5	223
ICE CREAM CONES & CUPS			
Comet Cups	1	0	20
Comet Sugar Cone	1	0	40
ICE CREAM, NON-DAIRY			
Mocha Mix Neapolitan	1/2 cup	7	130
ICE CREAM TOPPINGS			
Hot fudge topping (nonfat)	1 Tbsp	0	70

296

JAM

MILK

	Serving Size	Fat Grams	Calories
Swiss Milk Chocolate			
Fudge Topping (Smucker's)	2 Tbsp	1	140
JAM/ JELLY/ PRESERVES			
ALL FRUIT JAMS			
All Flavors, Simply Fruit			
Spread (Smucker's)	1 tsp	0	16
Blueberry Fruit Spread			
(Pritikin Foods)	1 tsp	0	14
Peach Fruit Spread			
(Pritikin Foods)	1 tsp	0	14
All Fruit Jams (LEAN & FREE)	2 Tbsp	t	32
JUICE (see *FRUIT JUICES*)			
KIDNEY BEANS			
CANNED	1 cup	1	216
Red, kidney	1	tr	46
KIWIFRUIT			
Kiwifruit	1 Tbsp	0	6
KETCHUP/CATSUP	1 Tbsp	0	15
LEMON JUICE			
Lemon (Seneca)	1 Tbsp	0	6
LENTILS			
CANNED			
Lentils; cooked	1 cup	tr	258
LETTUCE			
Iceberg	1 leaf	tr	3
Romaine; shredded	1/2 cup	tr	4
LOBSTER			
FROZEN			
Northern; cooked	1 cup	1	142
Home Recipe: Newburg	1 cup	27	485
LUNCHEON MEATS/COLD CUTS (See also *CHICKEN HAM, TURKEY*)			
Carl Budding Beef	1 oz.	2	40
Oscar Mayer Corned Beef	1 sl	tr	16
Oscar Mayer Honey Loaf	1 sl	1	32
Oscar Mayer Pastrami	1 sl	tr	16
Oscar Mayer Smoked Beef	1 sl	tr	14
MARGARINE			
REDUCED CALORIE			
Blue Bonnet Diet	1 Tbsp	6	50
Fleischmann's Diet	1 Tbsp	6	50
Kraft Spread	1 Tbsp	6	50
REGULAR			
Blue Bonnet	1 Tbsp	11	100
Fleischmann's	1 Tbsp	11	100
Parkay	1 Tbsp	11	100
MARSHMALLOW			
Campfire (Borden)	21g	0	40
Miniature (Kraft)	10	0	18
MAYONNAISE (See also *MAYONNAISE-TYPE SALAD DRESSING*)			
FAT FREE			
Kraft Free Nonfat Mayonnaise Dressing	1 Tbsp	0	12

	Serving Size	Fat Grams	Calories
REDUCED CALORIE			
Best Foods Light	1 Tbsp	5	50
REGULAR			
Best Foods Real	1 Tbsp	11	100
Best Foods Real	1 cup	175	1570
MAYONNAISE-TYPE SALAD DRESSINGS (See also *MAYONNAISE*)			
FAT FREE			
Kraft Free Miracle Whip Nonfat Dressing	1 Tbsp	0	12
REGULAR			
Miracle Whip Salad Dressing	1 Tbsp	7	70
Delicious Buttermilk Dressing (LEAN & FREE)	2 Tbsp	1	42
MELONS (See also *INDIVIDUAL NAMES*)			
FROZEN: Melon balls	1 cup	tr	55
MEXICAN FOOD (See also *CHIPS, DINNER, SNACKS*)			
CANNED			
Enchilada sauce, hot	1 oz	0	12
Enchilada sauce, mild	1 oz	0	12
Picante salsa	1 oz	0	10
Red taco sauce, mild	2 Tbsp	0	10
FROZEN			
3 Chicken Enchiladas (El Charrito)			
Shredded Beef Enchilada with Rice & Corn, Mexican	11 oz	13	440
Classic (Van De Kamp's)	14.75 oz	15	490
Tortillas, corn			
Tortillas, corn	2	1	95
Tortillas, flour	2	4	170
HOME RECIPE			
Taco salad	1 cup	20	292
MIX	1 1/2 cup	10	247
Taco meat seasoning, mild;	1 oz	1	90
as prepared with ground beef	3 oz	12	180
MILK (See also *CHOCOLATE, COCOA*)			
CANNED			
Carnation Evaporated	1/2 cup	10	170
Carnation Evaporated, Lowfat	1/2 cup	3	110
Carnation Evaporated, Skimmed	1/2 cup	tr	100
Carnation Sweetened, Condensed	1 oz	3	123
Carnation Sweetened, Condensed	1/3 cup	9	318
Eagle Sweetened, Condensed	1/3 cup	9	320
Pet 99 Evaporated, Skimmed	1/2 cup	0	100

MINERAL / BOTTLED WATER

	Serving Size	Fat Grams	Calories
DRIED			
Carnation Nonfat Dry;			
as prepared with water	8 oz	tr	80
Buttermilk, Sweet Cream	1 Tbsp	tr	25
LIQUID, LOWFAT			
1%	1 cup	3	102
2%	1 cup	5	121
Lactaid	1 cup	0	102
Buttermilk	1 cup	2	99
Whey, sweet	1 cup	1	66
LIQUID, REGULAR			
Goat milk	1 cup	10	168
Human milk	1 oz	14	21
Whole, 3.3% fat	1 cup	8	150
LIQUID, SKIM			
Skim	1 cup	tr	86
Skim, nonfat milk,			
solids added	1 cup	tr	90
MINERAL/BOTTLED WATER			
Artesian	7 oz	0	0
MOLASSES			
Brer Rabbit, Dark	1 Tbsp	0	60
MOUSSE			
Chocolate Mousse,			
No Bake Dessert;			
as prep (Jell-O)	1/2 cup	5	141
MUFFINS (LEAN & FREE)			
(see pages 259 through 263)			
MUFFIN MIXES			
Corn Muffin; as prepared			
(Dromedary)	1	4	120
Wild Blueberry; as prepared			
(Duncan Hines)	1	3	110
Oat Bran Raisin			
(Health Valley)	2 oz	3	140
MUSHROOMS			
CANNED			
Mushrooms (Libby)	1/4 cup	0	35
Fresh: raw; sliced	1/2 cup	tr	9
MUSTARD			
Grey Poupon Dijon	1 Tbsp	1	18
Kraft Pure Prepared	1 Tbsp	0	4
NECTARINES			
Fresh: nectarine	1	tr	67
NOODLES			
(See also *PASTA DINNERS*)			
CANNED			
Chow mein noodles	1/2 cup	5	228
DRY			
Chow mein noodles			
(La Choy)	1/2 cup	8	150
Egg Noodles			
(Creamette)	2 oz	3	221
Noodles & Sauce, Beef			
as prep (Lipton)	1/4 pkg	2	128

ORIENTAL FOOD

	Serving Size	Fat Grams	Calories
Ramen Noodles with Chicken			
Flavoring; as prepared			
(La Choy)	1/2pkg	7	190
Spinach egg noodles	2 oz	2	209
Whole wheat lasagna			
noodles	2 oz dry	2	210
Whole wheat spaghetti	2 oz dry	tr	200
noodles	1 cup cooked	tr	200
NUTS, MIXED			
(See also *INDIVIDUAL NAMES*)			
Mixed Nuts, Dry Roasted			
(Planters)	1 oz	15	170
OATS	1 oz	2	100
OIL	(1/3 cup)		
(See also *FAT*)			
Crisco	1 Tbsp	14	120
Mazola	1 Tbsp	14	120
Mazola No Stick Spray	2.5 sec spray	1	6
Planters Peanut	1 Tbsp	14	120
Puritan (canola)	1 Tbsp	14	120
Coconut	1 Tbsp	14	120
Corn	1 cup	218	1927
Cottonseed	1 Tbsp	14	120
Olive	1 Tbsp	14	119
Palm	1 Tbsp	14	120
Rapeseed (canola)	1 Tbsp	14	120
Safflower	1 Tbsp	14	120
Soybean	1 Tbsp	14	120
Sunflower	1 Tbsp	14	120
Sunflower	1/4 cup	54	482
Sunflower	1/2 cup	109	964
Sunflower	1 cup	218	1927
Wheat germ	1 Tbsp	14	120
ONIONS			
Fresh onion, chopped	1 cup	tr	48
OLIVES			
Ripe, Pitted, Large (S&W)	8 small	3	30
ORANGES			
FRESH, Orange	1	tr	62
FROZEN, Orange juice, prepared	1 cup	tr	112
Mandarin oranges in light syrup	1 cup	tr	125
ORIENTAL FOOD			
CANNED			
Chun King Divider Pak			
Beef Chow Mein	7 oz	2	100
Chun King Divider Pak			
Chicken Chow Mein	8 oz	4	120
Chun King Divider Pak			
Pork Chow Mein	7 oz	4	120
Chun King Divider Pak			
Shrimp Chow Mein	7 oz	2	100
La Choy Beef Pepper			
Oriental	3/4 cup	2	90
La Choy Chow Mein, Beef	3/4 cup	1	60

PANCAKES

	Serving Size	Fat Grams	Calories
La Choy Chow Mein, Chicken	3/4 cup	2	70
La Choy Chow Mein, Shrimp	3/4 cup	1	45
La Choy Sweet & Sour Oriental with chicken	3/4 cup	2	240
Chow mein noodles	1/2 cup	5	228
Chow mein with chicken	1 cup	tr	95
Chow Mein with pork (LEAN & FREE)	1 cup	8	302
Sweet and Sour Chicken (LEAN & FREE)	3/4 cup	4	396
FROZEN			
Birds Eye Chinese Style Stir-Fry Vegetable	1/2 cup	tr	36
Birds Eye Chow Mein Style International Recipe	1/2 cup	4	89
Chun King Imperial Chicken	13 oz	1	294
Chun King Szechuan Beef	13 oz	2	331
La Choy Shrimp Chow Mein	2/3 cup	1	70
La Choy Shrimp Egg Roll	3 sm	2	80
La Choy Fresh & Lite Beef Broccoli	11 oz	7	290
La Choy Fresh & Lite Sweet & Sour Chicken	10 oz	4	280
PANCAKES			
Krusteaz Whole Wheat & Honey Pancake Mix	3 4" pancakes	1	215
Krusteaz Buckwheat Pancake Mix	3 4" pancakes	3	215
LEAN & FREE(see pages 268 & 269)			
PANCAKE/WAFFLE SYRUP (see also *SYRUP*)			
Karo Pancake Syrup	1 Tbsp	0	60
Log Cabin Syrup, Buttered	1 oz	tr	106
PASTA (See also *NOODLES, PASTA DINNERS, PASTA SALAD*)			
DRY			
Elbow macaroni	2 oz	1	210
Lasagna, jumbo	2 oz	1	210
Lasagna, Whole Wheat	2 oz	1	170
Ribbon Pasta, Whole Wheat (Pritikin Foods)	2 oz	2	220
Spaghetti, regular & thin	2 oz	1	210
Spaghetti, Whole Wheat (Health Valley)	2 oz	1	170
COOKED			
Macaroni	1 cup	1	155
EGG NOODLES	1 cup	2	200
PASTA DINNERS (See also *PASTA SALAD*)			
Chef Boy.ar.dee ABC's & 1,2,3's in sauce	7.5 oz	1	160
Chef Boy.ar.dee Beef Ravioli	7 oz	5	180

PICKLES

	Serving Size	Fat Grams	Calories
Chef Boy.ar.dee Cheese Ravioli in Beef & Tomato Sauce	7.5 oz	3	200
Chef Boy.ar.dee Chicken Ravioli	7.5 oz	4	180
Chef Boy.ar.dee Dinosaurs in Spaghetti Sauce with Cheese Flavor	7.5 oz	1	155
Chef Boy.ar.dee Macaroni Shells in Tomato Sauce	7.5 oz	1	150
Franco-American PizzO's	7.5 oz	2	170
Franco-American Spaghetti-O's	7 3/8 oz	2	170
Mama Leone's Pasta Supreme Mini Lasagna	7.5 oz	1	170
DRY MIX			
Chef Boy.ar.dee Spaghetti Dinner with Mushroom Sauce	1 serving 7.9 oz	1	210
Lipton Pasta & Sauce, Cheddar Broccolli with Fusilli; as prepared	1/2 cup	2	137
Lipton Pasta & Sauce, Creamy Garlic; as prepared	1/2 cup	tr	144
Lipton Pasta & Sauce, Herb Tomato; as prepared	1/2 cup	tr	130
PASTA SALAD			
FROZEN			
Italian Pasta Salad (Hanover)	1/2 cup	0	60
Oriental Pasta Salad (Hanover)	1/2 cup	0	80
PEACHES			
CANNED, halves in juice	1 cup	tr	109
FRESH peach	1	tr	37
JUICE, Pure & Light (Dole)	6 oz	tr	102
PEANUT BUTTER			
Jif Creamy	2 Tbsp	16	190
Jif Crunchy	2 Tbsp	16	190
Skippy Creamy	2 Tbsp	17	190
Skippy Creamy	1 cup	135	1540
PEANUTS			
Dry roasted	1 oz	14	170
PEARS			
CANNED, halves in juice	1 cup	tr	123
halves in light syrup	1 cup	tr	144
FRESH, pear	1	0	98
PEAS			
CANNED, green	1/2 cup	tr	61
DRIED, split; cooked	1 cup	1	231
FROZEN, Chinese Pea Pods (Chun King)	6 oz	0	8
PECANS			
halves, dried	1 cup	73	721
PECTIN			
Sure-Jell Fruit Pectin	1/4 pkg	0	38
PEPPERS			
CANNED, green & red, sweet, chopped	1/2 cup	tr	13
PICKLES			

PIE   POTATO STARCH

	Serving Size	Fat Grams	Calories
Bread & Butter Sweet Butter Chips (Vlasic)	1 oz	0	30
Kosher Dill Spears (Vlasic)	1 oz	0	4
PIE			
(See also *PIE CRUST*)			
FROZEN			
Apple (Banquet)	3.33 oz	11	250
Cherry (Banquet)	3.33 oz	11	250
Lemon (Banquet)	2.33 oz	9	170
Peach (Banquet)	3.33 oz	11	245
Pumpkin (Banquet)	3.33 oz	8	200
Strawberry (Banquet)	2.33 oz	9	170
MIX			
Banana Cream; as prepared with whole milk (Jell-O)	1/6 of 8" pie	3	107
Coconut Cream; as prepared with whole milk (Jell-O)	1/6 of 8" pie	5	115
Key Lime Pie Filling; as prepared (Royal)	1/2 cup	3	160
Lemon; as prepared (Jell-O)	1/6 of 8" pie	2	180
Real Cheese Cake (No Bake)	1/8 pie	9	280
PIE CRUST			
(See also *PIE*)			
FROZEN			
Pie Shell (Mrs. Smith's)	1/8 of 9 5/8" Shell	8	130
Deep Dish (Pet-Ritz)	1/6 shell	8	130
Graham Cracker (Pet-Ritz)	1/6 shell	6	110
HOME RECIPE; pie crust	one 9" pie	60	900
PINE NUTS			
Pignolia, dried	1 Tbsp	5	51
PINEAPPLE			
CANNED			
All Cuts in Juice (Dole)	1/2 cup	tr	70
Crushed	1 cup	tr	140
FRESH; diced	1 cup	tr	77
FROZEN; pineapple juice	1 cup	tr	139
PINTO BEANS			
CANNED; pinto beans	1 cup	tr	186
PIZZA			
FROZEN; Canadian-style bacon	1 pizza 9.25 oz	26	550
Croissant Pastry Delux (Pepperidge Farm)	1 pizza	27	520
Cheese	1/7 of 10"	4	140
MIX			
Chef Boy.ar.dee 2 Complete Cheese Pizzas	1 serving 3.16 oz	5	210
SAUCE			
Ragu Pizza Quick Sauce, Chunky Style	3 Tbsp	2	45
Ragu Pizza Quick Sauce with Mushrooms	3 Tbsp	2	40

	Serving Size	Fat Grams	Calories
PIZZA WHEELS (LEAN & FREE) (see page 255)			
PLUMS			
CANNED, purple, in juice	3	tr	55
FRESH, plum	1	tr	36
POPCORN			
(See also *CHIPS, PRETZELS, SNACKS*)			
Jiffy Pop, Microwave Butter Flavor; as prepared	4 cups	7	140
Air popped	1 cup	tr	30
Microwave light butter flavor	3 cups	3	80
POT PIE			
Beef (Banquet)	7 oz	29	439
Chunky Chicken (Swanson)	10 oz	33	580
Hungry-Man Turkey (Swanson)	16 oz	38	690
POTATOES			
(See also *CHIPS*)			
Fresh Baked, Flesh & Skin	1(6.5oz)	tr	220
Cheddar Browns (Ore-Ida)	3 oz	2	90
Hash Browns, shredded (Ore-Ida) (uncooked)	3 oz	tr	70
Tater Tots (uncooked) (Ore-Ida)	3 oz	tr	140
Tater Tots, Microwave (uncooked) (Ore-Ida)	2 oz	9	200
MIX			
Mashed; not prepared	1/3 cup	0	70
Potato Salad, Classic Idaho; as prepared (Lipton)	1/2 cup	tr	94
Potato Salad, German; as prepared (Lipton)	1/2 cup	tr	99
Potatoes & Sauce Au Gratin; as prepared (Lipton)	1/2 cup	tr	108
Potatoes & Sauce, Beef & Mushroom; as prepared (Lipton)	1/2 cup	tr	95
Potatoes & Sauce, Cheddar Bacon; as prepared (Lipton)	1/2 cup	1	106
Potatoes & Sauce, Cheddar Broccoli; as prepared (Lipton)	1/2 cup	1	104
Potatoes & Sauce, Chicken Flavored Mushroom; as prepared (Lipton)	1/2 cup	tr	90
Potatoes, Italiano; as prepared (Lipton)	1/2 cup	2	107
Potatoes & Sauce; Nacho; as prepared (Lipton)	1/2 cup	1	103
Potatoes & Sauce, Scalloped; as prepared (Lipton)	1/2 cup	2	102
POTATO STARCH			
Potato starch	1 cup	0	570

	Serving Size	Fat Grams	Calories
PRETZELS			
(See also *CHIPS, POPCORN, SNACKS*)			
Twist, tiny	14 pieces	1	109
PRUNES			
Prunes, dried	10	tr	201
Prune, juice	1 cup	tr	181
PUDDING			
MIX			
Banana Cream, Instant (Jell-O)	1 pkg (3.6 oz)	tr	360
Butterscotch (Jell-O)	1 pkg (3.6 oz)	tr	364
Chocolate (Jell-O)	1 pkg (3.5 oz)	1	346
Chocolate Tapioca Americana (Jell-O)	1 pkg (3.5 oz)	2	378
French Vanilla, Instant (Jell-O)	1 pkg (3.5 oz)	tr	360
PUMPKIN			
CANNED, pumpkin	1/2 cup	1	40
RADISHES			
Fresh, raw	10	tr	7
RAISINS			
California seedless	1/2 cup	0	250
RASPBERRIES			
FRESH, red raspberries	1 cup	1	61
FROZEN, Red Raspberries, Whole in Lite Syrup (Birds Eye)	1/2 cup	tr	99
JUICE, Pure & Light (Dole)	6 oz	tr	87
RICE			
BROWN			
Brown, cooked	1/2 cup	tr	90
Birds Eye Rice & Peas with Mushrooms	2/3 cup	tr	108
Birds Eye Spanish Style International Rice	1/2 cup	tr	111
WHITE			
Long Grain, cooked	2 oz	0	61
RICE CAKES			
7 Grain Rice Cakes (Pritikin Foods)	1	0	35
ROUGHY			
Orange, raw	3 oz	6	107
SALAD			
(See also *PASTA SALAD*)			
HOME RECIPE			
Chef	1.5 cups	28	386
Tossed	1 cup	tr	32
SALAD DRESSING			
Buttermilk Farm Style; as prepared (Good Seasons)	1 Tbsp	6	58

	Serving Size	Fat Grams	Calories
READY-TO-USE, REDUCED CALORIE			
Bacon & Tomato (Kraft)	1 Tbsp	2	30
Buttermilk Creamy (Kraft)	1 Tbsp	3	30
Thousand Island (Kraft)	1 Tbsp	2	30
SALMON			
CANNED			
Pink (Bumble Bee)	3 oz	7	137
FRESH			
Salmon steak	3.5 oz	15	220
SAUSAGE			
Polish (Oscar Mayer)	1(2.7 oz)	20	229
Vienna, canned, beef & pork	1 sausage	4	45
SCALLOPS			
FROZEN			
Lightly Breaded Scallops (King & Prince)	3.5 oz	tr	120
SCONES			
Scone (home recipe)	1(1.4 oz)	6	130
SHRIMP			
CANNED			
Canned	1 cup	3	154
FROZEN			
Fried Shrimp (Mrs. Paul's)	3 oz	11	200
Gourmet Hand Breaded Shrimp Round (King & Prince)	3.5 oz	tr	150
Shrimp Pimavera (Mrs. Paul's)	11 oz	4	240
Shrimp Scampi (Gorton's)	1 pkg	24	350
HOME RECIPE			
Breaded & Fried	3 oz	10	206
SNACKS (nutritious snacks)			
(See also *CHIPS, NUTS, POPCORN, PRETZELS*)			
Cheddar Lites (Health Valley)	2 oz	2	40
Cheddar Lites with Green Onion (Health Valley)	2 oz	1	40
Wheat Snax (Estee)	1 oz	1	110
SNAPPER			
Cooked	1 fillet (6 oz)	3	217
SODA			
Apple Sparkling (Welch's)	12 oz	0	180
Root Beer (Hire's)	6 oz	0	90
Sprite	6 oz	0	71
SOLE			
FROZEN			
Au Natural Sole Fillets (Mrs. Paul's)	4 oz	2	90

SOUP

	Serving Size	Fat Grams	Calories
Today's Catch, Baby Sole (Van De Kamp's)	5 oz	1	100
SOUP			
SOUP, CANNED, READY-TO-SERVE			
Bean with Ham, Chowder (Hormel Micro-Cup Hearty),	9.5 oz	3	191
Bean with Ham (Campbell's Chunky Old Fashioned)	9.5 oz	8	250
Beef (Campbell's Chunky)	9.5 oz	4	170
Beef Hearty (Campbell's Home Cookin')	9.5 oz	3	130
Chicken (Campbell's Chunky Old Fashioned)	9.5 oz	4	150
Chicken Barley (Progresso)	9.5 oz	3	120
Chicken Broth	1 cup	1	39
Chicken with Noodles; (Campbell's Home Cookin')	9.5 oz	3	120
Chicken with Rice (Campbell's Chunky)	9.5 oz	4	140
Chicken Vegetable (Campbell's Chunky)	9.5 oz	6	170
Chili Beef (Campbell's Chunky)	9.75 oz	6	260
Clam Chowder, Manhattan (Campbell's Chunky)	9.5 oz	4	150
Lentil Hearty (Campbell's Home Cookin')	9.5 oz	1	150
Pea, Split with Ham (Campbell's Chunky)	9.5 oz	5	210
Pepper Steak (Campbell's Chunky)	9.5 oz	3	160
Steak and Potato (Campbell's Chunky)	9.5 oz	4	170
Tomato, Garden (Campbell's Home Cookin')	9.5 oz	3	130
Vegetable Beef (Campbell's Old Fashioned)	9.5 oz	5	160
SOUP, CANNED, CONDENSED AND PREPARED ACCORDING TO DIRECTIONS			
Bean w/Bacon (Campbell's)	8 oz	4	120
Beef, (Campbell's)	8 oz	2	80
Chicken Broth and Noodles (Campbell's)	8 oz	2	35
Chicken, Cream of (Campbell's)	8 oz	7	110
Mushroom, Cream of (Campbell's)	8 oz	7	100
Potato, Cream of (Campbell's)	8 oz	3	70
Tomato (Campbell's)	8 oz	2	90
HEALTHY REQUEST, (Campbell's)			
Bean with Bacon	8 oz	4	140
Cream of Chicken, prepared	8 oz	2	70
Cream of Chicken, condensed	10 3/4 oz	5.5	193
Cream of Mushroom, prepared	8 oz	2	60

SWEET POTATOES

	Serving Size	Fat Grams	Calories
Cream of Mushroom, condensed	10 3/4 oz	5.5	165
Vegetable	8 oz	2	90
Chicken Noodle	8 oz	2	60
Tomato	8 oz	2	90
SOUR CREAM			
(See also *SOUR CREAM SUBSTITUTES*)			
FAT FREE	1 Tbsp	0	10
	1 cup	0	160
Lean Cream (Land O' Lakes)	1 Tbsp	1	20
REGULAR			
Sour cream	1 Tbsp	3	26
Sour cream	1 cup	48	493
SOUR CREAM SUBSTITUTES			
Imitation, nondairy	1 cup	45	479
SPAGHETTI SAUCE			
(See also *PIZZA, TOMATO*)			
BOTTLED			
Chef Boy.ar.dee, Meatless	4 oz	1	60
Chef Boy.ar.dee with Ground Beef	4 oz	3	90
Chef Boy.ar.dee w/Mushrooms	4 oz	2	70
Econo-Sauce (LEAN & FREE)	3/4 cup	tr	62
Ragu Chunky Gardenstyle, Extra Tomatoes, Garlic, and Onions	4 oz	2	80
Ragu Homestyle with Mushrooms	4 oz	2	70
Spaghetti Econo-Sauce (LEAN & FREE)	3/4 cup	tr	62
SPINACH			
FRESH			
Cooked	1/2 cup	tr	21
Chopped, raw	1/2 cup	tr	6
SQUASH			
(See also *ZUCCHINI*)			
FRESH			
Acorn, cubed, baked	1/2 cup	tr	57
Summer, all varieties, raw, sliced	1/2 cup	tr	13
STRAWBERRIES			
FRESH, strawberries	1 cup	tr	45
STUFFING/DRESSING			
MIX			
Chicken (Stove Top)	1/2 cup	9	181
Corn Bread (Pepperidge Farm)	1 oz	1	110
Herb Seasoned (Pepperidge Farm)	1 oz	1	110
SUGAR			
Brown	1 cup	0	836
Powdered	1 cup	0	493
White	1 cup	0	770
SUNFLOWER SEEDS			
Sunflower (Planters)	1 oz	14	160
SWEET POTATOES			
CANNED, in syrup	1/2 cup	tr	106
Mashed	1/2 cup	tr	233

SYRUP　　　　　　　　　　　　　　　　　　　　　　　　**ZUCCHINI**

	Serving Size	Fat Grams	Calories
FRESH, baked in skin			
SYRUP	3.5 oz	tr	118
Maple			
TANGERINE	2 Tbsp	0	110
FRESH, tangerine			
TOMATO	1	tr	37
(See also *PIZZA, SPAGHETTI SAUCE*)			
CANNED			
Stewed Tomatoes (S&W)	1/2 cup	0	35
Red, whole	1 cup	tr	47
Tomato paste	1/2 cup	1	110
Tomato sauce	1 cup	tr	74
FRESH, tomato	1	tr	30
JUICE, tomato	6 oz	tr	32
TORTILLAS			
Corn	1	0	45
Taco shell	1	2	50
Flour	1	2	85
Taco salad shell	1	12	200
Whole wheat	1	2	93
TROUT			
Rainbow, cooked	1 fillet (2.1 oz)	3	94
TUNA			
CANNED			
Chunk Light in Oil (Bumble Bee)	3 oz	15	200
Chunk Light in Water (Bumble Bee)	3 oz	2	90
White in water	3 oz	2	116
TURKEY			
CANNED			
Turkey with broth	1/2 can (2.5 oz)	5	116
FRESH			
Ground Lean 90% Fat Free; cooked (Louis Rich)	3.5 oz	9	183
Dark meat with skin, roasted	3.6 oz	11	222
Dark meat without Skin, roasted	1 cup	10	260
Light Meat with skin, roasted	4.8 oz	10	260
Light meat without skin, roasted	1 cup	4	215
READY-TO-USE			
Breast, Honey Roasted (Louis Rich)	1 sl (29g)	tr	29
Breast, Oven Roasted (Louis Rich)	1 oz	tr	30
TURNIPS			
FRESH			
Cubed, raw	1/2 cup	tr	18
VANILLA EXTRACT			
Pure vanilla extract	1 tsp	0	10

	Serving Size	Fat Grams	Calories
VEGETABLES, MIXED			
(See also *INDIVIDUAL VEGETABLES*)			
FROZEN			
Brussels Sprouts, Cauliflower & Carrots, Farm Fresh Mixtures (Birds Eye)	3/4 cup	tr	40
Chinese Style Stir Fry Vegetable (Birds Eye)	1/2 cup	tr	36
VINEGAR			
Apple cider	2 Tbsp	0	4
WAFFLES			
FROZEN READY-TO-USE			
Raisins, Bran & Whole Grain Nutri-Grain (Eggo)	1	5	130
WATER CHESTNUTS			
Water Chestnuts (La Choy)	1/4 cup	tr	16
WATERMELON			
Diced	1 cup	tr	50
WHEAT			
Durum	1 cup	5	650
Hard red	1 cup	3	628
Hard white	1 cup	3	656
Soft white	1 cup	3	571
Bulgur, cooked	1 cup	tr	152
Sprouted	1 cup	1	214
WHIPPED TOPPING			
(See also *CREAM*)			
Cool Whip (non-dairy)	1 Tbsp	tr	11
Dream Whip as prepared	1 Tbsp	tr	9
YEAST			
Baker's Dry, Active	1 pkg (7g)	tr	20
YOGURT			
(See also *YOGURT, FROZEN*)			
Fruit, lowfat	1 cup	3	232
Fruit, nonfat	1 cup	0	200
Plain, lowfat	1 cup	3.5	144
Plain, skim milk	1 cup	tr	127
Vanilla, lowfat	1 cup	3	194
Vanilla, nonfat	1 cup	0	180
YOGURT, FROZEN			
Mixed Berries On-a Stick (Dannon)	1 bar	1	50
Vanilla (Colombo)	4 oz	2	99
ZUCCHINI			
FRESH			
Sliced; cooked	1/2 cup	tr	14
Siced, raw	1/2 cup	tr	9

SPECIAL NOTICE

These charts have been especially fine-tuned for your optimal health needs. They will heighten your awareness of foods you should eat abundantly and foods you should avoid or eat in moderation. These lists contain the vast majority of foods you'll be eating, so study them very carefully.

FOOD PERCENT FAT CHARTS

Find the calorie number across the top of the chart with your right index finger and find the number of fat grams along the left side with your left index finger. Follow your right finger down and your left finger across to the right. The number your two fingers meet on indicates the percentage of fat in that particular food.

INDIVIDUAL FOOD CALORIES

Fat Grams	10	20	30	40	50	60	70	80	90	100	110	120	130	140	150	160	170
1	90	45	30	23	18	15	13	11	10	9	8	8	7	6	6	6	5
2	100	90	60	45	36	30	26	23	20	18	16	15	14	13	12	11	11
3		100	90	68	54	45	39	34	30	27	25	23	21	19	18	17	16
4			100	90	72	60	51	45	40	36	33	30	28	26	24	23	21
5				100	90	75	64	56	50	45	41	38	35	32	30	28	26
6					100	90	77	68	60	54	49	45	42	39	36	34	32
7						100	90	79	70	63	57	53	48	45	42	39	37
8							100	90	80	72	65	60	55	51	48	45	42
9								100	90	81	74	68	62	58	54	51	48
10									100	90	82	75	69	64	60	56	53
11										99	90	83	76	71	66	62	58
12										100	98	90	83	77	72	68	64
13											100	98	90	84	78	73	69
14												100	97	90	84	79	74
15													100	96	90	84	79
16														100	96	90	85
17															100	96	90
18																100	95
19																	100

INDIVIDUAL FOOD CALORIES

Fat Grams	180	190	200	210	220	230	240	250	260	270	280	290	300	310	320	330
1	5	5	5	4	4	4	4	4	3	3	3	3	3	3	3	3
2	10	9	9	9	8	8	8	7	7	7	6	6	6	6	6	5
3	15	14	14	13	13	12	12	11	11	10	10	9	9	9	8	8
4	20	19	18	17	16	16	15	14	14	13	13	12	12	12	11	11
5	25	24	23	21	20	20	19	18	17	17	16	16	15	15	14	14
6	30	28	27	26	25	23	23	22	21	20	19	19	18	17	17	16
7	35	33	32	30	29	27	26	25	24	23	23	22	21	20	20	19
8	40	38	36	34	33	31	30	29	28	27	26	25	24	23	23	22
9	45	43	41	39	37	35	34	32	31	30	29	28	27	26	25	25
10	50	47	45	43	41	39	38	36	35	33	32	31	30	29	28	27
11	55	52	50	47	45	43	41	40	38	37	35	34	33	32	31	30
12	60	57	54	51	49	47	45	43	42	40	39	37	36	35	34	33
13	65	62	59	56	53	51	49	47	45	43	42	40	39	38	37	35
14	70	66	63	60	57	55	53	50	48	47	45	43	42	41	39	38
15	75	71	68	64	61	59	56	54	52	50	48	47	45	44	42	41
16	80	76	72	69	65	63	60	58	55	53	51	50	48	46	45	44
17	85	81	77	73	70	67	64	61	59	57	55	53	51	49	48	46
18	90	85	81	77	74	70	68	65	62	60	58	56	54	52	51	49
19	95	90	86	81	78	74	71	68	66	63	61	59	57	55	53	52
20	100	95	90	86	82	78	75	72	69	67	64	62	60	58	56	55
21		99	95	90	86	82	79	76	73	70	68	65	63	61	59	57
22		100	99	94	90	86	83	79	76	73	71	68	66	64	62	60
23			100	99	94	90	86	83	80	77	74	71	69	67	65	63
24				100	98	94	90	86	83	80	77	74	72	70	68	65
25					100	98	94	90	87	83	80	78	75	73	70	68
26						100	98	94	90	87	84	81	78	75	73	71
27							100	97	93	90	87	84	81	78	76	74
28								100	97	93	90	87	84	81	79	76
29									100	97	93	90	87	84	82	79
49										100	96	93	90	87	84	82
50											100	96	93	90	87	85
51												99	96	93	90	87
52												100	99	96	93	90
53													100	99	96	93
54														100	98	95
55															100	98
56																100

FAT GRAMS

FAT GRAMS

FAT GRAMS/CAL.

INDIVIDUAL FOOD CALORIES

	340	350	360	370	380	390	400	410	420	430	440	450	460	470	480	490	500
1	3	3	3	3	2	2	2	2	2	2	2	2	2	2	2	2	2
2	5	5	5	5	5	5	5	4	4	4	4	4	4	4	4	4	4
3	8	8	8	7	7	7	7	7	6	6	6	6	6	6	6	6	5
4	11	10	10	10	9	9	9	9	9	8	8	8	8	8	8	7	7
5	13	13	13	12	12	12	11	11	11	10	10	10	10	10	9	9	9
6	16	15	15	15	14	14	14	13	13	13	12	12	12	11	11	11	11
7	19	18	18	17	17	16	16	16	15	15	15	14	14	14	13	13	13
8	21	21	20	10	19	19	18	18	18	17	17	16	16	15	15	15	14
9	24	23	23	22	21	21	20	20	19	19	18	18	18	17	17	17	16
10	26	26	25	24	24	23	23	22	21	21	20	20	20	19	19	19	18
11	29	28	28	27	26	25	25	24	24	23	23	22	22	21	21	20	20
12	32	31	30	29	28	28	27	26	26	25	25	24	23	23	23	22	22
13	34	33	33	32	31	30	29	29	28	27	27	26	25	25	24	24	23
14	37	36	35	34	33	32	32	31	30	29	29	28	27	27	26	26	25
15	40	39	38	36	36	35	34	33	32	31	31	30	29	29	28	28	27
16	42	41	40	39	38	37	36	35	34	33	33	32	31	31	30	29	29
17	45	44	43	41	40	39	38	37	36	36	35	34	33	33	32	31	31
18	48	46	45	44	43	42	41	40	39	38	37	36	35	34	34	33	32
19	50	49	48	46	45	44	43	42	41	40	39	38	37	36	36	35	34
20	53	51	50	49	47	46	45	44	43	42	41	40	39	38	38	37	36
21	56	54	53	51	50	48	47	46	45	44	43	42	41	40	39	39	38
22	58	57	55	54	52	51	50	48	47	46	45	44	43	42	41	40	40
23	61	59	58	56	54	53	52	50	49	48	47	46	45	44	43	42	41
24	64	62	60	58	57	55	54	53	51	50	49	48	47	46	45	44	43
25	66	64	63	61	59	58	56	55	54	52	51	50	49	48	47	46	45
26	69	67	65	63	62	60	59	57	56	54	53	52	51	50	49	48	47
27	71	69	68	66	64	62	61	59	58	57	55	54	53	52	51	50	49
28	74	72	70	68	66	65	63	61	60	59	57	56	55	54	53	51	50
29	77	75	73	71	69	67	65	64	62	61	59	58	57	56	54	53	52
30	79	77	75	73	71	69	68	66	64	63	61	60	59	57	56	55	54
31	82	80	78	75	73	72	70	68	66	65	63	62	61	59	58	57	56
32	85	82	80	78	76	74	72	70	69	67	65	64	63	61	60	59	58
33	87	85	83	80	78	76	74	72	71	69	68	66	65	63	62	61	59
34	90	87	85	83	81	78	77	75	73	71	70	68	67	65	64	62	61
35	93	90	88	85	83	81	79	77	75	73	72	70	68	67	66	64	63
36	95	93	90	88	85	83	81	79	77	75	74	72	70	69	68	66	63
37	98	95	93	90	88	85	83	81	79	77	76	74	72	71	69	68	67
38	100	98	95	92	90	88	86	83	81	80	78	76	74	73	71	70	68
39		100	98	95	92	90	88	86	84	82	80	78	76	75	73	72	70
40			100	97	95	92	90	88	86	84	82	80	78	77	75	73	72
41				100	97	95	92	90	88	86	84	82	80	79	77	75	74
42					99	97	95	92	90	88	86	84	82	80	79	77	76
43					100	99	97	94	92	90	88	86	84	82	81	79	77
44						100	99	97	94	92	90	88	86	84	83	81	79
45							100	99	96	94	92	90	88	86	84	83	81
46								100	99	96	94	92	90	88	86	84	83
47									100	98	96	94	92	90	88	86	85
48										100	98	96	94	92	90	88	86
49											100	98	96	94	92	90	88
50												100	98	96	94	92	90
51													100	98	96	94	92
52														100	98	96	94
53															99	97	95
54															100	97	95
55																100	99
56																	100

Making Healthy Choices When Eating Out

"A" = Fat-Loss Choice
"B" = Coasting Choice
No Rating = "C","D", or "F" Choice

Ratings are based on the fat, cholesterol, complex carbohydrate, protein, sugar, and overall nutrient content of the foods listed. Many "B" and "C" Choices can be advanced to "A" and "B" Choices by omitting items such as butter, mayonnaise, oil, cheese, and sour cream. Always request no mayonnaise, no oil, and extra vegetables on fast food sandwiches. Also ask for whole-grain buns, if available.

		Serving Size	Fat Grams	Calories
ARBY'S				
	Junior Roast Beef	3 oz.	9	218
	Regular Roast Beef	5.2 oz.	15	353
	Beef 'n Cheddar	7 oz.	27	455
	Bac 'n Cheddar Deluxe	8 oz.	37	526
	Super Roast Beef	8.3 oz.	22	501
	Hot Ham 'n Cheese Sandwich	5.5 oz.	14	292
	Turkey Deluxe	7 oz.	17	375
	Fish Fillet Sandwich	7 oz.	32	580
	Philly Beef 'n Swiss	7 oz.	28	460
B+	Roasted Chicken Boneless Breast	5 oz.	7	254
A	Rice Pilaf	4 oz.	2	123
	Scandinavian Vegetables in Sauce	4 oz.	2	56
	Chicken Salad Sandwich	5.2 oz.	20	386
	Chicken Club Sandwich	7 oz.	32	621
	Chicken Salad & Croissant	5 oz.	36	472
	Chicken Salad with Tomato & Lettuce	9 oz.	36	515
A	Tossed Salad with Low Calorie Italian Dressing	8 oz.	1	57
A	Baked Potato, Plain	11 oz.	1	290
	Superstuffed Potato, Deluxe	11 oz.	38	648
	Superstuffed Potato Broccoli & Cheddar	12 oz.	22	541
	Superstuffed Potato Mushroom & Cheese	10.5 oz.	22	506
	Superstuffed Potato, Taco	15 oz.	27	619
	French Fries	2.5 oz.	10	215
	Potato Cakes	3 oz.	13	201
	Vanilla Shake	8.8 oz.	10	295
	Chocolate Shake	10.6 oz.	11	384
BURGER KING				
B–	BK Broiler		10	280
	Hamburger		12	275
	Cheeseburger		15	317
	Whopper Sandwich		36	628

	Serving Size	Fat Grams	Calories
Whopper with Cheese	1	43	711
Whaler Fish Sandwich	1	27	488
Ham & Cheese			
Specialty Sandwich	1	23	471
Chicken Specialty Sandwich	1	40	688
Chicken Tenders	6 pieces	10	204
Chicken Bundles	1 order	23	410
Chicken Bundles with Cheese	1 order	28	470
Burger Bundles	Serv of 3	18	435
Chef Salad	1 order	11	180
B+ Chicken Salad without			
Salad Dressing	1 salad	4	140
Shrimp & Pasta Salad	1 order	8	170
Onion Rings	1 serv	16	274
French Fries (Lightly Salted)	regular	13	227
A Salad Bar (Typical)			
without Dressing	1	0	28
Garden Salad	1	6	110
Salad Dressing	1 pkg	23-26	260-280
Reduced Calorie Italian			
Salad Dressing	1 pkg	2	30
Breakfast Croissan'wich	1	19	304
Bacon, Egg, Cheese			
Croissan'wich	1	24	355
Sausage, Egg, Cheese			
Croissan'wich	1	41	538
Ham, Egg, Cheese			
Croissan'wich	1	20	335
Scrambled Egg Platter	1	30	468
Scrambled Egg Platter			
with Sausage	1	52	702
Scrambled Egg Platter with Bacon	1	36	536
French Toast Sticks	1 serv	29	499
Bagel with Bacon, Egg, Cheese	1 bagel	19	438
Bagel with Ham, Egg, Cheese	1 bagel	15	418
Bagel with Sausage, Egg, Cheese	1 bagel	36	621
Vanilla Shake	1	10	321
Chocolate Shake	1	12	320
Apple Pie	1	12	305
Great Danish	1	36	500

		Serving Size		Fat Grams	Calories
CARL JR.'S					
	Famous Star Hamburger	231 g	1	36	590
	Super Star Hamburger	301 g	1	50	770
	Happy Star Hamburger	86 g	1	8	220
A	Charbroiler BBQ Chicken Sandwich	178 g	1	5	320
	Charbroiler Chicken Club Sandwich	234 g	1	22	510
B+	California Roast Beef 'n Swiss	209 g	1	8	360
	Fillet of Fish Sandwich	223 g	1	26	550
	Hot Dog with Chili	174 g	1	23	510
	Fiesta & Cheese Potato	432 g	1	23	550
	Broccoli & Cheese Potato	398 g	1	17	470
	Bacon & Cheese Potato	400 g	1	34	650
	Sour Cream & Chive Potato	294 g	1	13	350
	Cheese Potato	403 g	1	22	550
A	Lite Potato	278 g	1	tr	250
	French Fries, Regular	170 g	1 order	17	360
	Zucchini	121 g	1 order	16	300
	Onion Rings	90 g	1 order	15	310
	Reduced-Cal Italian Dressing	57 g	2 oz	10	90
	House Dressing	57 g	2 oz	17	186
	Soups:				
	Cream of Broccoli	186 g	1 order	6	140
	Boston Clam Chowder	186 g	1 order	8	140
A	Old Fashioned Chicken Noodle	186 g	1 order	1	80
	Lumber Jack Mixed Vegetable	186 g	1 order	3	70
	Hot Cakes with Margarine (Syrup not included)	156 g	1 order	12	360
	Sausage	44 g	1 patty	17	190
	Bacon	10 g	2 strips	4	50
	Hashed Brown Nuggets	85 g	1 order	9	170
	Bran Muffins	113 g	1	6	220
	Shakes	330 g	reg. size	7	353
CHICK-FIL-A					
A	Chick-Fil-A Sandwich, with bun	5.8 oz.	1	9	426
	Chick-Fil-A Nuggets	4 oz	8 pack	15	287
A	Hearty Breast of Chicken Soup	17.5 oz.	large	9	432

	Serving Size	Fat Grams	Calories
Chicken Salad Sandwich (Wheat)	5.7 oz.	1	26	449
Chicken Salad Plate	11.8 oz.	1	63	875
Chicken Salad Cup	4 oz.	1	28	309
Cole Slaw		1 cup	14	175
Potato Salad		1 cup	15	198
B Carrot-Raisin Salad		1 cup	5	116
Waffle, Potato Fries	3 oz.	regular	14	270
Icedream	4.5 oz.		5	134
Lemon Pie		1 slice	5	329
Fudge Brownies with nuts	2.8 oz.	1	5	369

COLOMBO

	Serving Size	Fat Grams	Calories
Lowfat Frozen Yogurt	4 fl oz.		2	99
B– Lite Nonfat Frozen Yogurt	4 fl oz.		0	95

DAIRY QUEEN

	Serving Size	Fat Grams	Calories
Single Hamburger	148 g	1	16	360
Double Hamburger	210 g	1	28	530
Double with cheese	239 g	1	37	650
Hot Dog	100 g	1	16	280
Fish Sandwich	170 g	1	17	400
Chicken Sandwich	200 g	1	41	670
Chicken Breast Fillet	202 g	1	34	608
All White Chicken Nuggets	99 g	1 order	18	276
Cone		regular	7	240
Mr. Misty		small	0	190
DQ Sandwich		1	4	140
Dilly Bar		1	13	210
Chocolate Malt		large	20	1060
Heath Blizzard		1	15	800
B– BREEZES *(Basic calories and fat grams change depending on what you add. Breezes are made with nonfat yogurt.)*				
		small	0	100+
		medium	0	150+
		large	0	200+

DOMINO'S PIZZA

	Serving Size	Fat Grams	Calories
B Cheese Pizza 16" (large)	5.5 oz.	2 sl	10	376
Pepperoni Pizza 16" (large)	5.5 oz.	2 sl	18	460

EATING OUT

	Serving Size	Fat Grams	Calories
Deluxe Pizza 16" (large) includes: sausage, pepperoni, onion, green pepper, mushrooms	5.5 oz.	2 sl	20	498
B– Ham Pizza 16" (large)	5.5 oz.	2 sl	11	417

GODFATHER'S PIZZA

	Serving Size	Fat Grams	Calories
B+ Original Pizza: Cheese Pizza—mini	79 g	1/4 of whole	4	190
B– Original Cheese Pizza— large, Hot Slice	156 g	1/8 of whole	11	370
Combo Pizza— large, Hot Slice	241 g	1/8 of whole	24	550
B– Thin Crust: Cheese Pizza—small	75 g	1/6 of whole	6	180
B– Thin Crust: Cheese Pizza—large	96 g	1/10 of whole	7	228
Thin Crust: Combo Pizza—large	152 g	1/10 of whole	16	336
B– Stuffed Pie: Cheese Pizza—small	124 g	1/6 of whole	11	310
Stuffed Pie: Combo Pizza—large	216 g	1/10 whole	26	521

GOLDEN CORRAL

	Serving Size	Fat Grams	Calories
Sirloin	104 g	5 oz	14	230
Ribeye	146 g	reg	35	450
Sirloin Tips with onions & peppers	233 g	1 order	13	290
B Golden Grilled Chicken	118 g	1 order	5	170
Golden Fried Chicken Fillets	155 g	1 order	19	370
Golden Fried Shrimp	87 g	1 order	12	250
A Baked Potato	219 g	1	2	220
Texas Toast	49 g	1 order	6	170

HARDEE'S

	Serving Size	Fat Grams	Calories
Hamburger	99 g	1	10	264
Cheeseburger	110 g	1	13	310
Big Deluxe	226 g	1	27	495
Bacon Cheeseburger	229 g	1	39	610

	Serving Size		Fat Grams	Calories
Mushroom 'N Swiss	197 g	1	28	516
Roast Beef Sandwich	141 g	1	15	338
B– Hot Ham 'N Cheese	140 g	1	10	316
Fisherman's Fillet	205 g	1	25	510
B– Turkey Club (Request no bacon or mayonnaise for an "A" Choice)	224 g	1	14	374
Chicken Fillet	183 g	1	16	416
Hot Dog	120 g	1	16	306
Chicken Stix	100 g	6 pieces	9	210
Garden Salad	241 g	1 salad	14	208
Side Salad	112 g	1	1	19
Chef Salad	294 g	1	15	248
Chicken Fiesta Salad	297 g	1	14	286
Regular French Fries	2.5 oz.	1	10	226
Rise 'N Shine Biscuit	84 g	1	19	319
Sausage & Egg Biscuit	150 g	1	37	530
Ham Biscuit	115 g	1	15	321
Ham, Egg Biscuit	155 g	1	22	404
Cinnamon 'N Raisin Biscuit	79 g	1	17	315
Canadian Rise 'N Shine Biscuit	159 g	1	28	478
Big Country Breakfast Sausage	313 g	1	74	1005
B+ Orange Juice	6 oz		tr	83
Apple Turnover	91 g	1	12	268
Big Cookie Treat	138 g	1	13	250
Cool Twist Cone, Chocolate	138 g	1	6	208
Cool Twist Cone, Vanilla	124 g	1	6	192
Shake, Chocolate	335 g	1	8	447

JACK-IN-THE-BOX

	Serving Size		Fat Grams	Calories
Hamburger	103 g	1	13	288
Cheeseburger	113 g	1	17	325
Jumbo Jack with Cheese	242 g	1	40	667
Ultimate Cheeseburger	280 g	1	69	942
B Club Pita without sauces	179 g	1	8	277
Chicken Supreme	231 g	1	36	575
Pizza Pocket	497 g	1	28	497
Moby Jack	137 g	1	25	444
Fish Supreme	228 g	1	32	554
Hot Club Supreme	213 g	1	28	524

		Serving Size	Fat Grams		Calories
	Sirloin Steak Dinner	334 g	1	27	699
	Chicken Strip Dinner	321 g	1	30	689
	Shrimp Dinner	301 g	1	37	731
	Taco Salad	358 g	1	24	377
	Pasta and Seafood Salad	417 g	1	22	394
	Side Salad	111 g	1	3	51
	Buttermilk House Dressing	35 g	1 pkg	18	181
	Bleu Cheese Dressing	35 g	1 pkg	11	131
	Reduced Calorie French Dressing	35 g	1 pkg	4	80
	Super Taco	135 g	1	17	288
	Cheese Nachos	170 g	1	35	571
	Supreme Nachos	338 g	1	45	787
B+	Fajita Pita	175 g	1	7	278
B	Chicken Fajita Pita	189 g	1	8	292
	French Fries	68 g	regular	12	221
	Chicken Strips	125 g	4 piece	14	349
	Shrimp	84 g	10 piece	16	270
	Supreme Crescent	146 g	1	40	547
	Hash Browns	62 g	1	7	116
	Mayo-Onion Sauce	21 g	1 pkg	15	143
	Mayo-Mustard Sauce	21 g	1 pk	13	124
	Hot Apple Turnover	119 g	1	24	410
	Cheesecake	99 g	1	18	309
	Vanilla Milk Shake	317 g	1	6	320
	Chocolate Milk Shake	322 g	1	7	330
	Pancake Platter	231 g	1	22	612

KENTUCKY FRIED CHICKEN

		Serving Size	Fat Grams		Calories
	Center Breast, Original Recipe	107 g	1	14	257
	Drumstick, Original Recipe	58 g	1	9	147
	Center Breast, Extra Crispy	120 g	1	21	353
	Kentucky Nuggets	96 g	6	17	276
	Buttermilk Biscuits	75 g	1	14	269
B–	Mashed Potatoes with gravy	86 g	1	1	62
	Kentucky Fries	119 g	1	13	268
A	Corn-on-the-Cob	143 g	1	3	176
	Cole Slaw	79 g	1	6	103
	Potato Salad	90 g	1	9	141
A	Baked Beans	89 g	1	1	105

		Serving Size	Fat Grams	Calories	
MCDONALD'S					
	Hamburger	102 g	1	10	257
	Cheeseburger	114 g	1	14	308
	Quarter Pounder	166 g	1	21	414
	Quarter Pounder w/Cheese	194 g	1	29	517
	Big Mac	215 g	1	32	562
	Fillet-O-Fish	142 g	1	26	442
	McD.L.T.	288 g	1	42	674
	Chicken Fajitas		1	8	185
	Chicken McNuggets	113 g	6	16	288
	French Fries	68 g	Regular	12	220
B+	Orange Juice	6 oz.		0	80
A–	Grapefruit Juice	6 oz.		0	80
	Chef Salad	283 g	1	14	231
B	Shrimp Salad	262 g	1	3	104
	Garden Salad	213 g	1	7	112
A	Chicken Salad Oriental	244 g	1	3	141
	Side Salad	115 g	1	3	57
	Croutons	11 g	11	2	52
	Bacon Bits	3 g	1	1	16
	Chow Mein Noodles	9 g	1	2	45
	Dressings:				
	Blue Cheese	.5 oz.		7	69
	French	.5 oz.		5	58
	Ranch	.5 oz.		9	83
	1000 Island	.5 oz.		8	78
	Lite Vinaigrette	.5 oz.		1	15
A	Oriental	.5 oz.		tr	24
	Egg McMuffin	138 g	1	12	293
	Scrambled Eggs	100 g	1	11	157
	Pork Sausage	48 g	1	16	180
	English Muffin w/butter	59 g	1	5	169
	Hash Brown Potatoes	53 g	1	7	131
	Biscuit with Biscuit Spread	75 g	1	13	260
	Biscuit with Sausage	123 g	1	29	440
	Biscuit with Sausage and Egg	180 g	1	35	529
	Biscuit with Bacon, Egg and Cheese	156 g	1	27	449
	Sausage McMuffin	117 g	1	22	372
	Sausage McMuffin with Egg	167 g	1	27	440
	Apple Pie	83 g	1	15	262

	Serving Size		Fat Grams	Calories
Soft Serve Cone	86 g	1	5	144
Vanilla Shake	303 g	1	10	354
Chocolate Shake	303 g	1	11	388
Strawberry Shake	303 g	1	10	384
Strawberry Sundae	171 g	1	7	283
Hot Fudge Sundae	169 g	1	9	313
Hot Caramel Sundae	174 g	1	9	343
McDonaldland Cookie	56 g	1 box	9	288
Chocolate Chip Cookie	56 g	1 box	16	325
Hot Cakes with Butter, Syrup	176 g	1	9	413
Apple Danish	115 g	1	18	389
Hot Cheese Danish	110 g	1	22	395
Cinnamon Raisin Danish	110 g	1	21	445
Raspberry Danish	117	1	16	414

PIZZA HUT

	Serving Size		Fat Grams	Calories
Thin-n-Crispy Pizza, Beef	1/2 of 10"	3 sl	19	490
Thin-n-Crispy Pizza, Pork	1/2 of 10"	3 sl	23	520
B– Thin-n-Crispy Pizza, Cheese	1/2 of 10"	3 sl	15	450
Thin-n-Crispy Pizza, Pepperoni	1/2 of 10"	3 sl	17	430
Thin-n-Crispy Pizza, Supreme	1/2 of 10"	3 sl	21	510
B Thick 'n Chewy Pizza, Cheese	1/2 of 10"	3 sl	14	560
B– Thick 'n Chewy Pizza, Pepperoni	1/2 of 10"	3 sl	18	560
B– Thick 'n Chewy Pizza, Supreme	1/2 of 10"	3 sl	22	640

PONDEROSA

	Serving Size	Fat Grams	Calories
Fish, baked Bake 'R Broil	5.2 oz.	13	230
Fish, Broiled			
A Halibut	6.0 oz.	3	170
B Roughy	5.0 oz.	5	139
A Salmon	6.0 oz.	3	192
B– Swordfish	5.9 oz.	10	271
A Trout	5.0 oz.	4	228
A Chicken Breast	5.5 oz.	2	98
Chopped Steak	5.3 oz.	22	296
Kansas City Strip	5 oz.	6	138
New York Strip, Choice	8 oz.	11	304
Porterhouse, Choice	16 oz.	31	640
Ribeye, Choice	6 oz.	14	282

	Serving Size		Fat Grams	Calories
Sirloin Tips, Choice	5 oz.		8	197
B– Steak Kabbobs (meat only)	3 oz.		5	153
A– Teriyaki Steak	5 oz.		3	174
T-Bone, Choice	10 oz.		18	444
Chicken Wings	2 pieces		9	213

RAX

	Serving Size		Fat Grams	Calories
Roast Beef Sandwich	226 g	large	35	570
BBC (Beef, Bacon, & Chicken Sandwich)	212 g	1	49	720
Turkey Bacon Club	254 g	1	43	670
B– BBQ Sandwich	162 g	1	14	420
A Potatoes: Plain Potato	250 g	1	tr	270
Cheese (3 oz & Bacon Potato)	364 g	1	28	780
Cheese (3 oz & Broccoli Potato)	192 g	1	26	760
BBQ Potato (2 oz Cheese)	406 g	1	24	730
Chili & Cheddar (2 oz Potato)	406 g	1	23	700
Drive-Thru Salads:				
Garden Salad without dressing	1 salad		11	160
Chef Salad without dressing	1 salad		14	230
A Chicken Noodle Soup	3.5 oz.		tr	40
Cream of Broccoli Soup	3.5 oz.		2	50

RED LOBSTER

	Serving Size		Fat Grams	Calories
Catfish	5 oz.		10	170
A Atlantic Cod	5 oz.		1	100
A Flounder	5 oz.		1	100
A Grouper	5 oz.		1	110
A Haddock	5 oz.		1	110
A Halibut	5 oz.		1	110
Mackerel	5 oz.		12	190
A Monkfish	5 oz.		1	110
B+ Atlantic Ocean Perch	5 oz.		4	130
A Pollock	5 oz.		1	120
A Red Rockfish	5 oz.		1	90
A Red Snapper	5 oz.		1	110
Norwegian Salmon	5 oz.		12	230
B+ Sockeye Salmon	5 oz.		4	160
A Blacktip Shark	5 oz.		1	150

LEAN & FREE 2000 PLUS

		Serving Size	Fat Grams	Calories
A–	Mako Shark	5 oz.	1	140
A	Lemon Sole	5 oz.	1	120
	Swordfish	5 oz.	4	100
A	Tilefish	5 oz.	2	100
	Rainbow Trout	5 oz.	9	170
B	Yellowfin Tuna	5 oz.	6	180
A	Cherrystone Clams	5 oz.	2	130
A	King Crab Legs	1 lb	2	170
A	Snow Crab Legs	1 lb	2	150
	Calamari, Breaded & Fried	5 oz.	21	360
B	Mussels	3 oz.	2	70
	Oysters	6 raw on 1/2 shell	4	110
A	Langostino	5 oz.	1	120
B–	Maine Lobster	1 1/4 lb	8	240
A–	Rock Lobster	1 tail	3	230
A–	Calico Scallops	5 oz.	2	180
A–	Deep Sea Scallops	5 oz.	2	130
B+	Shrimp	8-12 pieces	2	120
	Porterhouse Steak	18 oz.	131	1420
	Sirloin Steak	7 oz.	48	570
	Strip Steak	7 oz.	64	690
	Hamburger	1/3 lb	23	320
B+	Chicken Breast	4 oz.	3	120

SUBWAY SANDWICHES

		Serving Size	Fat Grams	Calories
A	Subway Club*	12"	12	668
A	Seafood Crab*	12"	14	686
B	Steak and Cheese*	12"	18	756
A	Turkey Breast*	12"	10	624
B	Roast Beef*	12"	12	660
B	Meatball*	12"	11	758
A	Tuna*	12"	10	624

All sandwiches are without salad dressing and oil.

TACO BELL

		Serving Size		Fat Grams	Calories
B–	Bean Burrito	191 g	1	11	359
	Beef Burrito	191 g	1	17	402
	Double Beef Burrito Supreme	255 g	1	22	451
	Tostada	156 g	1	11	243
	Beefy Tostada	196 g	1	20	322

	Serving Size	Fat Grams		Calories
Bellbeefer	177 g	1	13	312
Burrito Supreme	248 g	1	19	422
Combination Burrito	191 g	1	14	380
Enchirito	213 g	1	20	382
Taco	78 g	1	11	184
Taco Light Platter	488 g	1	58	1062
Burrito Supreme Platter	452 g	1	37	774
Cinnamon Crisps	47 g	1 order	16	266
Ranch Dressing	74 g	1 pkg	25	236
Guacamole	21 g	1 serving	2	34
Taco Salad without Beans	516 g	1	57	822
Taco Salad without Salsa	510 g	1	62	931
Taco Salad with Ranch Dressing	584 g	1	87	1167
Seafood Salad with Ranch Dressing	435 g	1	66	884
Seafood Salad without Dressing/Shell	291 g	1	11	217
Seafood Salad without Dressing	362 g	1	42	648
Cheesarito	115 g	1	13	312
Mexican Pizza	269 g	1	48	714
Taco Bellgrande Platter	488 g	1	51	1002
Pintos & Cheese (no cheese ="A–")	127 g	1 order	10	194
Nachos	106 g	1 order	18	346
Nachos Bellgrande	287 g	1 order	35	649
Taco Bellgrande	170 g	1	22	351
Taco Light	170 g	1	29	411
Soft Taco	92 g	1	12	228
Taco Salad with Salsa	601 g	1	62	949
Taco Salad without Shell	530 g	1	31	502
Taco Salad with Salsa, w/out Shell	530 g	1	31	520
Fajita Steak Taco (no sour cream and cheese = "B+")	142 g	1	11	235
Fajita Steak Taco with Sour Cream	163 g	1	15	281
Fajita Steak Taco with Guacamole	163 g	1	13	269
Chicken Fajita (no sour cream and cheese = "B+")	135 g	1	10	226

TCBY (YOGURT)

B– TCBY—All Flavors	5 oz.		3-4	150 to 169

WENDY'S

Single Hamburger Patty on White Bun	127 g	1	16	350
Double Hamburger Patty on White Bun	203 g	1	30	560

		Serving Size	Fat Grams	Calories
	Big Classic on Kaiser Bun	241 g	1	25	470
	Big Classic Double on Kaiser Bun	317 g	1	39	680
	Double with Cheese	221 g	1	36	620
	Bacon Cheeseburger	151 g	1	24	440
	Chicken Fried Steak	176 g	1	41	580
	Fish Fillet	92 g	1	11	210
A	Multi Grain Bun	48 g	1	3	140
B–	Chicken Breast on White Bun	138 g	1	12	340
A	Plain Baked Potato	250 g	1	2	250
	Bacon & Cheese Potato	350 g	1	30	570
	Broccoli & Cheese Potato	365 g	1	25	500
	Cheese Potato	350 g	1	34	590
	Chili & Cheese Potato (no cheese = "B+")	400 g	1	20	510
	Sour Cream & Chives Potato	310 g	1	24	460
	Cheese Sauce	2 oz.		12	140
	French Fries		regular	15	300
	Cheddar Chips	28 g	1 oz	11	160
	Crispy Chicken Nuggets		6 pieces	21	310
	Chicken Nuggets		9 pieces	32	465
	Chicken Nuggets		20 pieces	69	1023
B	Barbecue Sauce	28 g	1	tr	50
B	Sweet & Sour Sauce	28 g	1	tr	45
B	Sweet Mustard	28 g	1	1	50
	Cheese Sauce	963 g	2 oz	12	140
	Tartar Sauce	14 g	1 Tbsp	9	80
B–	Chili	256 g	9 oz	9	230
	Taco Salad	791 g	1 prepared	37	660
B	Taco Sauce		1 pkg	tr	10
	Pick-up Window Salad	570 g	1	6	110
	Garden Salad (take out)	277 g	1	5	102
	Chef Salad (take out)	331 g	1	9	180
	Cole Slaw	57 g	1/4 cup	5	80
	Pasta Salad	57 g	1/4 cup	6	130
	Salad Dressings (1 ladle equals 2 tablespoons)				
	Bleu Cheese	15 g	1 Tbsp	7	60
	Celery Seed	15 g	1 Tbsp	6	70
	French Style	16 g	1 Tbsp	5	70
	Golden Italian	16 g	1 Tbsp	4	50

318

	Serving Size		Fat Grams	Calories
Ranch	15 g	1 Tbsp	6	50
1000 Island	15 g	1 Tbsp	7	70
Oil	14 g	1 Tbsp	14	120
A Wine Vinegar	15 g	1 Tbsp	tr	2
Reduced Calorie Dressings:				
Bacon/Tomato	15 g	1 Tbsp	4	45
Creamy Cucumber	15 g	1 Tbsp	5	50
Italian	15 g	1 Tbsp	2	25
1000 Island	15 g	1 Tbsp	4	45
A Old Fashioned Corn Relish	57 g	1/4 cup	tr	35
A Deluxe Three Bean Salad	57 g	1/4 cup	tr	60
Red Bliss Potato Salad	57 g	1/4 cup	9	110
A Pasta Deli Salad	57 g	1/4 cup	tr	35
California Coleslaw	57 g	2 oz	6	60
Omelet, Ham, Cheese and/or Mushroom	114 g	1	21	290
Omelet, Mushroom, Green Pepper, Onion	114 g	1	15	210
Omelet, Ham, Cheese, Onion, Green Pepper	128 g	1	19	280
Breakfast Sandwich	129 g	1	19	370
Breakfast Sandwich with Sausage		1	37	570
Breakfast Sandwich with Bacon		1	23	430
French Toast	135 g	2 sl	19	400
Apple Topping	70 g	1	tr	130
Blueberry Topping	70 g	1	tr	60
Breakfast Potatoes	103 g	1 serving	22	360
Buttermilk Biscuit	94 g	1	17	320
Sausage Patty	45 g	1	18	200
Sausage Gravy	214 g	6 oz	36	440
Eggs—Scrambled	91 g	2 eggs	12	190
Bacon	6 g	1 strip	2	30
B+ Orange Juice	185 g	6 oz	tr	80
White Toast	69 g	2 sl	9	250
Cheese or Cinnamon Raisin Danish	95 g		21	430
Apple Danish	95 g		14	360
Frosty Dairy Dessert	243 g	Small	14	400
Chocolate Chip Cookie	64 g	1	17	320

Cookbook Sampler Alphabetical Index

Cookbook Sampler Topical Index

● **Dana's *WHERE DO I START?* Video**
Don't be overwhelmed! Learn step by step from Dana how to adapt LEAN & FREE to your own personal lifestyle. This video will answer your questions.

● **The *DANA, I NEED TO KNOW* Video Support Group**
You'll be inspired and motivated when you join Dana's own support group on video. Learn first hand from Dana and others just like you who have struggled with excess body fat and health problems. Strengthen your own resolve as they share their stories, discuss their new-found hope, and tell how they discovered the best within themselves while gaining control of their bodies and lives. Dana's LEAN & FREE Support Group can tremendously accelerate *your* success!

● **Dana's *ENJOYING THE FREEDOM* Aerobic Video**
Dana takes her eleven years as a sought-after aerobics instructor and incorporates it into this revolutionary approach to FUN AND FAT LOSS. This tape can encourage your body to burn more fat even 24 hours after your workout with Dana. It is like two workouts in one, including a 20 and a 60 minute aerobic workout. Dana highlights an extra-low, low, medium, and advanced level to meet your individual needs. A must for your LEAN & FREE success!

● **Dana's *LEAN & FREE 2000 PLUS Book* on Audio Cassette**
Perfect for reinforcing LEAN & FREE principles again and again—while you drive, exercise, or work around the house or yard!

● **Dana's LEAN & FREE *LECTURE SERIES* on Audio Cassette**
In response to thousands of requests, Dana has recorded her *live,* eleven-session lecture series on audio cassette. These cassettes are packed full of invaluable information that greatly expands upon Dana's book and videos.

WE WANT TO HEAR FROM YOU

Dear LEAN & FREE Participant,

Please send me your comments, suggestions, and the following research information. I am very interested in knowing how the LEAN & FREE LIFESTYLE is working for you so that further enhancements can be made to better meet your *individual* needs.

Sincerely, Dana Thornock

Please fill out the following Personal Progress Form and send it to:
Danmar Health Corporation
P.O. Box 2000
Kaysville, Utah 84037

Personal Progress Form

Name:_____

Date: _____ Age: _____

Sex:_____ Race: _____

Address: _____

City: _____ State: _____ Zip Code: _____

Phone No. : (_____)_____

1. When did you start the program?_____
2. How often do you eat as the program recommends?
   (circle) Time: 100%   75%   50%   25%   0%
3. Approximately how many calories did you eat
   in a day before starting this program? (circle)
   0 to 500 / 500 to 1000 / 1000 to 1500 / 1500 to 2000
   2000 to 2500 / 2500 to 3000 / 3000 to 4000 / 4000 plus
4. Approximately how many calories do you *now* eat
   in a day? (circle)
   0 to 500 / 500 to 1000 / 1000 to 1500 / 1500 to 2000
   2000 to 2500 / 2500 to 3000 / 3000 to 4000 / 4000 plus
5. What type of exercise do you do?_____
   How often?_____
6. Do you feel you can achieve optimal health and
   leanness by following the LEAN & FREE 2000 PLUS
   principles? Yes___No___
7. What eating disorders have you experiencd, if any?
   _____ Have they improved? Yes ___ No ___
8. What changes have you experienced?

	Starting	Current	
Energy	5 4 3 2 1	5 4 3 2 1	5 = Excellent
Disposition	5 4 3 2 1	5 4 3 2 1	3 = Fair
Self-Esteem	5 4 3 2 1	5 4 3 2 1	1 = Poor
Skin Tone	5 4 3 2 1	5 4 3 2 1	
Health	5 4 3 2 1	5 4 3 2 1	

9. Please list any changes in the following areas:

	Starting	Current
Depression	_____	_____
Body % Fat	_____	_____
Inches*:		
Chest	_____	_____
Waist	_____	_____
Hips	_____	_____
Thigh (right)	_____	_____
Pant Size	_____	_____
Cholesterol	_____	_____
Blood Pressure	_____	_____
Weight	_____	_____

10. How often do you practice positive body talk?
    (circle) Time: 100% 75% 50% 25% 0%
11. What medical problems have you experienced
    in the past and at present, if any? Past:_____
    Present:_____
12. What medications are you currently taking,
    if any?_____
13. List foods and substances you are allergic to,
    if any?_____
14. How do you feel about the LEAN & FREE 2000
    PLUS program? _____

*Measure the chest, hips, and thigh at the largest
circumference. Measure the waist at the smallest
circumference.*

DANMAR
Health Corporation™

Permission granted to copy this form.
Please send one completed copy to us annually.

THE RIGHT-BRAIN SUCCESS PLANNER

NAME:_____ DATE:_____

Simply follow the LEAN & FREE MENUS and check each completed box. Boxes vary in size according to the foods you should be eating the most of. If you miss a food at a meal, just include it with your next snack and check it off. Snacks are not essential, but are very helpful for increasing metabolism.

BREAKFAST

WATER: ☐

GRAIN: ☐
PROTEIN: ☐
FRUIT: ☐

SNACK

WATER: ☐
VEGGIE + ☐)

LUNCH

WATER: ☐
VEGGIE + ☐
GRAIN: ☐
PROTEIN: ☐
FRUIT: ☐

Today I exercised aerobically (nonstop, entire-body, rhythmic movement) for:

(CHECK ONE)
15 minutes: ☐
30 minutes: ☐
45 minutes ☐
60 minutes: ☐

SNACK

WATER: ☐
VEGGIE+ ☐)

DINNER

WATER: ☐
VEGGIE + ☐
GRAIN: ☐
PROTEIN: ☐
FRUIT: ☐

Today I practiced positive body talk. I like myself today!

YES ☐
NO ☐

SNACK

WATER: ☐
VEGGIE+ ☐)

All Appropriate Boxes Checked = A+, Healthy, High-Energy, Fat-Burning Habits

Permission granted to enlarge and copy this page.

© Dana Thornock 1994

THE RIGHT-BRAIN SUCCESS PLANNER

NAME:_____ DATE:_____

Simply follow the LEAN & FREE MENUS and check each completed box. Boxes vary in size according to the foods you should be eating the most of. If you miss a food at a meal, just include it with your next snack and check it off. Snacks are not essential, but are very helpful for increasing metabolism.

BREAKFAST

WATER: ☐

GRAIN: ☐

PROTEIN: ☐

FRUIT: ☐

SNACK

WATER: ☐

VEGGIE + (☐)

Veggie + hand diagram labeled: WATER, VEGGIE, GRAIN, PROTEIN, FRUIT

LUNCH

WATER: ☐

VEGGIE + ☐

GRAIN: ☐

PROTEIN: ☐

FRUIT: ☐

SNACK

WATER: ☐

VEGGIE+ (☐)

Today I exercised aerobically (nonstop, entire-body, rhythmic movement) for:

(CHECK ONE)
15 minutes: ☐
30 minutes: ☐
45 minutes ☐
60 minutes: ☐

DINNER

WATER: ☐

VEGGIE + ☐

GRAIN: ☐

PROTEIN: ☐

FRUIT: ☐

SNACK

WATER: ☐

VEGGIE+ (☐)

Today I practiced positive body talk. I like myself today!

YES ☐
NO ☐

All Appropriate Boxes Checked = A+, Healthy, High-Energy, Fat-Burning Habits

Permission granted to enlarge and copy this page.

LEAN&FREE 2000 PLUS™

THE LEFT-BRAIN PLANNER

NAME: _____ DATE: _____

1 . K N O W L E D G E		
2 . C O M M I T M E N T		
3 . N U R T U R I N G		
4 . N O U R I S H M E N T		
5 . M O T I O N		
6 . S E R V I C E		
7. PLAN	♥	8. ACTION

PLAN	Points 5__	Breakfast	
		Lunch	
		Dinner	
		Snacks	
		Exercise	
		Failure Avoidance	Today, I foresee and resolve any problem that could cause me to fail.*

KNOWLEDGE	5__	Knowledge	Today I studied or reinforced LEAN&FREE . principles. This knowledge empowers my success.*
COMMITMENT	5__	Commitment	Today I am realizing and enjoying signs of success and feel a passion to be LEAN&FREE . .*
NURTURING	5__	Nurturing	I am practicing positive body talk. I am a friend and partner with my body.*

				FG/Cal
NOURISHMENT	5__	Comfortable Satisfaction	**BREAKFAST**	XXXXX
	1__	Water		
	1__	Grain		
	1__	Protein		
	1__	Fruit		
	2__	Water & Snack		
	5__	Comfortable Satisfaction	**LUNCH**	XXXXX
	1__	Water		XXXXX
	1__	Vegetable		
	1__	Grain		
	1__	Protein		
	1__	Fruit		
	2__	Water & Snack		
	5__	Comfortable Satisfaction	**DINNER**	XXXXX
	1__	Water		XXXXX
	1__	Vegetable		
	1__	Grain		
	1__	Protein		
	1__	Fruit		
	2__	Water & Snack		
	5__	Fat Grams	Score 5 points if fat grams are about 20% of total calories. (Record calories once a week.) Total FG/Cal ►	
	10__	Stressors* A. B. C. D.	Score 10 points for avoiding ALL of the following fat-storing stressors—0 points otherwise. Alcohol, unnecessary drugs (smoking & caffeine), and artificial sweeteners. Excessive amounts of refined flour, sugar, and salt. Desserts and sweets, except after comfortable satisfaction on W.V.G.P.F. Extreme anger with self or others.	

			TYPE (Non-stop aerobic)	MINUTES (Goal 30 - 60)	PULSE (110 - 180 per minute)
MOTION	15__ 5__	Exercise Adequate sleep	Score 15 points for meeting your exercise goal and recording your exercise pulse*. Score 5 points for receiving adequate sleep. (Hours slept:_____)		

SERVICE	10__	Personal Service	Today, I used my increased health and energy in service to myself and others.*

ACTION		Do It Now!	Action enables you to feel LEAN&FREE success daily and get on with living a happy, fulfilled life. Take it just ONE DAY at a time. Get Excited! Go for it!

DAILY SCORE	100 Total	Scoring	"A" Day = 90 to 100 pts. = Superior day for physical and mental health. "B" Day = 80 TO 89 pts. = Very good "coasting" day. "A" Week = 630 to 700 pts. "B" Week = 560 to 629 pts.

* You may want to record your feelings and observations in your Journal Entry on the back.

Permission granted to enlarge and copy this page.

LEAN&FREE 2000 PLUS™

JOURNAL ENTRY

1. KNOWLEDGE
2. COMMITMENT
3. NURTURING
4. NOURISHMENT
5. MOTION
6. SERVICE
7. PLAN
8. ACTION

LEAN&FREE 2000 PLUS™

THE LEFT-BRAIN PLANNER

NAME: _____ DATE: _____

```
1. KNOWLEDGE
2. COMMITMENT
3. NURTURING
4. NOURISHMENT
5. MOTION
6. SERVICE
7.            8.
PLAN ♥ ACTION
```

PLAN	Points / 5___	Breakfast		
		Lunch		
		Dinner		
		Snacks		
		Exercise		
		Failure Avoidance	Today, I foresee and resolve any problem that could cause me to fail.*	

KNOWLEDGE 5___	Knowledge	Today I studied or reinforced LEAN&FREE. principles. This knowledge empowers my success.*
COMMITMENT 5___	Commitment	Today I am realizing and enjoying signs of success and feel a passion to be LEAN&FREE . .*
NURTURING 5___	Nurturing	I am practicing positive body talk. I am a friend and partner with my body.*

NOURISHMENT

			FG/Cal
5___	Comfortable Satisfaction	**BREAKFAST**	XXXXX
1___	Water		
1___	Grain		
1___	Protein		
1___	Fruit		
2___	Water & Snack		
5___	Comfortable Satisfaction	**LUNCH**	XXXXX
1___	Water		XXXXX
1___	Vegetable		
1___	Grain		
1___	Protein		
1___	Fruit		
2___	Water & Snack		
5___	Comfortable Satisfaction	**DINNER**	XXXXX
1___	Water		XXXXX
1___	Vegetable		
1___	Grain		
1___	Protein		
1___	Fruit		
2___	Water & Snack		
5___	Fat Grams	Score 5 points if fat grams are about 20% of total calories. (Record calories once a week.)	Total FG/Cal ➤

10___	Stressors* A. B. C. D.	Score 10 points for avoiding ALL of the following fat-storing stressors—0 points otherwise. Alcohol, unnecessary drugs (smoking & caffeine), and artificial sweeteners. Excessive amounts of refined flour, sugar, and salt. Desserts and sweets, except after comfortable satisfaction on W.V.G.P.F. Extreme anger with self or others.

MOTION

TYPE (Non-stop aerobic)	MINUTES (Goal 30 - 60)	PULSE (110 - 180 per minute)

15___ / 5___	Exercise / Adequate sleep	Score 15 points for meeting your exercise goal and recording your exercise pulse*. Score 5 points for receiving adequate sleep. (Hours slept:_____)

SERVICE 10___	Personal Service	Today, I used my increased health and energy in service to myself and others.*

ACTION	Do It Now!	Action enables you to feel LEAN&FREE success daily and get on with living a happy, fulfilled life. Take it just ONE DAY at a time. Get Excited! Go for it!

DAILY SCORE 100 Total	Scoring	"A" Day = 90 to 100 pts. = Superior day for physical and mental health. "B" Day = 80 TO 89 pts. = Very good "coasting" day. "A" Week = 630 to 700 pts. "B" Week = 560 to 629 pts.

* You may want to record your feelings and observations in your Journal Entry on the back.

Permission granted to enlarge and copy this page.

© Dana Thornock 1994

LEAN&FREE
2000 PLUS™
JOURNAL ENTRY

1.KNOWLEDGE
2.COMMITMENT
3.NURTURING
4.NOURISHMENT
5.MOTION
6.SERVICE

7.
PLAN

8.
ACTION

LEAN&FREE 2000 PLUS™

DAILY SUCCESS MENU

Date:_____

FG/CAL

Breakfast

Water
Grain

Protein

Fruit

Snack

Water
Veggie+

Lunch

Water
Vegetable

Grain

Protein

Fruit

Snack

Water
Veggie+

Dinner

Water
Vegetable

Grain
Protein

Fruit

Snack

Water
Veggie+

DAY'S TOTAL ▶

Calories: _____
Fat Grams: _____
Percent Fat: _____

LEAN&FREE 2000 PLUS™

DAILY SUCCESS MENU

Date:____

		FG/CAL

Breakfast

Water
Grain

Protein

Fruit

Snack

Water
Veggie+

Lunch

Water
Vegetable

Grain

Protein

Fruit

Snack

Water
Veggie+

Dinner

Water
Vegetable

Grain
Protein

Fruit

Snack

Water
Veggie+

DAY'S TOTAL ►

Calories: _____
Fat Grams: _____
Percent Fat: _____

Permission granted to enlarge and copy this page.

© Dana Thornock 1994